PULMONARY EMBOLISM

Edited by **Ufuk Çobanoğlu**

Pulmonary Embolism
Edited by Ufuk Çobanoğlu

Published by InTech

Janeza Trdine 9, 51000 Rijeka, Croatia

Publishing Process Manager Anja Filipovic

Technical Editor Teodora Smiljanic

Cover Designer InTech Design Team

Additional hard copies can be obtained from orders@intechopen.com

Pulmonary Embolism, Edited by Ufuk Çobanoğlu
p. cm.
ISBN 978-953-51-0233-5

For EU product safety concerns:
IN TECH d.o.o., Prolaz Marije Krucifikse Kozulić 3, 51000 Rijeka, Croatia,
info@intechopen.com or visit our website at intechopen.com.

Meet the editor

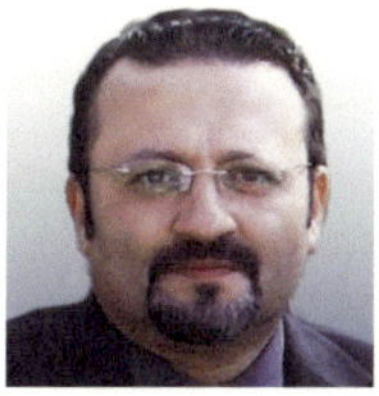

Dr Ufuk Çobanoğlu was born on August 26, 1964 in Çorum, Turkey. He graduated from Atatürk University School of Medicine. He completed his residency in the Thoracic Surgery Department of Yüzüncü Yıl University School of Medicine. Currently he is working as an academician in the same clinic.

Contents

Preface

Pulmonary embolism is a serious, potentially life-threatening cardiopulmonary disease that occurs due to partial or total obstruction of the pulmonary arterial bed. Pulmonary embolism constitutes 5-25% of in-hospital deaths, and mortality is decreased from 30% to 8% with early treatment. Therefore, risk factors should be identified and treatment should be planned to decrease the risk of mortality. Clinical findings, routine laboratory data, electrocardiogram, chest X-ray, and arterial blood gases are not sufficient to diagnose or rule out pulmonary embolus. The presence of some nonspecific findings such as dyspnea, pleuritic chest pain, tachypnea, and tachycardia, and one or more risk factors for venous thromboembolism raise suspicion for pulmonary embolus. However, it is not possible to diagnose pulmonary embolus with these factors. Recently, new improvement occurred in the diagnosis and treatment of the disease. The aim of this disease is to re-review pulmonary embolism in the light of new developments. In this book, in addition to risk factors causing pulmonary embolus, a guide for systematic approaches to lead the risk stratification for decision making is also presented. In order to provide a maximum length of active life and continuation of functional abilities as the aim of new interventional gerontology, the risk factors causing pulmonary embolus in elderly individuals are evaluated, and the approach to prevention and treatment is defined. The risk of the development of deep vein thrombosis and pulmonary embolism, combined with obesity due to immobility, the disease of this era, irregular and excessive eating, and treatment management are highlighted. Non-thrombotic pulmonary emboli are also covered and an attempt is made to constitute an awareness of this picture that can change the treatment and prognosis of the disease to a considerable extent. In addition to the pathophysiological definition of pulmonary embolus, the priority goal of quick and definitive diagnosis is emphasized, and diagnostic strategies are discussed in the book. A numerical analysis of the vena cava filters, which is a current approach to prevent pulmonary emboli recurrences, is presented in the last chapter.

I would like to thank the authors of all chapters for their intense labor and efforts in the preparation of this book. It is our belief that the new opinions and approaches presented will be beneficial to the readers.

Dr. Ufuk Çobanoğlu
Yüzüncü Yıl University, School of Medicine
Chief of Department of Thoracic Surgery
Turkey

1

Risk Factor for Pulmonary Embolism

Ufuk Çobanoğlu
The University of Yuzuncu Yil
Turkey

1. Introduction

Pulmonary embolism (PE) is a common disease with high morbidity and mortality, yet it is a disorder that is difficult to diagnose (Stein & Matta, 2010). 90% of the clinical PE originates from the proximal deep veins of the lower extremities. An ultrasonographic study involving patients diagnosed with pulmonary embolism detected thrombus in 29% of the deep veins (Anderson et al., 1991). Failure to demonstrate the presence of deep vein thrombosis (DVT) in many patients with pulmonary embolism results from the detachment of the emerging blood clot or the inability of ultrasonography to show minor clots (Anderson et al., 1991). Besides DVT, immobilization after fracture or surgical procedures, pregnancy, delivery and usage of estrogen containing oral contraceptives are the other predisposing factors for pulmonary emboli (Quinn et al., 1992). The predisposing factors were first described by Virchow in 1856 as consisting of three major phenomena (Table 1) (Anderson et al., 1991; Quinn et al.,1992): the "Virchow triad", that is, the triad of the three factors that induce the process of vascular clotting: endothelial injury, hypercoagulability and lower extremity stasis (Carson et al., 1992).

In 75% of pulmonary embolism cases, the acquired and/or hereditary factors that lead to one of these predisposing factors are detected; in half of the hereditary thrombophilia cases, an accompanying acquired risk factor is also present (White, 2003). Stasis in the lower extremities usually results from slow blood flow occurring in the patient groups with decreased mobility. In patients with endothelial injury, causes such as trauma and surgery trigger this process while hypercoagulation is a mechanism observed in cases of hereditary thrombophilia (White, 2003). Table 2 presents the acquired and hereditary risk factors.

2. Genetic risk factors

Among the hereditary risk factors leading to a predisposition to thrombosis, antithrombin deficiency was first shown to create predisposition to thrombosis in 1965, followed by the description of protein C deficiency in 1981 and protein S in 1984. These three deficiencies represent only 15% of hereditary thrombophilias. The description of the active protein C (APC) resistance by Dahlback et al in 1993 (Dahlback, 1995) and of the factor V Leiden mutation by Bertina in 1994 (Bertina, 1999) enabled elucidation of the etiology in 20% of patients with thrombosis and in 50% of families with thrombophilia. Similarly, hyperhomocysteinemia and a mutation in the prothrombin gene were shown to cause hereditary thrombophilia in 1994 and 1996, respectively (Makris et al., 1997). In patients with genetic thrombophilia, the predisposition to thrombotic and recurrent venous thromboembolism (VTE) in the early stages of life is increased.

HYPERCOAGULABILITY	VENOUS STASIS	VASCULAR INJURY
Malignancy	Atrial fibrillation	Trauma or surgery
Pregnancy and peri-partum period	Left ventricular dysfunction	Venepuncture
Oestrogen therapy	Immobility or paralysis	Chemical irritation
Trauma or surgery of lower extremity, hip, abdomen or pelvis	Venous insufficiency or varicose veins	Heart valve disease or replacement
Inflammatory bowel disease	Venous obstruction from tumour, obesity or pregnancy	Atherosclerosis
Nephrotic syndrome		Indwelling catheters
Sepsis		
Thrombophilia		

CLOT FORMATION

Table 1. Virchow's triad/ venous thromboembolism risk factors

Genetic risk factors	Acquired risk factors
Antithrombin III deficiency	Advanced age
Protein C deficiency	Obesity
Protein S deficiency	Long haul air travel
Activated Protein C resistance and Factor V Leiden Mutation	Immobilization
Factor II G20210A Mutation:	Major surgery
Hyperhomocysteinemia	Trauma
Increase in Factor VIII Levels	Congestive cardiac failure / Myocardial infraction
Congenital Dysfibrinogenemia	Smoking
Plasminogen deficiency	Stroke
Factor VII deficiency	Malignity/ Chemotherapy
Factor XII deficiency	Central venous catheter
Factor IX increase	Pregnancy/puerperality
	The use of Oral contraceptives and hormone replacement
	Previous pulmonary emboli and deep vein thrombosis
	Antiphospholipid syndrome
	Chronic obstructive pulmonary disease (COPD)
	Medical Conditions requiring hospitalization

Table 2. Risk factor for pulmonary embolism

2.1 Antithrombin III deficiency

Antithrombin III (AT III) deficiency is among the first described thrombophilias. It is one of the most important natural protease inhibitors and a glycoprotein that is synthesized in the liver, which exhibits anticoagulant efficacy through inhibition of thrombin and the other serine proteases (factor IX a, X a, XI a, XIIa and kallikrein). Owing to these properties, it is accepted to be one of the most potent physiologic inhibitors of the fibrin formation. There are two types of antithrombin III deficiencies: type I involves reduction in the synthesis while type II involves functional inactivity. Type I AT III deficiency is characterized by both a functional and an immunological reduction in AT III. Type II AT deficiency involves variant AT III molecules (Thaler & Lechner, 1981). When the serum concentration of antithrombin III is mildly decreased, factor Xa, IXa, XIa and XIIa and thrombin cannot be inactivated, leading to thrombus formation. In addition to congenital deficiency, the antithrombin level is also decreased in cases of diffuse intravascular clotting, oral contraceptive (OC) use, and liver and kidney diseases. In antithrombin III deficiency, thrombotic events occur mostly in the mesenteric and lower extremity deep veins, leading to an increased predisposition to pulmonary embolism. A trial detected a rate of AT III deficiency at 1/600 in healthy individuals (Tait et al., 1994). In another trial, this figure was 1.5% in patients diagnosed with VTE (Bauer& Rosenberg, 1991).

2.2 Protein C deficiency

Protein C (PC) is a glycoprotein synthesized in the liver. Its deficiency exhibits autosomal dominant or autosomal recessive inheritance. Protein C deficiency has two subtypes. Type I protein C deficiency: protein C antigen level is low due to genetic defect while the protein C activity is normal. Type II protein C deficiency involves the presence of an abnormal protein C molecule. Protein C antigen is normal while the protein C activity is low (Hoshi et al., 2007). Protein C is activated after the thrombin binds to the endothelial receptors. Activated PC binds to the factor Va and factor VIIIa and inactivates these factors, thereby inhibiting the clot formation.

In the general population, protein C deficiency prevalence is between 1/16000 and 36000. The fact that the protein C deficiency rate is 10% in patients with previous VTE below 40 years of age and that it increases the VTE risk 6-fold, protein C level should be investigated in all young patients with previous VTE (Folsom et al., 2002).

2.3 Protein S deficiency

Protein S is a glycoprotein that is vitamin K-dependently synthesized, exhibits an autosomal dominant inheritance and activates protein C as a cofactor. Protein S exhibits anticoagulant efficacy through both the inactivation of factor Va and factor VIIIa by Protein C that is activated as a cofactor and directly through inhibition of the interaction of prothrombin with factor Va and Xa; therefore, protein S deficiency is considered a significant risk factor for thrombosis formation (Bertina, 1999). Protein S deficiency has three subtypes. Type I protein S deficiency involves a reduction in the total protein S antigen level. The free protein S antigen level and activity is low. Type II protein S deficiency involves the presence of a functionally abnormal protein S molecule. The total and free protein S antigens are normal but the protein S activity is decreased. Type III protein S deficiency involves a normal total protein S antigen but a decreased free protein S antigen level and activity (Dykes et al., 2001). Protein S deficiency is observed at a rate of 0.03%-0.13 (Dykes et al., 2001) and 6% in healthy individuals and families with thrombophilia (Bertina 1999). The trials performed demonstrated a 6 to 10-fold increased VTE risk in heterozygous Protein S gene carriers (Bauer& Rosenberg, 1991). As well as leading to thrombus formation in the deep (axillary, femoral etc), mesenteric, cerebral and superficial veins, it also causes PE and arterial thrombus formation. It is also one of the causes of recurrent VTE attacks. Pregnancy, OC or estrogen replacement use, nephritic syndrome, disseminated intravascular coagulation, HIV infection and liver diseases may also result in acquired protein S deficiency (Bauer& Rosenberg, 1991).

2.4 Activated protein C resistance and factor V Leiden mutation

In cases of activated partial thromboplastin time (aPTT) changes, an addition of activated Protein C to the plasma is expected to cause the prolongation of bleeding time. However, Dahlback et al detected no prolongation in some patients with VTE in 1993 (Dahlback, 1995); this phenomenon was described as the activated protein C resistance (APCR). Activated Protein C resistance is clearly associated with an increase in thrombosis incidence. The subsequent studies detected this phenotype in 20-50% of the patients with VTE (Dahlback, 1995). In many cases of hereditary APCR, aG→A transition causes translocation of the amino acids (glutamine and arginine) at 506 location in the position 1691 nucleotide as a result of the activated function of the point mutation in factor V (site of cleavage for the activated PC in the factor V molecule). This point mutation was first described in 1994 and named as Factor V Leiden (FVL), FVR Q or FV: Q (Rosendaal et al., 1995). Factor V mutation notably increases the predisposition to VTE, causes hypercoagulability and neutralizes activated PC-mediated resistance. The risk of VTE is increased 3 to 8-fold in individuals heterozygous for factor Leiden mutation; as for homozygous individuals, the increase in the thrombotic risk is 50 to 100-fold (Rosendaal et al., 1995). The incidence of factor V Leiden carriers is 1-15% in the population (Rosendaal et al., 1995). Factor V Leiden is present in 10-50% of the cases with VTE. Factor V Leiden abnormality results from a single mutation. In APCR without factor V Leiden mutation, the VTE risk is increased (Rosendaal et al., 1995).

2.5 Factor II G20210A mutation

A new genetic factor was discovered in the etiology of VTE in 1996. The G→A transition (Factor II G20210A) of the nucleotides at 20120 location in the region of the coagulation factor II gene not undergoing 3′-translation is associated with hyperprothrombinemia. G→A transition increased the prothrombin synthesis at the level of mRNA and protein synthesis. In heterozygous carriers of this mutation, the prothrombin level is increased 1.3-fold while it is increased 1.7-fold in homozygous carriers. The increase in the plasma prothrombin level results in a predisposition to thrombosis. This mutation was detected in 1-3% of the general population and 6-18% of the patients with VTE (Poort et al. 1996). Factor II G20210A diagnosis is only established by gene analysis. It is the second most common genetic abnormality, secondary to thrombophilia. In the case of factor II G20210A, there is no increase in the risk of VTE (Miles et al., 2001).

2.6 Hyperhomocysteinemia

It is the only hereditary cause of thrombophilia that has been proven to lead to arterial and venous thrombosis. Hyperthrombosis is believed to trigger the development of thrombosis via various mechanisms; there are in vitro studies showing that it affects the endothelial cells by causing the formation of reactive oxygen forms, such as superoxide, hydrogen peroxide and hydroxyl radicals, it causes proliferative response by affecting the smooth muscle cells and increasing collagen production, it affects the clotting system by increasing tissue factor production in the monocytes, creating acquired APC resistance and increasing the synthesis of thromboxane in the platelets (Miletich et al., 1987). Hyperhomocysteinemia is an established risk factor for VTE and is usually associated with a 2 to 4-fold increased thrombotic risk. Plasma homocysteine concentration is affected by genetic and acquired factors and thus known as the mixed risk factor (Miletich et al., 1987). Vitamin B12, vitamin B6 and folate deficiency, advanced age, chronic renal failure and malnutrition involving anti-folic drug use represent acquired factors in hyperhomocysteinemia. Gene defects in two enzymes involved in the intracellular metabolism, methyltetrahydrofolate reductase (MTHFR) and cystathionine B-synthase (CBS) result in hyperhomocysteinemia and enzyme deficiency. Various mutations have been defined in methyltetrahydrofolate reductase and CBS to date; most are rare and lead to clinical outcomes in homozygous cases only. This condition is characterized by multiple neurological deficiency, physicomotor retardation, seizures, skeletal abnormalities, lens dislocation, premature arterial disease and VTE (Weisberg et al., 1999). Methyltetrahydrofolate reductase 677 C→T is associated with high-prevalence polymorphism in the general population and reduced enzyme activity in homozygous cases. Methyltetrahydrofolate reductase 1298 A→C is not considered to be associated with hyperhomocysteinemia and not considered a thrombotic risk factor.

However, MTHFR results in reduced enzyme activity and increased homocysteine levels in heterozygous cases of 677 C→T (Weisberg et al., 1999). 68-bp insertion in the cystathionine B-cynthase gene (844ins68) is a common mutation in various populations. This gene change has no effect on the risk of DVT or homocysteine levels. Hyperhomocysteinemia is not defined as a genetic abnormality for VTE but as an independent risk factor (Kluijtmans et al., 1997).

2.7 Increase in factor VIII levels

Factor VIII is an entity with a gene localized on the 10th chromosome, which activates the factor X by forming a complex with factor IXa and phospholipids in the coagulation cascade. The increase in factor VIII is included among the thrombotic risk factors since it further increases formation of thrombin from prothrombin by factor X activation (Schambeck et al., 2004). The increased factor was detected in 3-9.4% of healthy individuals and in 11.3% of patients with VTE (Schambeck et al., 2004). A high FVIII level was reported to increase the VTE risk approximately 5-fold compared to individuals with a normal level (Schambeck et al., 2004). In addition, the factor VIII level was demonstrated to be an independent risk factor for VTE (Kraaijenhagen et al., 2000) (21) and to be correlated with the PE recurrence (Kyrle et al., 2000).

2.8 Congenital dysfibrinogenemia

The impairment in the formation of fibrin from fibrinogen secondary to the changes in the structure of fibrinogen is called dysfibrinogenemia. Dysfibrinogenemia is a dominant disease group characterized by qualitative abnormal fibrinogen formation. Various fibrinogen abnormalities are assessed within this group. Approximately 300 abnormal fibrinogen have been defined (Schorer et al., 1995). The most common structural defects are detected in fibrinopeptides and their sites of cleavage. Each dysfibrinogenemia affects thrombin time and clotting in a different way. While some dysfibrinogenemias do not have the effect of bleeding or thrombosis, some may cause abnormal bleeding and even thrombosis (Schorer et al., 1995).

2.9 Plasminogen deficiency

Plasminogen (plg) plays an important role in intravascular and extravascular fibrinolysis, wound healing, cell migration, tissue remodeling, angiogenesis, and embryogenesis (Castellino & Ploplis, 2005).

Plasminogen deficiency shows an autosomal dominant inheritance.

Plasminogen deficiency is classified into two groups: one is type I deficiency characterized by the parallel reduction of both activity and antigen, and the other is dysplasminogenemia (type II) characterized by reduced activity with a normal antigen level (Schuster et al., 2001).

Hypoplasminogenemia (type I plg deficiency): No significantly increased risk of deep venous thrombosis. In hypoplasminogenemia, or type I plg deficiency, the level of immunoreactive plg is reduced in parallel with its functional activity. The specific plg activity is normal.

Some further case reports and family studies had originally suggested that heterozygous hypoplasminogenemia might be a risk factor for venous thrombosis (Leebeek et al., 1989). The relationship between hypoplasminogenemia and venous thrombosis has more recently been called into question, mainly based on two lines of evidence. Dysplasminogenemia (type II plg deficiency): in dysplasminogenemia, or type II plg deficiency, the level of immunoreactive plg is normal (or only slightly reduced), whereas the specific functional plg activity is markedly reduced because of abnormalities in the variant plg molecule (Robbins, 1990).

2.10 Factor VII deficiency

Inherited factor VII (FVII) deficiency is the most widespread of the rare inherited bleeding disorders, with an estimated prevalence of 1 in 400 000 Caucasians (Mariani et al., 2005). It is characterized by a wide heterogeneity as regards clinical, biological and genetic parameters. Clinical features are extremely variable, ranging from mild cutaneo-mucosal bleeding to lethal cerebral haemorrhages, and are poorly correlated with residual FVII coagulant activity (FVII:C). Moreover, several patients remain asymptomatic (Aynaoğlu et al., 2010), even under conditions of high haemorrhagic challenge. Notably, in some rare cases, patients have a history of arterial (Escoffre et al., 1995) or venous (Mariani & Bernardi, 2009) thromboses. The mechanisms accounting for the association of FVII deficiencies with thrombosis remain unclear. FVII deficiency is characterized by a wide heterogeneity, even amongst those patients presenting with rare thrombotic events. In a few case reports, thrombosis can occur in "usual" sites, such as the deep veins of the lower limbs or pulmonary embolism, or in atypical sites, such as the sinus veins (Lietz et al., 2005). The first series of FVII deficiency associated with thrombosis included seven cases of venous thrombosis, localized primarily in typical sites (lower limbs and pulmonary embolism) (Mariani et al., 2005).

2.11 Factor XII deficiency

Severe FXII deficiency (FXII activity <1%) shows an autosomal recessive inheritance and patients are detected to have a prolonged aPTZ time. Despite this prolongation in the active partial thromboplastin time, patients do not have bleeding diathesis. In contrast, these patients develop VTE and myocardial infarction. While the incidence of thrombosis secondary to factor XII deficiency was not well-established, it was reported to be 8% approximately (Goodnough et al., 1983).

2.12 Factor IX increase

Factor IX plays a key role in hemostasis; it is a vitamin K–dependent glycoprotein, which is activated through the intrinsic pathway as well as the extrinsic pathway (B. Furie & BC. Furie, 1988). Factor IX, when activated by factor XIa or factor VIIa-tissue factor, converts factor X into Xa and this eventually leads to the formation of a fibrin clot. This conversion is accelerated by the presence of the nonenzymatic cofactor factor VIIIa, calcium ions, and a phospholipid membrane (van Dieijen et al., 1981). In healthy individuals, factor IX activity and antigen levels vary between 50% and 150% of that in pooled normal plasma (B. Furie & BC. Furie, 1988; van Dieijen et al., 1981). Individuals who have high levels of factor IX (>129 U/dL) have a more than 2-fold increased risk of developing a first DVT compared with individuals having low levels of factor IX. The risk of thrombosis increased with increasing plasma levels of factor IX (dose response). At factor IX levels of more than 125 U/dL, an increase of the risk can already be observed compared with the reference category (factor IX levels ≤100 U/dL). Individuals with a factor IX level over 150 U/dL have a more than 3-fold increase in the risk of thrombosis when compared with the reference category.

3. Acquired risk factors

3.1 Advanced age

The VTE incidence increases linearly with the age. Above 50 years of age, the PE incidence was detected to be higher in women. This increase is also associated with other comorbidities (cancer, myocardial infarction) that increase with age (Stein et al., 1999).

3.2 Obesity

The risk of PE by obesity is correlated with the body mass index. While the relative risk of pulmonary embolism is 1.7 for those with a body mass index of 25-28.9 kg/m^2, it is increased 3.2-fold for those with a BMI ≥29 (Goldhaber et al., 1997). Obesity is correlated with VTE, particularly in women. It was reported to be an independent risk factor in women with a body mass index ≥ 29. However, there are controversial study results on this subject (Goldhaber et al., 1997).

3.3 Long haul air travel

Air travel is a risk factor for PE. In a trial by Lapostolle et al, severe pulmonary embolism was detected in 56 of 135.29 million passengers from 14 countries. The assessment of the results revealed a rate of 1.5 in one million cases in those flying more than 5000 km and a rate of 4.8 in one million cases in those flying more than 10000 km, leading to the reported result that PE risk was correlated with flight distance. Conditions that lead to hemoconcentration during air travel, such as dehydration, lower oxygen pressure and foot swelling are believed to induce venous stasis (Lapostolle et al., 2001).

3.4 Immobilization

Immobility is a condition that is most commonly observed in PE, which may concomitantly exist with other risk factors (Stein et al., 1999). Long-term absence of mobilization results in a weakening of the muscles that provide an upward flow of the blood in the leg veins. The blood accumulates backwards; thus, among the activated platelets and clotting factors, thrombin in particular accumulates locally, leading to the formation of thrombus. Even if for a short time, for example one week, in the postoperative period, immobilization increases the risk of VTE (Stein et al., 1999).

3.5 Major surgery

Surgical intervention is one of the most significant acquired risk factors that cause PE. The decreased mobility during the operation, hypercoagulation secondary to local trauma and endothelial injury, the prothrombotic process that may be caused by the general anesthesia administered increase the risk of PE (Rosendaal, 1999). The presence of operation history within a 45-90 day period increases the risk of thromboembolism 6 to 22-fold (Rosendaal, 1999); 25% of these emboli occur after discharge from the hospital (Huber et al., 1992). Surgeries of the hip, knees, and the abdominopelvic region represent the most risky operations for venous thromboembolism development (Huber et al., 1992).

3.6 Trauma

Trauma is also a risk factor for PE development; the localization of the trauma is very important with respect to venous thrombus development (Geerts et al., 1996). VTE occurs in 50% of chest or abdomen traumas, 54% of head traumas and 62% of spinal cord injuries, and 69% of lower extremity orthopedic traumas (Geerts et al., 1996). The incidence of venous thromboembolism increases proportionally with time after the traumatic event. While the rate of PE confirmed by autopsy was 3.3% in those who survived less than 24 hours after trauma, this rate was 5.5% in those who survived up to seven days. PE was reported at a rate of 18.6% in individuals who survived longer (Geerts et al., 1996). Patients over 45, a requirement of more than three days bed rest, a previous history of VTE, fractures of the lower extremity, pelvis, spine, the development of coma and plegia, a requirement for blood transfusion and surgery further increase the risk of DVT and PE, therefore, effective and safe prophylactic anticoagulant treatment is recommended in traumatic patients unless contraindicated (Shackford et al., 1990).

3.7 Congestive cardiac failure/myocardial infraction

The presence of congestive cardiac failure or arrhythmia underlying heart disease further increases the risk of PE. In cardiac failure, the risk of mortality from PE is increased due to decreased cardiopulmonary reserve (Anderson & Spencer, 2003). The increase of factor VIII, fibrinogen and fibrinolysis in the acute phase following acute myocardial infarction leads to PE (Anderson & Spencer, 2003). Nearly all of the PEs occurring in acute myocardial infarction result from deep vein thrombosis in the lower extremity. Very rarely, they result from mural thrombi occurring in the infraction site in the right ventricle (Anderson & Spencer, 2003).

3.8 Smoking

Smoking may increase the risk of VTE through a number of mechanisms:

1. Smoking is a well established, potent risk factor for a number of diseases, including cancer and cardiovascular diseases (stroke and coronary heart diseases); these, in turn, are associated with an increased risk of VTE. Therefore, smoking might be associated with the risk of provoked VTE.

2. Smoking is associated with a higher plasma concentration of fibrinogen (Yanbaeva et al., 2007; Lee & Lip, 2003).
3. Smoking is associated with reduced fibrinolysis (Lee & Lip, 2003; Yarnell et al., 2000).
4. Smoking is associated with inflammation (Yanbaeva et al., 2007; Yarnell et al., 2000).
5. Smoking increases the viscosity of the blood (Yanbaeva et al., 2007; Lee & Lip, 2003).

3.9 Stroke

Most patients with acute ischemic stroke or intracranial hemorrhage survive the initial event. Early in-hospital mortality has been attributed not only to swelling of the brain and enlargement of hematoma but also to aspiration pneumonitis, sepsis, and severe heart disease (Brandstater et al., 1992). Pulmonary embolism after a stroke has received some attention, but the incidence is considered small. The incidence of clinical PE reported in the absence of heparin prophylaxis varies considerably, depending on the methodology of the studies. In the International Stroke Trial, the incidence was 0.8% at 2 weeks (International Stroke Trial Collaborative Group [ISTCG], 1997). Similarly, in a retrospective study of 607 patients who had acute stroke, PE was reported in 1% during the period of hospitalization (Davenport et al., 1996). However, prospective studies that focused specifically on venous thromboembolic complications reported incidences of clinically apparent PE of 10% to 13% (excluding pulmonary emboli identified in autopsy that were asymptomatic during life) (Warlow et al., 1972). In a retrospective study of 363 patients who did not receive heparin prophylaxis and entered a rehabilitation unit four weeks after stroke, 4% developed PE (confirmed by VQ scanning) on average 11 days after entering the unit (Subbarao & Smith, 1984). Only one small study has prospectively screened for PE by using VQ scintigraphy. Dickmann et al (Dickmann et al., 1988) studied a group of 23 patients 10 days after hemorrhagic stroke and found evidence of PE in 39%, though the proportion with symptoms was not stated. Autopsy studies show that half of the patients who die in hospital after the first 48 hours post stroke have evidence of PE, (McCarthy & Turner, 1986) which suggests that pulmonary emboli are often subclinical and/or unrecognized after stroke.

3.10 Malignity/chemotherapy

Cancer patients have a higher risk of complications and recurrence compared to patients without cancer. This risk is more marked especially in the pancreas, pulmonary disease, gastrointestinal system and mucinous carcinoma patients (Er & Zacharski 2006). Different mechanisms were proposed for the development of thrombotic predisposition in cancer patients. Development of procoagulant activity by the tumor products, coagulatory macrophage activation, endothelial cell injury and platelet activation secondary to interaction with the tumor cells are among these mechanisms. Some malignities (pancreas, colon, lungs and promyelocytic leukemias) systemically result in activation of the clotting system, leading to thrombotic complications. In cancer patients, the serum concentrations of the clotting factors, such as factors V, VIII, VII and fibrinogen are increased. Again, in these patients, local or systemic coagulation may occur secondary to vascular wall injury and factor X is activated (Falanga & Zacharski, 2005). The chemotherapeutical agents used for DVT after chemotherapy are significantly involved in this process due to the endothelial injury occurring in the vein to which these agents are administered (Nightingale et al., 1997).

3.11 Central venous catheter

Jugular, subclavian and femoral venous catheters lead to vascular injury and represent a focus for thrombus formation. Although less common, these patients may develop symptomatic PE caused by the catheter-associated upper extremity thrombi (Haire & Lieberman 1992). In approximately 10-20% of the cases with pulmonary emboli, the emboli results from the thrombus in the site of the superior vena cava. Recently, upper extremity venous thrombus has been commonly known to occur as a result of invasive diagnostic and therapeutical procedures (intravascular catheter and intravenous chemotherapeutical agents) (Haire & Lieberman 1992).

3.12 Pregnancy/puerperality

Compared to the age-matched individuals, the risk of VTE is 5-fold higher in pregnant women. While 75% of the deep vein thrombi occur in the pre-delivery period, 66% of the PEs develop after the delivery. The risk is 20-fold higher in the postpartum period relative to the antepartum period (Kovacevich et al., 2000; Greer, 2003). Venous stasis secondary to dilated uterus in pregnancy, hormonal venous atonia, increased levels of thrombin and various clotting factors (fibrinopeptide A), increased platelet activation, decreased acquired protein S, antithrombin deficiency, the decreased APC response due to factor VIII increase are the risk factors. There are no trials using objective diagnostic techniques to show that cesarean section involves an additional thrombotic risk relative to normal delivery. The risk of a thrombotic event is higher in patients who are on mandatory bed rest due to premature action or preterm premature membrane rupture (Kovacevich et al., 2000). Since oral anticoagulation is risky for the fetus, low-molecule weight heparin treatment with a lower osteoporosis risk relative to the conventional heparin that will be maintained at least until puerperality appears to be an appropriate choice (Greer, 2003).

3.13 The use of oral contraceptives and hormone replacement

Oral contraceptive (OC) use was shown to increase the risk of PE approximately 3-7-fold. Oral contraceptives result in PE by increasing the levels of coagulation factors, such as prothrombin, factor VII, factor VIII, factor X and fibrinogen, and decreasing the levels of the coagulation factors, such as antithrombin III and protein S (Spitzer et al., 1996). Compared to the persons who are not on oral contraceptives, the risk was detected to be 3.4 for low-estrogen levonorgestrel and 7.3 and 10.2 for the 3rd generation progesterone desogestrel and gestodene (World Health organization [WHO], 1995). Third generation OC use increases the VTE risk particularly in Factor V Leiden mutation carriers and those with a positive familial history (Bloemenkamp et al., 1995). In women, hormone replacement therapy used in the postmenopausal period is reported to be a risk factor for PE (Cushman et al., 2004). This risk is higher in patients with coronary artery disease. The risk is higher at the start of treatment and disappears upon discontinuation of the hormone replacement therapy. The mechanism involved in the increase of thrombosis by estrogen alone or in combination with progesterone is not known. However, recent trials report that OCs cause a reduction in the sensitivity to activated protein C irrespective of the type of drug used and that this reduction is higher with 3rd generation monophasic OCs relative to 2nd generation drugs (Rosing et al., 1997).

3.14 Previous pulmonary emboli and deep vein thrombosis

Hospitalized patients with a history of pulmonary emboli have a significant risk of recurrence. More than 50% of patients with a history of venous thromboembolism undergoing surgery develop postoperative DVT if no prophylaxis is administered. The rate of recurrence within 5 years after the first DVT is 21.5% (Hansson et al., 2000). Jeffrey et al (Jeffrey et al., 1992) detected the PE recurrence as 8.3% and reported that recurrence occurred mostly within the first week of treatment. In addition, mortality was 45% in these patients.

3.15 Antiphospholipid syndrome

Antiphospholipid syndrome (APS) characterized by arterial and venous thrombosis predisposition, repeated miscarriage and the presence of antiphospholipid antibodies is one of the leading causes of acquired thrombophilia. While the pathogenesis of the syndrome is not elucidated clearly, the negatively charged phospholipids and the phospholipid antibodies developing against the phospholipid protein complexes (lupus anticoagulant-LA and anticardiolipin antibodies-AKLA) are believed to be responsible for clinical manifestations. In AFS, the most important factor affecting mortality and morbidity is thromboembolic complications. Thromboses can both involve the arterial and the venous system and may be observed in each tissue and organ. The recurring tendency of the thromboses and the high risk of consecutive thrombotic complications involving the same system (for example, recurrent arterial thrombosis in a case with previous arterial thrombosis) are interesting. Approximately 2/3 of the cases develop venous thromboembolism and 1/3 develop arterial thrombosis. In venous thrombosis, DVT and PE rank first while ischemic cerebral attack ranks first in arterial thrombosis followed by myocardial infarction and digital thromboses. Thrombosis in abnormal regions is common in antiphospholipid syndrome (thrombosis in upper extremity veins, intra abdominal veins and the veins inside the head) (Hanly, 2003).

3.16 Chronic Obstructive Pulmonary Disease (COPD)

COPD is a major health burden worldwide. It is the fourth-leading cause of mortality, accounting for > 3 million deaths annually; and by 2020, COPD will be the third-leading cause of death, trailing only ischemic heart disease and stroke. Most COPD-related deaths occur during periods of exacerbation (Sapey & Stockley, 2006). Previous studies (Sidney et al., 2005) estimate that 50 to 70% of all COPD exacerbations are precipitated by an infectious process, while 10% are due to environmental pollution. Up to 30% of exacerbations are caused by an unknown etiology Sapey & Stockley, 2006). Exacerbations are characterized by increase in cough and dyspnea. A study (Sidney et al., 2005) suggests that patients with COPD have approximately twice the risk of PE and other venous thromboembolic events (VTE) than those without COPD. Since thromboembolic events can lead to cough and dyspnea (just like infectious events), PE may be another common cause of COPD exacerbations (Tapson, 2008). However, dissimilar to infectious etiologies, which are effectively treated by antimicrobials and systemic corticosteroids, thromboembolic diseases require anticoagulant therapy and significant delays in treatment are associated with poor outcomes (Hull et al., 1997). Owing to multiple perfusion and ventilation abnormalities frequently observed in COPD lungs (even in the absence of VTE), noninvasive diagnosis of PE using imaging modalities was a significant challenge until quite recently. With the advent of contrast-enhanced (multidetector) CT, it is now possible to reliably diagnose PE in COPD subjects with minimal discomfort or risk to the patients. The primary purpose of this review was to determine the reported prevalence of PE in patients with COPD who required hospitalization for their disease.

3.17 Medical conditions requiring hospitalization

The incidence of thromboembolic diseases in inpatients is reported to be different depending on the type of disease. While the risk is reported to be 3% in patients without risk factors, it is reported to be 50% in patients with previous VTE. Massive PEs account for 4-8% of inpatient mortality (Rubinstein et al., 1988). The VTE risk is higher in patients with neurological and cardiac diseases during hospitalization compared to other patient groups (Nicolaides et al., 2001). There are certain diseases that have been proven to increase the risk of venous thromboembolism complications; these include SLE, inflammatory intestinal diseases, nephritic syndrome, paroxysmal nocturnal hemoglobinuria, myeloproliferative diseases, Behcet's disease, Cushing syndrome and sickle cell syndrome. The number of DVT cases is larger in these diseases relative to the general population.

4. References

Anderson, FA. Jr., & Spencer, FA. (2003). Risk Factor for Venous Thromboembolism. *Circulation,* Vol.107, No. [Suppl I].I-9, (Jun), pp.(1-16), ISSN: (Print) 0009-7322, (Electronic)1524-4539.

Anderson, FA. Jr., Wheeler, HB., Goldberg, RJ., Hosmer, DW., .Patwardhan, NA., Jovanovic, B., Forcier, A., & Dalen JE. (1991). A population-based perspective of the hospital incidence and case-fatality rates of deep vein thrombosis and pulmonary embolism. The Worcester DVT study. *Arch Intern Med,* Vol.151, No.5, (May) pp.(933-938), ISSN: (Print) 0003-9926, (Electronic)1538-3679.

Aynaoğlu, G., Durdağ, GD., Ozmen, B., Söylemez, F. (2010). Successful treatment of hereditary factor VII deficiency presented for the first time with epistaxis in pregnancy: a case report. *J Matern Fetal Neonatal Med,* Vol.23, No.9, (Sep), pp.(1053-1055), ISSN: (Print) 1476-7058, (Electronic) 1476-4954.

Bauer, KA., & Rosenberg, RD. (1991). Role of antithrombin III as a regulator of in vivo coagulation. Semin Hematol, Vol.28, No.1, (Jan), pp.10-18, ISSN: (Print) 0037-1963, (Electronic)1532-8686.

Bertina, RM. (1999). Molecular risk factors for thrombosis. *Thromb Haemost,* Vol.82, No.2, (Aug), pp.(601-609), ISSN: (Print) 0340-6245, (Electronic) 0340-6245.

Bloemenkamp, KW., Rosendaal, FR., Helmerhorst, FM., Bumer, HR., & Voldenbroucke JP. (1995). Enhancement by factor V Leiden mutation of risk of deep vein thrombosis associated with oral contraceptives containing a third generation progestagen. *Lancet,* Vol.346, No.8990, (Dec), pp.(1593-1596), ISSN: (Print) 0140-6736, (Electronic)1474-547X.

Brandstater, ME., Roth, EJ., & Siebens, HC. (1992). Venous thromboembolism in stroke: literatüre revievv and implica- tions for clinical practice. *Arch Phys Med Rehabil,* Vol.73, No. (5-S) (Study Guide), (May), pp.(379-391), ISSN: (Print) 0003-9993, (Electronic) 1532-821X.

Carson, JL., Kelley, MA., Duff, A., Weg, JG., Fulkerson, WJ., Palevsky, HI., Schwartz, JS., Thompson, BT., Popovich, J., Jr., Hobbins, TE., Spera, MA., Alavi, A., & Terin ML. (1992). The clinical course of pulmonary embolism. *N Engl J Med,* Vol.326, No.19, (May), pp. (1240-1245), ISSN: (Print):0028-4793, (Electronic):1533-4406.

Castellino, FJ., & Ploplis, VA. (2005). Structure and function of the plasminogen/plasmin system. *Thromb Haemost,* Vol.93, No.4, (Apr), pp. (647–654), ISSN: (Print) 0340-6245, (Electronic) 0340-6245.

Cushman, M., Kuller, LH., Prentice, R., Prentice, R., Rodabough, RJ., Psaty, BM., Stafford, Rs., & Rosendaal, FR.(2004),. Estrogen plus progestin and risk venous thrombosis. *JAMA,* Vol. 292, No.13, (Oct), pp.(1573-1580), ISSN: (Print) 0098-7484, (Electronic) 1538-3598.

Dahlback, B. (1995). Inherited Thrombophilia: resistance to activated protein C as a pathogenetic factor of venous thromboembolism. *Blood,* Vol.85, No.3, (Feb), pp.(607-614), ISSN: (Print) 0006-4971, (Electronic) 1528-0020.

Davenport, RJ., Dennis, MS., Wellwood, I.,& Warlow, CP. (1996). Complications after acute stroke. *Stroke,* Vol.27, No.3, (Mar), pp.(415-420), ISSN: (Print) 0039-2499, (Electronic) 1524-4628.

Dickmann, U., Voth, E., Schicha, H., Henze, T., Prange, H., & Emrich, D. (1988). Heparin therapy, deep vein thrombosis and pulmonary embolism after intracerebral haemorrhage. *Klin Wochenschr,* Vol.66, No.23, (Dec), pp.(1182-183), ISSN: (Print) 0023-2173, (Electronic) 0023-2173.

Dykes, AC., Walker, ID., McMahon, AD., Islam, SI., & Tait RC. (2001). A study of protein S antigen levels in 3788 healthy volunteers: Influence of age, sex and hormone use, and estimate for prevalence of deficiency state. *Br J Haematol,* Vol.113, No.3, (Jun). pp.(636-641, ISSN: (Print) 00071048, (Electronic) 13652141.

Er, O., & Zacharski, L. (2006). Management of cancer-associated venous thrombosis. *Vasc Health Risk Manag,* Vol.2, No.4, (Dec), pp.(351–356), ISSN: (Print) 1176-6344, (Electronic) 1178-2048.

Escoffre, M, Zini, JM., Schliamser, L., Mazoyer, E., Soria, C., Tobelem, G., & Dupuy, E.(1995). Severe arterial thrombosis in a congenitally factor VII deficient patient. *Br J Haematol,* Vol. 91, No.3, (May), pp.(739–741), ISSN: (Print) 0007-1048, (Electronic) 1365-2141.

Falanga, A., & Zacharski, L. (2005). Deep vein thrombosis in cancer: the scale of the problem and approaches to management. *Annals of Oncology,* Vol 16, No.5, (May), pp.(696-701), ISSN: (Print) 0923-7534, (Electronic) 1569-8041.

Furie, B., & Furie, BC. (1988). The molecular basis of blood coagulation. *Cell,* Vol.53, No.4, (May), pp. (505-518), ISSN: (Print) 0092-8674.

Folsom, AR., Aleksic, N., Wang, L., Cushman, M., Wu, KK., & White, RH. (2002). Protein C, antithrombin, and venous thromboembolism incidence: a prospective population-based study. *Arterioscler Thromb Vasc Biol,* Vol.22, No.6, (Jun), pp.(1018-1022). ISSN: (Print) 1079-5642, (Electronic) 1524-4636.

Geerts, W., Jay, RM., Code, KI., Chen, E., Szalai, JP., Saibil, AE., & Hamilton, PA. (1996). A comparison of low-dose heparin with low-molecular-weight heparin as prophylaxis against venous thromboembolism after major trauma. *N Engl J Med,* Vol.335, No.10, (Sep), pp.(701-707), ISSN: (Print):0028-4793, (Electronic):1533-4406.

Greer, IA. (2003). Prevention and management of venous thromboembolism in pregnancy. *Clin Chest Med,* Vol. 24, No.1, (Mar), pp.(123-137),ISSN: (Print) 0272-5231, (Electronic) 1557-8216.

Goldhaber, SZ., Grodstein, F., Stampfer, MJ., Manson, JE., Colditz, GA., Speizer, FE., Willett, WC., & Hennekens, CH. (1997). A prospective study of risk factors for pulmonary embolism in women. *JAMA,* Vol.277, No.8. (Feb), pp. (642-645), ISSN: (Print) 0098-7484, (Electronic) 1538-3598.

Goodnough, LT., Saito, H., & Ratnoff, OD. (1983). Thrombosis or myocardial infarction in congenital clotting factor abnormalities and chronic thrombocytopenias: a report of 21 patients and a review of 50 previously reported cases. *Medicine (Baltimore),* Vol.62, No.4, (Jul), pp. (248-255), ISSN: (Print) 0025-7974, (Electronic) 1536-5964.

Haire, WD., & Lieberman, RP. (1992). Thrombosed central venous catheters: restoring function with 6-hour urokinase infusion after failure of bolus urokinase. *J Parenter Enteral Nutr,* Vol.16, No.2, (Mar-Apr), pp. (129-132), ISSN: (Print) 0148-6071.

Hanly, JG. (2003). Antiphospholipid syndrome: an overview. *CMAJ,* Vol.168, No.13, (Jun), pp. (1675-1682), ISSN: (Print) 0820-3946, (Electronic) 1488-2329.

Hansson, P., Sorbo, J., Erikson, H. (2000). Recurrent Venous Thromboembolism After Deep Vein Thrombosis. *Arch Intern Med,* Vol.160, No.6, (March), pp.(769-774), ISSN: (Print) 0003-9926, (Electronic) 1538-3679.

Hoshi, S., Hijikata, M., Togashi, Y., Aoyagi, T., Kono, C., Yamada, Y., Amano, H., Keicho, N., & Yamaguchi, T. (2007). Protein C deficiency in a family with thromboembolism and identified gene mutations. *Intern Med,* Vol.46, No.13, (Jul), pp. (997-1003), ISSN:(Print) 0918-2918; (Electronic) 1349-7235.

Huber, O., Bounameaux, H., Borst, F., & Rohner, A. (1992). Postoperative pulmonary embolism after hospital discharge. An underestimated risk. *Arch Surg,* Vol.127, No.3, (Mar), pp. (310-313). ISSN: (Print) 0004-0010, (Electronic) 1538-3644.

Hull, RD., Raskob, GE., Brant, RF., Pineo, GF., & Valentine, KA. (1997). The importance of initial heparin treatment on long-term clinical outcomes of antithrombotic therapy: the emerging theme of delayed recurrence. *Arch Intern Med,* Vol.157, No.20, (Nov), pp. (2317–2321), ISSN: (Print) 0003-9926, (Electronic) 1538-3679.

International Stroke Trial Collaborative Group. (1997). The International Stroke Trial (IST): a randomised trial of aspirin, subcutaneous heparin, both, or neither among 19435 patients with acute ischaemic stroke. *Lancet,* Vol.349, No.9065, (May), PP. (1569–1581). ISSN: (Print) 0140-6736, (Electronic)1474-547X.

Jeffrey, LC., Kelley, AM.,& Duff, A.(1992). The Clinical Course of Pulmonary Embolism. *N Engl J Med,* Vol.326, No.19, (May), pp.(1240-1245), ISSN: (Print) 0028-4793, (Electronic) 1533-4406.

Kluijtmans, LA., Boers, GH., Trijbels, FJ., van Lith-Zanders, HM., van den Heuvel, LP, & Blom, HJ. (1997). A common 844INS68 insertion variant in the cystathionine beta-synthase gene. *Biochem Mol Med,* Vol. 62. No.1, (Oct), pp. (23-25), ISSN: (Print)1077-3150, (Electronic) 1077-3150.

Kovacevich, GJ., Gaich, SA., Lavin, JP., Hopkins, MP., Crane, SS., Stewart, J., Nelson, D, & Lavin, LM. (2000). The prevalenee of thromboembolie events among women with extended bed rest prescribed as part of the treatment for premature labor or preterm premature rupture of membranes. *Am J Obstet Gynecol,* Vol.182, No.5 (May), pp.(1089-1092), ISSN: (Print) 0002-9378, (Electronic) 1097-6868.

Kraaijenhagen, RA., in't Anker, PS., Koopman, MMW., Reitsma, PH., Prins, MH., van den Ende, A., & Buller, HR. (2000). High plasma concentration of factor VIIIc is a major risk factor for venous thromboembolism. *Thromb Haemost,* Vol.83, No.1, (Jan), pp. (5-9), ISSN: (Print) 0340-6245, (Electronic) 0340-6245.

Kyrle, PA., Minar, E., Hirschl, M, Bialonczyk, C., Stain, M., Schneider, B., Weltermann, A., Speiser, W., Lechner, K., & Eichinger, S. (2000). High plasma levels of factor VIII and the risk of recurrent venous thromboembolism. *N Engl J Med,* Vol.343, No.7, (Aug), pp. (457-462), ISSN: (Print):0028-4793, (Electronic)1533-4406.

Lapostolle, F., Surget, V., Borron, SW., Desmaizieres, M., Sordelet, D., Lapandry, C., Cupa, M., & Arnet, F. (2001). Severe pulmonary embolism associated with air travel. *New Eng J Med,* Vol.345, No.11, (Sep), pp. (779-783), ISSN: (Print):0028-4793, (Electronic):1533-4406.

Lee, KW., & Lip, GY. (2003). Effects of lifestyle on hemostasis, fibrinolysis, and platelet reactivity: a systematic review. *Arch Intern Med,* Vol.163, No.19, (Oct), pp.(2368-2392), ISSN: (Print) 0003-9926; (Electronic) 1538-3679.

Leebeek, FW., Knot, EA., Ten Cate, JW., & Traas, DW. (1989). Severe thrombotic tendency associated with a type I plasminogen deficiency. *Am J Hematol,* Vol.30, No.1, (Jan), pp.(32–35),. ISSN: (Print) 1939-6163, (Electronic) 1939-6163.

Lietz, K., Kuehling, SE., & Parkhurst, JB. (2005). Hemorrhagic stroke in a child with protein S and factor VII deficiencies. *Pediatr Neurol,* Vol.32, No.3, (Mar), pp.(208–210), ISSN: (Print) 0887-8994, (Electronic) 1873-5150.

Makris, M., Rosendaal, FR., & Preston, FE. (1997). Familial thrombophilia: Genetic risk factors and management. J *Int Med Suppl,* Vol.740, (Jan), pp. (9-15), ISSN: (Print) 0955-7873, (Electronic) 0955-7873.

Mariani, G, & Bernardi, F. (2009). Factor VII Deficiency. *Semin Thromb Hemost,* Vol.35, No.4, (Jun), pp.(400-406), ISSN: (Print) 0094-6176, (Electronic) 1098-9064.

Mariani, G., Herrmann, FH., Dolce, A., Batorova, A., Etro, D., Peyvandi, F., Wulff, K., Schved, JF., Auerswald, G., Ingerslev, J., & Bernardi, F; International Factor VII Deficiency Study Group. (2005). Clinical phenotypes and factor VII genotype in congenital factor VII deficiency. *Thromb Haemost,* Vol.93, No.3, (Mar), pp.(481–487), ISSN: (Print) 0340-6245, (Electronic) 0340-6245.

McCarthy, ST., & Turner, J. (1986). Low dose subcutaneous heparin in the prevention of deep vein thrombosis and pulmonary emboli following acute stroke. *Age Ageing,* Vol.15, No.2, (Mar), pp.(84–88). ISSN: (Print) 0002-0729, (Electronic) 1468-2834.

Miles, JS., Miletich, JP., Goldhaber, SZ., Hennekens, CH., & Ridker, PM. (2001). G20210 A mutation in the prothrombin gene and the risk of recurrent venous thromboembolism. *J Am Coll Cardiol,* Vol.37, No.1, (jun), pp.(215–218), ISSN: (Print) 0735-1097, (Electronic)1558-3597.

Miletich, JP., Sherman, L., & Broze, GJJ. (1987). Absence of Thrombosis in Subjects with Heterozygous Protein C Deficiency. *N Engl J Med,* Vol.317, No.16, (Oct), pp.(991–996), ISSN:(Print):0028-4793, (Electronic):1533-4406.

Nicolaides, AN., Breddin, HK., Fareed, J., Goldhaber, S., Haas, S., Hull, R., Kalodiki, E., Myers, K., Samama, M., & Sasahara, A. (2001). Cardiovascular Disease Educational and Research Trust and the International Union of Angiology. Prevention of venous thromboembolism. International Consensus Statement. Guidelines compiled in accordance with the scientific evidence. *Int Angiol,* Vol.20, No.1, (Mar), pp. (1-37), ISSN:(Print) 1061-1711, (Electronic) 1615-5939.

Nightingale, C.E., Norman, A., Cunningham, D., Young, J., Webb, A., & Filshie, J. (1997). A prospective analysis of 949 long-term central venous Access catheters for ambulatory chemotherapy in patients with gastrointestinal malignancy. *Eur J Cancer,* Vol.33, No.3, (Mar), pp.(398-403), ISSN: (Print) 0959-8049, (Electronic) 1879-0852.

Poort, SR., Rosendaal, FR., Reitsma, PH., & Bertina, RM. (1996). A common genetic variation in the 3′-untranslated region of the prothrombin gene is associated with elevated plasma prothrombin levels and an increase in venous thrombosis. *Blood,* Vol.88, No.10, (Nov), pp. (3698–3703), ISSN: (Print) 0006-4971, (Electronic) 1528-0020.

Quinn, DA., Thompson, BT., Terrin, ML., Thrall, JH., Athanasoulis, CA., McKusick, KA., Stein, PD., & Hales, CA. (1992). A prospective investigation of pulmonary embolism in women and men. *JAMA,* Vol.268, No.13, (Nov). pp. (1689-1696). ISSN: (Print) 0098-7484, (Electronic) 1538-3598.

Robbins, KC. (1990). Classification of abnormal plasminogens: dysplasminogenemias. *Semin Thromb Hemost,* Vol.16, No.3, (Jul), pp. (217–220), ISSN: (Print) 0094-6176, (Electronic) 1098-9064.

Rosendaal, FR. (1999). Risk factors for venous thrombotic disease. *Thromb Haemost,* Vol.82, No.2, (Aug), pp. (610-619), ISSN: (Print) 0340-6245, (Electronic) 0340-6245.

Rosendaal, FR., Koster, T., Vandenbroucke, JP., Reitsma, PH. (1995). High risk of thrombosis in patients homozygous for factor V Leiden (activated protein C resistance). *Blood,* Vol.85, No.6, (Mar), pp.(1505–1508), ISSN: (Print) 0006-4971, (Electronic) 1528-0020.

Rosing, J., Tans, G., Nicolaes, GA., Thomassen, MC., van Oerle, R., van der Ploeg, PM., Heijnen, P., Hamulyak, K., & Hemker, HC. (1997). Oral contraceptives and venous thrombosis: different sensitivities to activated protein C in women using second and third generation oral contraceptives. *Br J Haematol,* Vol. 97, No.1, (Apr), pp. (233-238), ISSN: (Print) 0007-1048, (Electronic) 1365-2141.

Rubinstein, I., Murray, D., & Hoffstein, V. (1988). Fatal pulmonary emboli in hospitalized patients. An autopsy study. *Arch Intern Med,* Vol.148, No.6, (Jun), pp. (1425-1426), ISSN: (Print) 0003-9926, (Electronic) 1538-3679.

Sapey, E., & Stockley, RA. (2006). COPD exacerbations: 2. Aetiology. *Thorax,* Vol.61, No.3, (Marc), pp. (250–258), ISSN: (Print) 0040-6376, (Electronic)1468-3296.

Schambeck, C., Grossmann, R., Zonnur, S., Berger, M., Teuchert, K., Spahn, A., & Walter U. (2004). High factor VIII (FVIII) levels in venous thromboembolism: role of unbound FVIII. *Thrombosis and haemostasis,* Vol. 92, No.1, (July), pp.(42-46), ISSN: (Print) 0340-6245, (Electronic) 0340-6245.

Schorer, AE., Singh, J., & Basara, ML. (1995). Dysfibrinogenemia: a case with thrombosis (fibrinogen Richfield) and an overview of the clinical and laboratory spectrum. *Am J Hematol,* Vol.50, No.3, (Nov), pp.(200-208), ISSN: (Print) 1939-6163, (Electronic) 1939-6163.

Schuster, V., Zeitler, P., Seregard, S., Ozcelik, U., Anadol, D., Luchtman, JL., Meirc, F., Mingers, AM., Schambeck, C., & Krelh, HW. (2001). Homozygous and compound-heterozygous lype I plasminogen deficiency is a common cause of ligneous conjunctivitis. *Thromb Haemost,* Vol.85, No.6, (Jun), pp.(1004-1010), ISSN: (Print) 0340-6245, (Electronic) 0340-6245.

Shackford, SR., Davis, JW., Hollingsworth-Fridlund, P., Brewer, NS., Hoyt, DB., & Mackersie, RC. (1990). Venous thromboembolism in patient with major trauma. *Am J Surg,* Vol.159, No.4, (Apr), pp.(365-369), ISSN: (Print) 0002-9610, (Electronic) 1879-1883.

Sidney, S., Sorel, M., Quesenberry, CP Jr., DeLuise, C., Lanes, S.,& Eisner MD. (2005). COPD and incident cardiovascular disease hospitalizations and mortality: Kaiser Permanente Medical Care Program. *Chest,* Vol.128, No.4, (Oct), pp.(2068–2075), ISSN: (Print) 0012-3692, (Electronic) 1931-3543.

Spitzer, WO., Lewis, MA., Heinemann, LA., Thorogood, M., & MacRae, KD. (1996). Third generation oral contraceptives and risk of venous thromboembolic disorders: an international case-control study. Transnational Research Group on Oral Contraceptives and the Health of Young Women. *Br Med J,* Vol.312, No.7023, pp. (83-88), ISSN: (Print) 0959-8138, (Electronic) 1468-5833.

Stein, PD., Huang, HI., Afzal, A., & Noor, HA. (1999). Incidence of acute pulmonary embolism in a general hospital: relation to age, sex, and race. *Chest,* Vol.116, No.4, (Oct), pp.(909-913), ISSN: (Print) 0012-3692, (Electronic) 1931-3543.

Stein, PD., & Matta, F. (2010). Acute pulmonary embolism. *Curr Probl Cardiol,* Vol.35, No.7, (Jul), pp.(317-376), ISSN: (Print) 0146-2806, (Electronic)1535-6280.

Subbarao, J., & Smith J. Pulmonary embolism during stroke rehabilitation. (1984). *IMJ Ill Med J,* Vol.165, No.5, pp.(328-332), (May), ISSN: (Print) 0019-2120, (Electronic) 0019-2120.

Tait, RC., Walker, ID., Perry, DJ., Islam, SI., Daly, ME., McCall, F., Conkie, JA., & Carrell, RW. (1994). Prevalence of antithrombin deficiency in the healthy population. *Br J Haematol,* Vol.87, No.1, (May), pp.(106-112), ISSN: (Print) 0007-1048, (Electronic) 1365-2141.

Tapson, VF. (2008). Acute pulmonary embolism. *N Engl J Med,* Vol.358, No.11, (Mar), pp.(1037–1052), ISSN: (Print):0028-4793, (Electronic):1533-4406.

Thaler, E., Lechner, K. (1981). Antithrombin III deficiency and thromboembolism. *Clin Haematol,* Vol.10, No.2, (Jun), pp.(369-90), ISSN: (print) 0308-2261, (Electronic) 0308-2261.

van Dieijen, G., Tans, G., Rosing, J., & Hemker, HC. (1981). The role of phospholipid and factor VIIIa in the activation of bovine factor X. *J Biol Chem,* Vol.256, No.7, (Apr), pp. (3433 3442), ISSN: (Print) 0021-9258, (Electronic) 1083- 351X.

Warlow, C., Ogston, D., & Douglas, AS. (1972). Venous thrombosis following strokes. *Lancet,* Vol.1, No.7764, (Jun), pp.(1305–1306), ISSN: (Print) 0140-6736, (Electronic) 1474-547X.

Weisberg, I., Tran, P., Christensen, B., Sibani, S., & Rozen R. (1998). A second genetic polymorphism in methylenetetrahydrofolate reductase (MTHFR) associated with decreased enzyme activity. *Mol Genet Metab,* Vol.64, No.3, (Jul). Pp.(511–512), ISSN: (Print)1096-7192, (Electronic) 1096-7206.

White, RH. (2003). The epidemiology of venous thromboembolism. *Circulation,* Vol.107, No. (23 Suppl 1), (Jun), pp.(14-18), ISSN: (Print) 0009-7322, (Electronic)1524-4539.

World Healt organization collaborative study of cardiovascular disease and steroid hormone contraception. (1995). Effect of different progestagens in low oestrogen oral contraseptives on venous thromboembolic disease. *Lancet,* Vol.346, No.8890, (Dec), pp.(1582-1588), ISSN: (Printed) 0140-6736, (Electronic)1474-547X.

Yanbaeva, DG., Dentener, MA., Creutzberg, EC., Wesseling, G., & Wouters, EF. (2007), Systemic effects of smoking. *Chest,* Vol.131, No.5, pp.(1557-1566), ISSN: (Print) 0012-3692, (Electronic) 1931-3543.

Yarnell, JW., Sweetnam, PM., Rumley, A., & Lowe, GD. (2000). Lifestyle and hemostatic risk factors for ischemic heart disease : the Caerphilly Study. *Arterioscler Thromb Vasc Biol,* Vol.20, No.1, (Jan), pp.(271-279), ISSN: (Print) 1079-5642, (Electronic)1524-4636.

2

Risk Stratification of Patients with Acute Pulmonary Embolism

Calvin Woon-Loong Chin
National Heart Center Singapore
Singapore

1. Introduction

Acute pulmonary embolism (PE) is an under-diagnosed but potentially fatal condition. This condition presents with a wide clinical spectrum, from asymptomatic small PE to life-threatening one causing cardiogenic shock.

Depending on the estimated risk of an adverse outcome, treatment with thrombolysis or embolectomy may be indicated in high-risk individuals. Conversely, early hospital discharge or even home treatment with anti-coagulation may be considered in low risk PE.

Thus, a systematic approach to risk stratification is essential in guiding the management of patients diagnosed with acute PE. Evidence-based prognostic tools such as clinical scores, echocardiography, computed tomography scans, and cardiac biomarkers will be discussed.

2. Hemodynamic consequences of acute pulmonary embolism

Anatomically massive PE has been defined as having more than 50% obstruction of the pulmonary vasculature or the occlusion of two or more lobar arteries (Urokinase Pulmonary Embolism Study Group, 1970). In a unique situation, a large embolus may lodge at the bifurcation of the main pulmonary artery, i.e. saddle embolus. Although it was once regarded as a severe form of PE, a saddle PE shares a similar clinical course with a non-saddle PE, and low in-hospital mortality (Pruszczyk et al., 2003; Kaczyńska et al., 2005; Ryu et al., 2007).

An anatomically massive PE in a patient with adequate cardiopulmonary reserve and a submassive PE in a patient with poor reserve may manifest similar hemodynamic outcomes. The hemodynamic response to an acute PE depends not only the size of the embolus and the degree of pulmonary vasculature obstruction, but also on the physiologic reaction to the neurohumoral factors released and the underlying cardiopulmonary status of the patient.

Normally, the RV faces low resistance as it empties into a low-pressure system of the pulmonary vasculature. In acute PE, both mechanical obstruction and hypoxic vasoconstriction increase pulmonary vascular resistance, and this initiates a series of hemodynamic derangements leading to RV dysfunction (Figure 1). The release of humoral factors, such as serotonin from platelets, thrombin from plasma and histamine from tissue also contribute to pulmonary artery vasoconstriction. As a consequence of the elevated pulmonary resistance, the highly compliant RV dilates acutely.

Initially, compensatory maintenance of cardiac output is achieved by catecholamine-driven tachycardia and vasoconstriction. The left atrial contraction also contributes more than usual to left ventricular filling. Eventually, with persistent pressure overload and wall stress, RV systolic function begins to fall. Cardiac output is decreased further by impaired distensibility of the left ventricle (LV) from the leftward shift and flattening of the interventricular septum during systole/early diastole, and impaired LV filling during diastole.

Myocardial ischemia also worsens RV function by increased oxygen demands due to elevated wall stress and decreased oxygen supply from elevated right-sided pressures (Goldhaber et al., 2003; Wood, 2002).

The hemodynamic cascade provides an appreciation in understanding the roles the various imaging modalities and biomarkers play in the risk assessment of patients with acute PE.

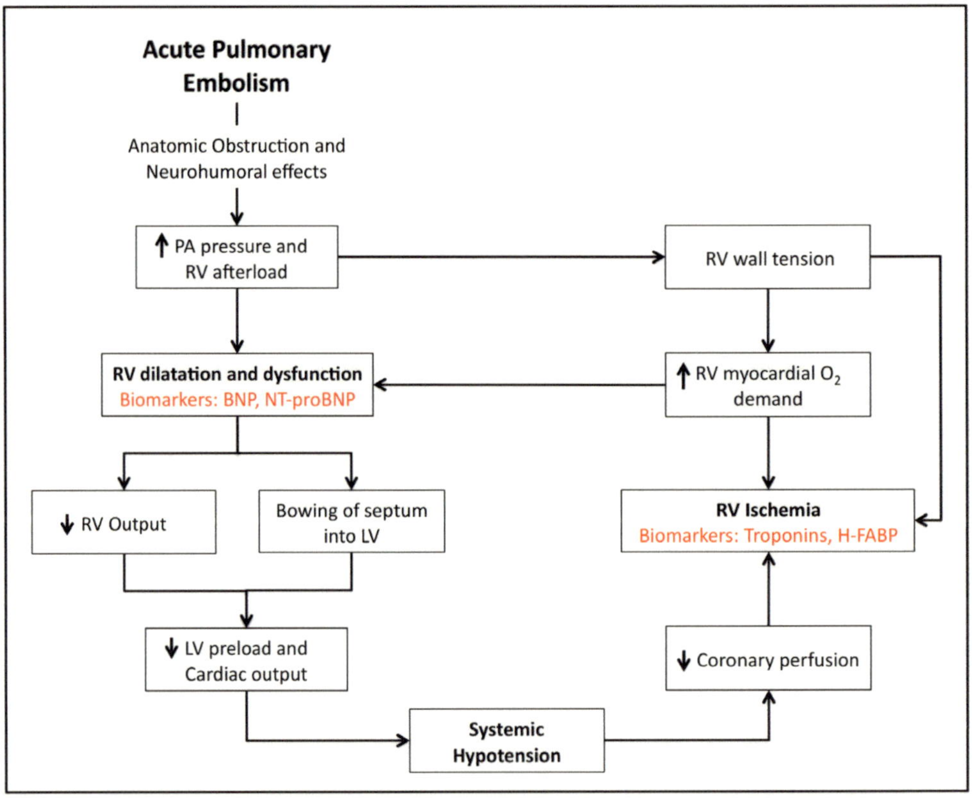

Fig. 1. Hemodynamic consequences due to acute pulmonary embolism and mechanism of biomarkers detection (PA, pulmonary artery; RV, right ventricle; LV, left ventricle; BNP, brain natriuretic peptide; NT-proBNP, NT-pro brain natriuretic peptide; H-FABP, heart-type fatty acid binding protein)

3. Classification of risk

The prognosis of acute PE correlates most directly with the degree of hemodynamic compromise and RV dysfunction.

The European Society of Cardiology recommends an individual risk assessment of early PE-related deaths (Torbicki et al, 2008). Based on the clinical presentation, presence of RV dysfunction and elevated biomarkers, high-risk PE has a short-term (in-hospital or 30-day) mortality risk of > 15%. Non high-risk patients are more heterogenous and are further stratified into intermediate risk (short term mortality risk of 3 to 15%) and low risk (short term mortality risk of less than 1%) (Figure 2).

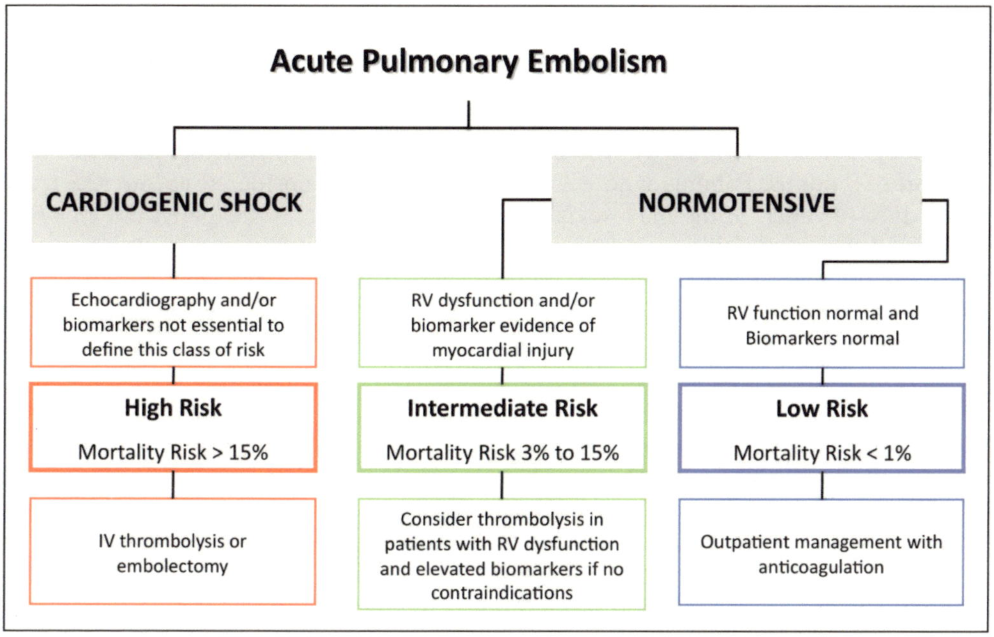

Fig. 2. Risk stratification based on pulmonary embolism-related adverse outcomes

4. Risk assessment based on clinical parameters and risk models

The presence of co-morbidities increases the risk of adverse events, even with a small PE. Advanced age (more than 70 years old), congestive heart failure, cancer, or chronic lung disease were identified as independent predictors of 3-month mortality from PE (Goldhaber, 1999).

The clinical manifestations of acute PE are non-specific and often overlap with other cardiac and pulmonary conditions. Chest pain is one of the most frequent presentations of PE. Pleuritic chest pain, with or without dyspnea, is usually caused by pleural irritation due to distal emboli which may be associated with pulmonary infarction. Individuals may also present with retrosternal angina-like chest pain, reflecting right ventricular ischemia. Isolated dyspnea of a rapid onset is suspicious of a more central and hemodynamically significant PE. Occasionally, the onset of dyspnea is more insidious especially in patients with co-existing heart failure or pulmonary disease.

Cardiogenic shock occurs in less than 5% of acute PE, and these patients have a high risk of death. Conversely, patients with non-massive PE present with stable blood pressure and have a lower risk of death. In the International Cooperative Pulmonary Embolism Registry, the death rate was about 58% in hemodynamically unstable patients and about 15% in patients who were hemodynamically stable (Goldhaber et al., 1999).

Despite the limited sensitivity and specificity of individual symptoms, and signs, clinical risk models consisting of a combination of clinical variables makes it possible to identify patients with suspected PE into risk categories. The Geneva prognostic index and the Pulmonary Embolism Prognostic Index (PESI) are two standardized prognostic scores that incorporated systolic blood pressure, amongst other clinical parameters, to predict risk of PE-related adverse outcomes. These scores have been well validated to identify low-risk, clinically stable patients for outpatient treatment.

The Geneva prognostic index is based mainly on findings from the past medical history and the clinical examination (Table 1). Risk stratification was performed using the score with a maximum of 8 points. Patients with a score of 2 or less are considered at low risk for PE-related adverse events. Of the 180 low risk patients identified, only 4 experienced an adverse outcome at 3 months (Wicki et al., 2000).

The PESI score uses 11 weighted clinical parameters commonly available on presentation (Table 2). Patients are stratified by their scores into five classes of increasing risk of death and adverse outcomes. Patients classified as low risk (score of 85 or less corresponding to PESI Class I or II) have a 30-day mortality of 1.0% (Aujesky et al., 2006).

Of the two, the PESI score appears to be more accurate at predicting low-risk patients. In a head-to-head comparison, the two models were retrospectively applied in a cohort of 599 patients with PE. The 30-day mortality in the Geneva low-risk patients was 5.6% compared to the PESI low-risk mortality rate of 0.9%. The PESI score classified fewer patients as low-risk than the Geneva model (36% vs. 84%), but the area under the receiver operating curve was higher for the PESI (0.76 vs. 0.61) (Jiménez et al., 2007).

Unfortunately, the major limitation of the PESI is the difficulty to apply in a busy clinical environment. There are many variables to be considered, each with its own weight. To address this limitation, a simplified PESI has been developed with similar prognostic accuracy (Jiménez et al., 2010). However, prospective validation of the simplified PESI is lacking.

Risk Factor	Geneva Risk Scale (Points)
Active cancer	2
Systolic blood pressure < 100mmHg	2
Concomitant deep venous thrombosis at diagnosis	1
History of venous thromboembolism	1
Congestive heart failure	1
Hypoxia (arterial PaO_2 < 60mmHg)	1
Geneva Risk Categories Low risk: 2 or fewer points; High risk: 3 or more points	

Table 1. Geneva Pulmonary Embolism Prognostic Index

Variable	Points
Age	1 point/year
Male gender	10
Cancer	30
Congestive heart failure	10
Chronic lung disease	10
Heart rate > 110/min	20
Systolic blood pressure < 100mmHg	30
Respiratory rate ≥ 30/min	20
Body temperature < 36°	20
Disorientation, lethargy, stupor or coma	60
Oxygen saturation < 90%(pulsoximetry)	20

Risk category	Points	30-day mortality risk
Class I	< 65	0 %
Class II	66 to 85	1.0 %
Class III	86 to 105	3.1 %
Class IV	> 125	24.4 %

Table 2. Pulmonary Embolism Severity index (Low risk = Class I and II)

5. Risk assessment based on presence of right ventricular dysfunction

The majority of patients with acute PE are stable at time of diagnosis, but this may not necessarily imply a benign course. Patients may appear stable initially because the development of RV failure and cardiogenic shock can be delayed as the vicious cycle of elevated pulmonary resistance, RV dilatation, and the RV hypokinesis unfolds. In stable patients with acute PE, the presence of RV dysfunction is associated with a high mortality rate (Sanchez et al., 2008).

In addition, RV dysfunction in acute PE predicts recurrent thromboembolic events. During a mean follow-up of three years, patients with persistent RV dysfunction were more likely to have a recurrent PE, deep venous thrombosis or higher PE-related deaths compared with patients without RV dysfunction or had RV dysfunction that resolved at discharge (Grifoni et al., 2006).

5.1 Echocardiography

Echocardiography is non-invasive and able to provide very useful information promptly. However, it is not recommended as a routine imaging test to diagnose PE because an echocardiogram can appear normal in about 50% of the patients with suspected PE. Despite its limitations, a bedside echocardiogram in a hemodynamically unstable patient is an invaluable first-line tool to diagnose other conditions that mimic an acute PE such as myocardial infarction, proximal aortic dissection or a pericardial tamponade. These emergency conditions require management very different from an acute PE.

More importantly, the main role of echocardiography in the setting of an acute PE is to identify a sub-group of stable, non-high-risk patients with RV dysfunction for more aggressive management. The prognostic implications of RV dysfunction detected with echocardiography, even in stable acute PE patients, are clear and this has been illustrated in two separate meta-analyses. In all studies, patients with normal RV function have very good prognosis, with low in-hospital mortality (ten Wolde et al., 2004; Sanchez et al., 2008). Unfortunately, unlike the left ventricle, the anatomy of the RV is complex and assessment of RV function is challenging. Thus, the criteria of RV dysfunction are not well established and differ among published studies (Table 3).

Echocardiography detects both direct and indirect hemodynamic consequences of acute PE (Figure 1). Direct evidence of RV dysfunction includes a dilated RV cavity as compared to the LV. More convincingly, the concomitant presence of RV hypokinesis suggests a failing RV. However, qualitative assessment of RV wall motion is subjective and insufficient in this era of standardization. There is a distinctive two-dimensional echocardiographic finding of regional RV dysfunction that has been described in acute PE. This abnormality is characterized by the presence of normal or hyperdynamic RV apex despite moderate to severe RV free-wall hypokinesis (McConnell sign, Figure 3). Echocardiography may also show flattened inter-ventricular septum or paradoxical motion towards the LV during systole to suggest RV pressure overload (Figure 4).

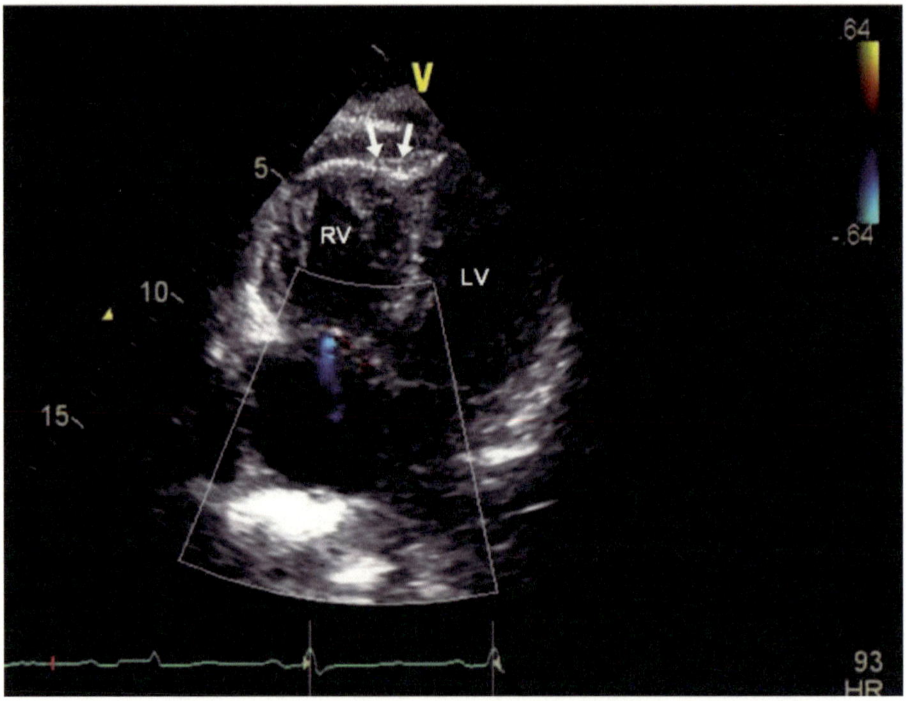

Fig. 3. Apical four-chamber view demonstrating McConnell sign: hypokinesis of the right ventricle (RV) free wall sparing the apex (arrows). The RV is markedly dilated.

Authors	Definition of RV dysfunction
Goldhaber et al, 1993, 1999 Ribeiro et al, 1997, Jerjes-Sanchz et al, 2001, Kucher et al, 2003, 2005	RV hypokinesis by qualitative assessment of the RV wall motion
Kasper et al, 1997	Dilated RV cavity (qualitative assessment of RV compared to left ventricle) or RVEDD > 30mm; or when 2 of the following were present: 1. TR velocity > 2.8m/s 2. TR velocity > 2.5m/s in the absence of inspiratory collapse of the IVC 3. Dilated RPA (> $12mm/m^2$) 4. RV wall thickness > 5mm 5. Loss of inspiratory collapse of the IVC
Grifoni et al, 2000, 2001	Presence of any 1 of the following: 1. Dilated RV (RVEDD/LVEDD > 1 or RVEDD > 30mm) 2. Septal dyskinesis 3. Pulmonary hypertension (Doppler PAT <90ms or RV-RA gradient >30mmHg) 4. Absence of RV hypertrophy (thickness > 7mm)
Pieralli et al, 2006	Presence of any 1 of the following: 1. Dilated RV (RVEDD/LVEDD > 1 or RVEDD > 30mm) 2. Septal dyskinesis 3. Pulmonary hypertension (Doppler PAT <90ms or RV-RA gradient >30mmHg)
Vieillar-Baron et al, 2001	RVEDA/LVEDA > 0.6 with septal dyskinesis
Kostrubiec et al, 2005	Presence of any 1 of the following: 1. RVEDD/LVEDD > 0.6 with RV hypokinesis 2. Pulmonary hypertension (Elevated TVPG >30mmHg with PAT <80ms)

(RVEDD/LVEDD, right to left end-diastolic diameter ratio; RVEDA/LVEDA, right to left ventricular end-diastolic area ratio; RV-RA gradient, right ventricular-right atrial gradient; PAT, pulmonary arterial flow acceleration time; TVPG, tricuspid valve pressure gradient; IVC, inferior vena cava; TR, tricuspid regurgitation).

Table 3. Studies evaluating RV dysfunction with echocardiography

Indirect evidence of RV dysfunction from echocardiography includes raised pulmonary artery systolic pressure (PASP). This can be estimated from the right ventricular systolic pressure (RVSP) according to the formula: PASP = RVSP + estimated right atrial pressure (Figure 5). The RVSP is obtained from the velocity of the tricuspid regurgitant jet (v), such that RVSP = $4v^2$ and the right atrial pressure is estimated from the size and respiratory variation of the inferior vena cava.

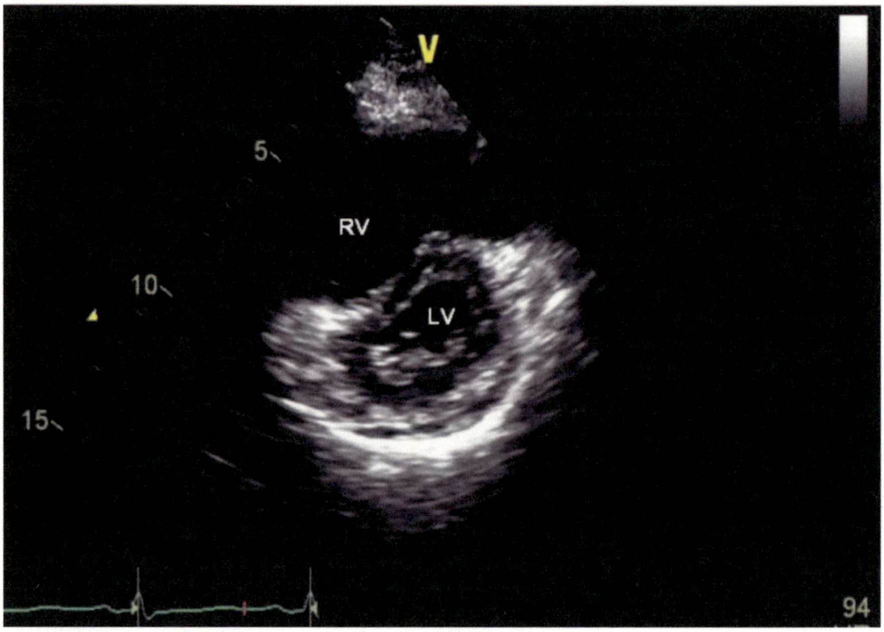

Fig. 4. Parasternal short axis view showing an enlarged right ventricle (RV) with a "D" shaped septum, suggesting RV pressure overload.

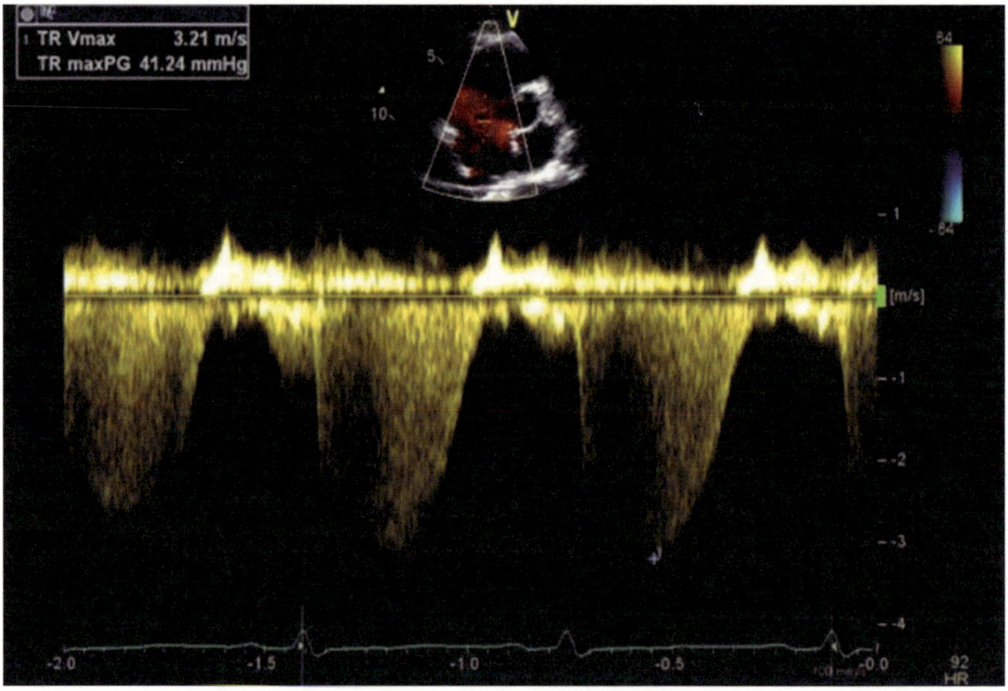

Fig. 5. Continuous wave Doppler demonstrating peak tricuspid velocity of 3.2m/s, corresponding to a right ventricular systolic pressure of 41mmHg.

An elevated pulmonary artery systolic pressure of more than 50mmHg at time of diagnosis is associated with persistent pulmonary hypertension at 1 year (Ribeiro et al., 1999). In patients with acute PE, the absence of any significant tricuspid regurgitation makes the severe pulmonary hypertension less likely.

Besides the evidence of RV dysfunction and elevated pulmonary arterial pressures, other echocardiographic features with prognostic implications include:

1. A right-to-left shunt, such as a patent foramen ovale (PFO). In a prospective study of 139 consecutive patients with acute PE, PFO was diagnosed in 48 patients by contrast echocardiography. Evidence of a PFO in patients with acute PE was associated with higher mortality rate (33% vs. 14%) and higher incidence of peripheral thromboembolic events (Konstantinides et al., 1998). These patients are particularly prone to paradoxical embolism due to increased right-to-left shunt from elevated right-sided pressures.
2. A free-floating right heart thrombus (Figure 6). The prevalence of patients with a right heart thrombus visualized during echocardiography was about 4% (Torbicki et al., 2003). Thrombus from the right heart usually arises from the lower limb veins. These thrombi are highly mobile and often described as having the appearance of a worm, or snake. Free-floating thrombus can embolize at any time and have a dismal prognosis regardless of therapeutic option (Chin et al., 2010). The mortality rate of about 20% within 24 hours of diagnosis, and mortality is significantly linked with the occurrence of cardiac arrest (Chartir et al., 1999).

5.2 Computed tomography

Contrast enhanced computer tomography (CT) of the pulmonary arteries is increasingly used as a first-line imaging modality for PE diagnosis. The anatomical distribution and burden of embolic occlusion of the pulmonary arterial bed can be assessed easily by CT (Figure 7). However, the anatomical assessment seems less relevant for risk stratification than assessment based on functional (hemodynamic) consequences of PE.

Most scanners allow reconstruction of standardized cardiac views and direct measurements of ventricular dimensions can be made. RV enlargement based on RV-to-LV dimension ratio, RV_d/LV_d, (Figure 8) on the reconstructed CT four-chamber view correlated with RV dysfunction on echocardiogram. Using $RV_d/LV_d > 0.9$ as cut-off, the sensitivity and specificity for predicting PE-related adverse events were 83% and 49% on the reconstructed CT, respectively. Comparatively, the sensitivity and specificity of $RV_d/LV_d > 0.9$ on echocardiography were 71% and 56%, respectively (Quiroz et al., 2004).

In addition to having good correlation with RV dysfunction on echocardiography, assessment of RV enlargement on chest CT in acute PE also predicted patients at risk of death from RV failure (Van der Meer et al., 2005; Schoepf et al., 2004). The greatest role appears to be the identification of low-risk patients due to its high negative predictive value (Table 4).

Author	CT equipment (Cutoff)	Sensitivity (%)	Specificity (%)	NPV (%)	PPV (%)
Van der Meer et al., 2005	SDCT (RV/LV >1)	100	45	100	10
Schoepf et al., 2004	4 - 16 MDCT (RV/LV > 0.9)	78	38	92	16

Table 4. Trials reporting RV/LV diameter ratio assessed by CT as a risk marker for 30-day all cause mortality in acute pulmonary embolism.

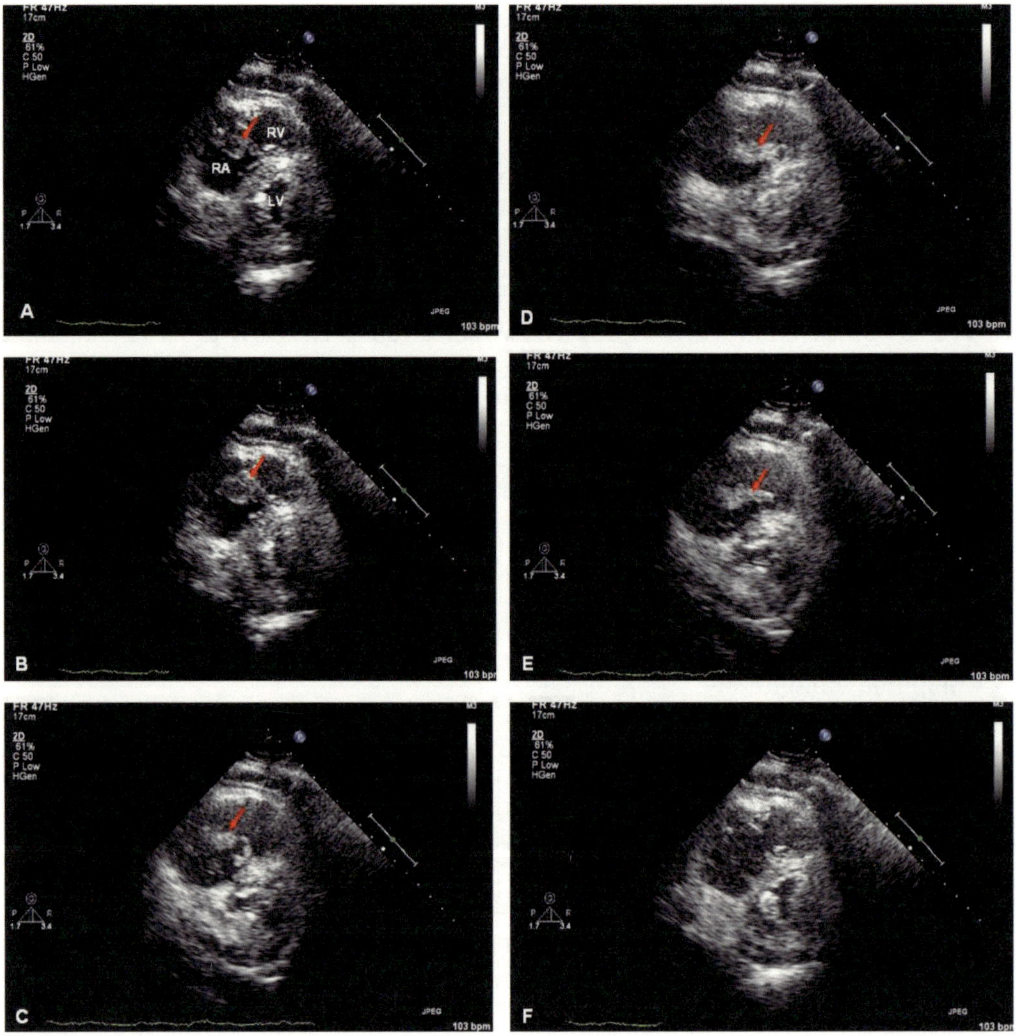

Fig. 6. Free floating thrombus (red arrow) transiting from the RA causing acute pulmonary embolism (RA, right atrium; LA, left atrium; LV, left ventricle).

Other CT-derived parameters have also been investigated. The presence of interventricular septal bowing is predictive of PE-related deaths but has low sensitivity and high inter-observer variability (Araoz et al., 2007), scores to quantify the extent and location of pulmonary artery obstruction have been developed but not shown to be of prognostic relevance yet (Qanadil et al., 2001; Ghanima et al., 2007).

5.3 Ventilation-perfusion scintigraphy

Lung ventilation-perfusion scintigraphy (V/Q scan) is a well-established diagnostic test used in patients suspected of PE. Interpretation of the scans can vary, depending on the algorithms used (PIOPED criteria, modified PIOPED criteria, McMaster Clinical criteria and PisaPED criteria) and the experience of the reader. The diagnostic roles and limitations of V/Q scan are beyond the scope and will not be discussed in this chapter.

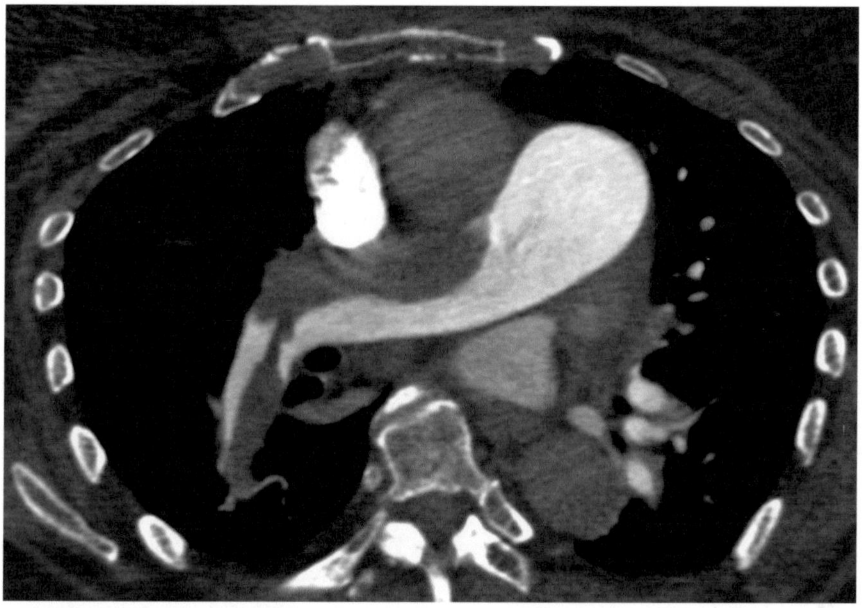

Fig. 7. Computed tomography pulmonary angiogram showing a large embolus within the right main pulmonary artery, extending to the main right upper lobe.

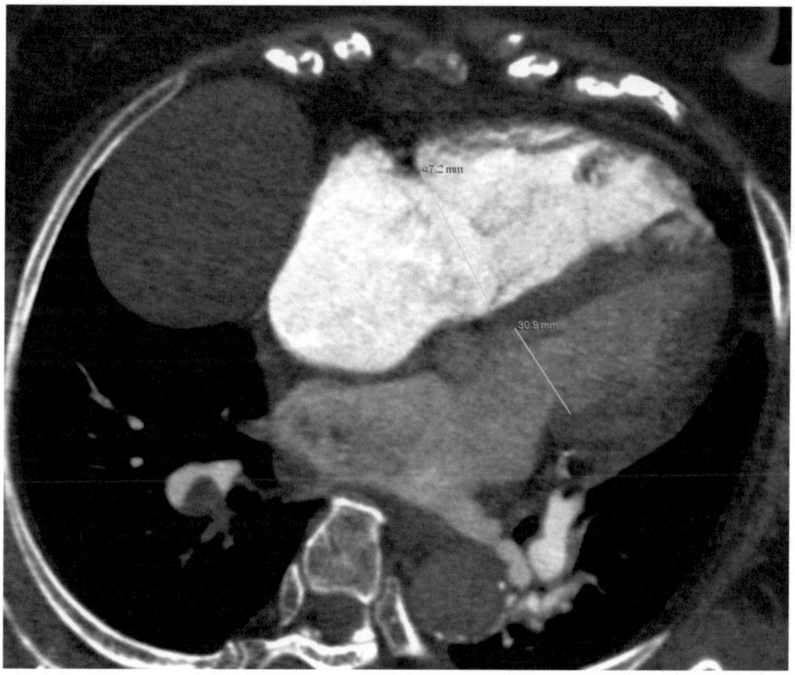

Fig. 8. Measurement of the short axes of the RV (47 mm) and LV (39 mm) on computed tomography pulmonary angiogram of the same patient (RV, right ventricle; LV, left ventricle)

Perfusion defects due to PE increase with the number and size of emboli, without corresponding ventilation compromise ("mismatch" defects). However, the prognostic implications of the number and size of defects on a V/Q scan have not been investigated.

6. Risk assessment based on biomarkers of myocardial injury

Cardiac troponins I and T as well as NT-pro brain natriuretic peptide (NT-proBNP) and brain natriuretic peptide (BNP) have emerged as promising tools for risk stratification.

6.1 Cardiac troponins

Cardiac troponins may be increased in patients with PE, even in the absence of coronary artery disease. The presumed mechanism is acute right heart overload attributed to myocardial ischemia and from oxygen supply-demand mismatch. The elevation usually resolves within 40 hours following PE in contrast to more prolonged elevation after an acute myocardial infarction. The peak level is usually lower than in acute myocardial infarction (Müller-Bardorff et al., 2002).

Patients with an elevated troponin I or troponin T levels had an increased risk for short-term mortality (OR 5.24, 95% CI 3.28 - 8.38) or PE-related deaths (OR 9.44, 95% CI 4.14 - 21.49). Elevated troponin levels even among patients who are hemodynamically stable are associated with higher mortality (Becattini et al., 2007; Jimenez et al., 2008).

Irrespective of various methods and cut-off values applied, most trials reported a low positive predictive value for PE-related mortality in the range of 12% to 44%, but with a very high negative predictive value between 99% and 100%.

6.2 Brain natriuretic peptide

Right ventricular dysfunction is associated with increased myocardial stretch which leads to the release of BNP and its amino terminal portion, NT-proBNP.

In acute PE, increasing levels of BNP or NT-proBNP predict the severity of RV dysfunction and mortality (Cavallazzi et al., 2008; Klok et al., 2008; Lega et al., 2009). Although elevated concentrations are related to worse outcome, the positive predictive value is low. On the other hand, low levels of BNP or NT-proBNP can be used reliably to identify patients with a good prognosis (Table 5).

6.3 Novel biomarker

Heart-type fatty acid binding protein (H-FABP), a protein released earlier than troponins during myocardial ischemia, has been evaluated as a prognostic marker in acute PE. The studies have reported a high sensitivity (78% to 100%) and negative predictive value (96% to 100%), but these studies are small and such measurements are not widely available (Puls et al., 2007; Kaczynska et al., 2006).

6.4 Summary of evidence on the prognostic value of biomarkers

Many studies did not perform an extensive comparison between all the available biomarkers, thus it remains debatable which biomarker will yield the best prognostic value.

Another limitation is biomarker thresholds were determined retrospectively, thus no consistent cut-off values were used in the studies. Despite this, it appears BNP/NT-proBNP and cardiac troponins could be used as rule-out tests.

Author	Test used (Threshold)	Outcome Definition	Sensitivity (%)	Specificity (%)	NPV (%)	PPV (%)
Ten Wolde et al, 2003	BNP Shionoria[a] (21.7 pmol/L)	PE-related deaths	86	71	99	17
Kucher et al, 2003a	NT-proBNP[b] (500 pg/mL)	In-hospital death or adverse events[e]	95	57	97	45
Kucher et al, 2003b	BNP Triage[c] (50 pg/mL)	In-hospital death or adverse events[e]	95	60	97	48
Pruszczyk et al, 2003	NT-proBNP[b] (600 pg/mL)	In-hospital mortality	100	33	100	23
Binder et al, 2005	NT-proBNP[b] (1000 pg/mL)	In-hospital mortality	100	49	100	10
Kostrubiec et al, 2007	NT-proBNP[b] (7500 pg/mL)	30-day all cause mortality	65	93	94	61

([a-c]Tests used: [a]Shionoria, CIS Bio International; [b]Elecsys, Roche Diagnostics; [c]Triage, Biosite Technologies. [e]Adverse events include the need for resuscitation, mechanical ventilation, inotropic support, thrombolytics, or embolectomy)

Table 5. Prognostic value of BNP or NT-proBNP in acute pulmonary embolism

Due to the high negative predictive value for PE-related mortality and adverse events, a potential approach consists of a combination of biomarker testing and echocardiography. In the setting of an acute PE, further risk stratification with echocardiography is warranted in patients with elevated cardiac biomarkers due to limited specificity of the assays for predicting RV dysfunction. Conversely, in patients with levels below cut-off, echocardiography will likely not add prognostic information.

This approach was demonstrated in a prospective study of 124 patients diagnosed with acute PE. The presence of RV dysfunction on echocardiography in patients with elevated NT-proBNP (cut-off of 1000 pg/mL) or cardiac troponins (cut-off of 0.04 ng/mL) is associated with a 10-fold increase in complication risk compared with patients biomarker levels below threshold (Binder et al., 2005).

7. Risk of recurrence

Recurrent PE can occur despite adequate anticoagulation therapy in patients who had survived an acute PE.

Patients with unprovoked PE (PE occurring in the absence of established risk factors or predisposing illnesses) are at a higher risk for recurrent PE compared to patients with risk factors for PE. In contrast, patients with risk factors of PE have a higher mortality risk (Klok et al., 2010). In addition, patients who presented with a first symptomatic PE are at a 4-fold increased risk of recurrent symptomatic PE compared to patients who presented with deep venous thrombosis without symptoms of PE (Eichinger et al., 2004).

In patients with recurrent PE or progressive deep venous thrombosis (DVT) despite adequate anticoagulation therapy, inferior vena cava (IVC) filters may be indicated. IVC filter placement is generally accepted in patients with massive PE or limited cardiopulmonary reserve and DVT. Current evidence indicates that IVC filters are largely effective, with breakthrough PE occurring in only 0% to 6.2% cases. Recurrent PE, IVC thrombosis, filter migration, filter fracture, or penetration of caval wall can sometimes occur with long-term use (Chung et al., 2008).

8. Conclusion

Risk stratification of acute PE is fundamental not only to select an appropriate treatment strategy, but also to potentially reduce costs of management (Figure 2). An appropriate risk stratification algorithm would include clinical, imaging and biomarkers. High risk PE is diagnosed in the presence of shock or persistent hypotension and should warrant urgent management. Thrombolysis with alteplase (rtPA), streptokinase, or urokinase is the recommended therapy. Embolectomy could represent an alternative therapy for patients with shock in the acute setting when thrombolysis has been unsuccessful.

Hemodynamically stable patients without RV dysfunction or myocardial injury are at low-risk for PE-related adverse events. These patients may be eligible for early hospital discharge or even outpatient treatment.

In the remaining normotensive patients, a plausible strategy is to combine biomarkers with echocardiography. The presence of RV dysfunction and myocardial injury identifies patients at intermediate risk.

Whether intermediate risk patients will have any survival benefit with early initiation of reperfusion therapy (and what type of therapy) is not well accepted. Current recommendations proposed thrombolysis be instituted in selected patients at high risk for adverse events without contraindications (Grade IIB ESC and ACCP VIII Edition), and intravenous unfractionated heparin should be reserved to conditions in which thrombolysis is contraindicated (Grade IA ESC and ACCP VIII Edition). An ongoing study assessing the benefit of thrombolysis as compared with anticoagulation in hemodynamically stable patients with evidence of RV dysfunction and an elevated troponin levels will hopefully provide some insights (NCT00639743).

9. References

Araoz PA, Gotway MB, Harrington JR, Harmsen WS, Mandrekar JN. Pulmonary embolism: prognostic CT findings. Radiology 2007;242:889.

Aujesky D, Roy PM, Le Manach CP, Verschuren F, Meyer G, Obrosky DS et al. Validation of a model to predict adverse outcomes in patients with pulmonary embolism. Eur Heart J 2006;27:476–481.

Becattini C, Vedovati MC, Agnelli G. Prognostic value of troponins in acute pulmonary embolism: a meta-analysis. Circulation 2007;116(4):427.

Binder L, Pieske B, Olschewski M, Geibel A, Klostermann B, Reiner C, Konstantinides S. N-terminal pro-brain natriuretic peptide or troponin testing followed by echocardiography for risk stratification of acute pulmonary embolism. Circulation. 2005 Sep 13;112(11):1573-9. Epub 2005 Sep 6.

Cavallazzi R, Nair A, Vasu T, Marik PE. Natriuretic peptides in acute pulmonary embolism: a systematic review. Intensive Care Med. 2008;34(12):2147.

Chartier L, Bera J, Delomez M, Asseman P, Beregi JP, Bauchart JJ, Warembourg H, Thery C. Free floating thrombi in the right heart: diagnosis, management, and prognostic indexes in 38 consecutive patients. Circulation 1999;99:2779-83.

Chin C, Lim ST, Ho KW, et al. Free Floating Thrombus in the Right Heart Causing Pulmonary Embolism. Postgraduate Medical Journal 2010;86:307.

Chung J, Owen RJ. Using inferior vena cava filters to prevent pulmonary embolism. Can Fam Physician. 2008 Jan;54(1):49-55.

Eichinger S, Weltermann A, Minar E, Stain M, Schönauer V, Schneider B, Kyrle PA. Symptomatic pulmonary embolism and the risk of recurrent venous thromboembolism. Arch Intern Med. 2004 Jan 12;164(1):92-6.

Ghanima W, Abdelnoor M, Holmen LO, Nielssen BE, Sandset PM. The association between the proximal extension of the clot and the severity of pulmonary embolism (PE): a proposal for a new radiological score for PE. J Intern Med. 2007;261:74.

Goldhaber SZ, Elliott CG. Acute pulmonary embolism: part 1. Epidemiology, pathophysiology, and diagnosis. Circulation 2003;108:2726.

Goldhaber SZ, Haire WD, Feldstein ML, et al. Alteplase versus heparin in acute pulmonary embolism: randomised trial assessing right-ventricular function and pulmonary perfusion. Lancet. 1993;341:507-511.

Goldhaber SZ, Visani L, De Rosa M. Acute pulmonary embolism: clinical outcomes in the International Cooperative Pulmonary Embolism Registry (ICOPER). Lancet 1999;353:1386.

Goldhaber SZ, Visani L, De Rosa M. Acute pulmonary embolism: clinical outcomes in the International Cooperative Pulmonary Embolism Registry (ICOPER). Lancet. 1999;353:1386-1389.

Grifoni S, Olivotto I, Cecchini P, et al. Short-term clinical outcome of patients with acute pulmonary embolism, normal blood pressure, and echocardiographic right ventricular dysfunction. Circulation. 2000;101:2817-2822.

Grifoni S, Olivotto I, Pieralli F, et al. Long-term clinical outcome of patients with pulmonary embolism with or without right ventricular dysfunction [abstract]. Thromb Haemost. 2001;86(suppl). Abstract P2231.

Grifoni S, Vanni S, Magazzini S, Olivotto I, Conti A, Zanobetti M, Polidori G, Pieralli F, Peiman N, Becattini C, Agnelli G. Association of persistent right ventricular dysfunction at hospital discharge after acute pulmonary embolism with recurrent thromboembolic events. Arch Intern Med. 2006;166(19):2151.

Jerjes-Sanchez C, Ramirez-Rivera A, Arriaga-Nava R, et al. High dose and short term streptokinase infusion in patients with pulmonary embolism: prospective with seven-year follow-up trial. J Thromb Thrombolysis. 2001;12:237-247

Jimenez D, Aujesky D, Moores L, Gomez V, Lobo Jose, et al. Simplification of the pulmonary embolism severity index for prognostication in patients with acute symptomatic pulmonary embolism. Arch Intern Med 2010;170:1383-1389.

Jiménez D, Díaz G, Marín E, Vidal R, Sueiro A, Yusen RD. The risk of recurrent venous thromboembolism in patients with unprovoked symptomatic deep vein thrombosis and asymptomatic pulmonary embolism. Thromb Haemost. 2006 Mar;95(3):562-6.

Jiménez D, Díaz G, Molina J, Martí D, Del Rey J, García-Rull S, Escobar C, Vidal R, Sueiro A, Yusen RD. Troponin I and risk stratification of patients with acute nonmassive pulmonary embolism. Eur Respir J. 2008 Apr;31(4):847-53. Epub 2007 Dec 19.

Jiménez D, Yusen RD, Otero R, Uresandi F, Nauffal D, Laserna E, Conget F, Oribe M, Cabezudo MA, Díaz G. Prognostic models for selecting patients with acute pulmonary embolism for initial outpatient therapy. Chest. 2007;132(1):24-30.

Kaczyńska A, Pacho R, Bochowicz A et al. Does saddle embolism influence short-term prognosis in patients with acute pulmonary embolism? Kardiol Pol, 2005; 62: 119–127.

Kaczynska An, Pelsers MM, Bochowicz A, Kostrubiec M, Glatz JF, Pruszczyk P. Plasma heart-type fatty acid binding protein is superior to troponin and myoglobin for rapid risk stratification in acute pulmonary embolism. Clin Chim Acta. 2006;371:117.

Kasper W, Konstantinides S, Geibel A, Tiede N, Krause T, Just H. Prognostic significance of right ventricular afterload stress detected by echocardiography in patients with clinically suspected pulmonary embolism. Heart. 1997;77:346-349.

Klok FA, Mos IC, Huisman MV. Brain-type natriuretic peptide levels in the prediction of adverse outcome in patients with pulmonary embolism: a systematic review and meta-analysis. Am J Respir Crit Care Med. 2008;178(4):425.

Klok FA, Zondag W, van Kralingen KW, van Dijk AP, Tamsma JT, Heyning FH, Vliegen HW, Huisman MV. Patient outcomes after acute pulmonary embolism. A pooled survival analysis of different adverse events. Am J Respir Crit Care Med. 2010 Mar 1;181(5):501-6. Epub 2009 Dec 3.

Konstantinides S, Geibel A, Kasper W, Olschewski M, Blumel L, Just H. Patent foramen ovale is an important predictor of adverse outcome in patients with major pulmonary embolism. Circulation 1998;97:1946.

Kostrubiec M, Pruszczyk P, Kaczynska A, Kucher N. Persistent NT-proBNP elevation in acute pulmonary embolism predicts early death. Clin Chim Acta 2007;382:124.

Kucher N, Printzen G, Doernhoefer T, Windecker S, Meier B, Hess OM. Low pro-brain natriuretic peptide levels predict benign clinical outcome in acute pulmonary embolism. Circulation 2003;107:1576–1578.

Kucher N, Printzen G, Goldhaber SZ. Prognostic role of brain natriuretic peptide in acute pulmonary embolism. Circulation 2003;107:2545.

Kucher N, Rossi E, De Rosa M, et al. Prognostic role of echocardiography in patients with acute PE and a systemic arterial pressure of 90mmHg or higher. Arch Intern Med 2005;165:1777.

Lega JC, Lacasse Y, Lakhal L, Provencher S. Natriuretic peptides and troponins in pulmonary embolism: a meta-analysis. Thorax. 2009;64(10):869.

McConnell MV, Solomon SD, Rayan ME, Come PC, Goldhaber SZ, Lee RT. Regional right ventricular dysfunction detected by echocardiography in acute pulmonary embolism. Am J Cardiol. 1996 Aug 15;78(4):469-73.

Müller-Bardorff M, Weidtmann B, Giannitsis E, Kurowski V, Katus HA. Release kinetics of cardiac troponin T in survivors of confirmed severe pulmonary embolism. Clin Chem. 2002;48(4):673-5.

Pieralli F, Olivotto I, Vanni S, Conti A, Camaiti A, Targioni G, Grifoni S, Berni G. Usefulness of bedside testing for brain natriuretic peptide to identify right ventricular dysfunction and outcome in normotensive patients with acute pulmonary embolism. Am J Cardiol 2006;97:1386–1390.

Pruszczyk P, Kostrubic M, Bochowicz A, Styczynski G, Szulc M, Kurzyna M et al. N terminal pro-brain natriuretic pepetide in patients with acute pulmonary embolism. Eur Respir J 2003;22:649.

Pruszczyk P, Pacho R, Ciurzynski M et al. Short term clinical outcome of acute saddle pulmonary embolism. Heart 2003; 89: 335–336.

Puls M, Dellas C, Lankeit M, et al. Heart-type fatty acid-binding protein permits early risk stratification of pulmonary embolism. Eur Heart J 2007;28:224.

Qanadli SD, El Hajjam M, Viellard-Baron A, et al. New CT index to quantify arterial obstruction in pulmonary embolism: comparison with angiographic index and echocardiography. Am J Roentgenol 2001;176:1415.

Quiroz R, Kucher N, Schoepf UJ, Kipfmueller F, Solomon SD, Costello P, et al. Right ventricular enlargement on chest computed tomography: prognostic role in acute pulmonary embolism. Circulation 2004;109:2401.

Ribeiro A, Lindmarker P, Johnsson H, Juhlin-Dannfelt A, Jorfeldt L. Ribeiro A, Lindmarker P, Johnsson H, Juhlin-Dannfelt A, Jorfeldt L. Pulmonary embolism: one-year follow-up with echocardiography doppler and five-year survival analysis. Circulation. 1999 Mar 16;99(10):1325-30.

Ribeiro A, Lindmarker P, Juhlin-Dannfelt A, Johnsson H, Jorfeldt L. Echocardiography Doppler in pulmonary embolism: right ventricular dysfunction as a predictor of mortality rate. Am Heart J. 1997;134:479-487.

Ryu JH, Pelikka PA, Froehling DA, Peters SG, Aughenbaugh GL. Saddle pulmonary embolism diagnosed by CT angiography: frequency, clinical features and outcome. Respir Med 2007;101:1537.

Sanchez O, Trinquart L, Colombet I, Durieux P, Huisman MV, Chatellier G, Meyer G. Prognostic value of right ventricular dysfunction in patients with hemodynamically stable pulmonary embolism: a systemic review. Eur Heart J 2008;29:1569.

Schoepf UJ, Kucher N, Kipfmueller F, Quiroz R, Costello P, Goldhaber SZ. Right ventricular enlargement on chest computed tomography: a predictor of early death in acute pulmonary embolism. Circulation. 2004 Nov 16;110(20):3276-80. Epub 2004 Nov 8.

Ten Wolde M, Söhne M, Quak E, Mac Gillavry MR, Büller HR. Prognostic value of echocardiographically assessed right ventricular dysfunction in patients with pulmonary embolism. Arch Intern 2004;164:1685.

Ten Wolde M, Tulevski II, Mulder JW, Sohne M, Boomsma F, Mulder BJ et al. Brain natriuretic peptide as a predictor of adverse outcome in patients with pulmonary embolism. Circulation 2003;107:2082.

The urokinase pulmonary embolism trial. JAMA 1970; 214:2163-72

Torbicki A, Galie N, Covezzoli A, Rossi E, De Rosa M, Goldhaber SZ. Right heart thrombi in pulmonary embolism: results from the International Cooperative Pulmonary Embolism Registry. J Am Coll Cardiol 2003;41:2245.

Torbicki A, Perrier A, Konstantinides S, et al., Guidelines on the diagnosis and management of pulmonary embolism. European Heart Journal 2008;29:2276-2315.

van der Meer RW, Pattynama PM, van Strijen MJ, van den Berg-Huijsmans AA, Hartmann IJ, Putter H, de Roos A, Huisman MV Right ventricular dysfunction and pulmonary obstruction index at helical CT: prediction of clinical outcome during 3-month follow-up in patients with acute pulmonary embolism. Radiology. 2005 Jun;235(3):798-803. Epub 2005 Apr 21.

Vieillard-Baron A, Page B, Augarde R, Prin S, Qanadli S, Beauchet A, Dubourg O, Jardin F. Acute cor pulmonale in massive pulmonary embolism: incidence, echocardiographic pattern, clinical implications and recovery rate. Intensive Care Med 2001;27:1481–1486.

Wicki J, Perrier A, Perneger TV, et al. Predicting adverse outcome in patients with acute pulmonary embolism: a risk score. Thromb Haemost 2000;84:548.

Wood KE. Major pulmonary embolism: review of a pathophysiologic approach to the golden hour of hemodynamically significant pulmonary embolism. Chest 2002;121:877–905.

3

Pulmonary Embolism in the Elderly – Significance and Particularities

Pavel Weber, Dana Weberová, Hana Kubešová and Hana Meluzínová
Department of Internal Medecine, Geriatrics and Practical Medicine
Masaryk University and University Hospital, Brno
Czech Republic

1. Introduction

The development of civilization and extreme technical progress leads to increasing hope of longer survival and makes the average life expectancy longer. Both in absolute and relative numbers the amount of the elderly, very old and long-aged people are increasing (Blackburn & Dulmus, 2007; Ratnaike, 2002). This tendency will continue and it will be emphasized by ageing volumes of people born after the World War 2 in the years 2010 -2015 (Kalvach et al., 2004). The basic survey and knowledge of geriatric medicine will be necessary in the future, especially for professionals such as doctors, nurses, psychologists, social workers, physio- and occupational therapists etc.

Knowledge of at least basic extraordinarities and specifics of geriatric medicine will be of huge practical significance, because in the year 2050 there will live 2 billions of people older than 60 years on the Earth. (Moody, 2009). From this fact it is obvious, that there is an objective need to master the basic knowledge of gerontology and geriatry among professionals (including doctors of all medical branches).

In this brief chapter it is not possible to include the whole issue dealing with the medical care of old-aged patients with PE, even if this issue deserves the attention because of its practical meaning and close relationship with other branches (internal medicine, surgery etc.). The emergency situations together with polymorbidity and exhaustion of functional reserves in advanced age (Campbell et al., 2008; Friedman et al., 2008) will be more frequent in all of the organ systems - cardiovascular, respiratory, GI (gastrointestinal) tract, endocrine, immune etc. (Bongard & Sue, 2003; Roberts & Hedges, 2009). We refer to the study of the clinical picture description (incl.therapy) of each of critical states in the old age in appropriate specialized chapters in this monograph and in other gerontologic literature (Hall et al., 2005; Stone & Humphries, 2004).

General knowledge of these aspects can substantially influence an approach of intensivists who face an increasing number of old patients in their practice (Brunner-Ziegler et al., 2008; Pathy et al., 2006). Among the aspects we would like to mention there are: global situation, specific problem of geriatric medicine, pharmacotherapy in the elderly, at last but not least problems of ageing organism as reflected in particularities and pitfalls of medical treatment in multi-morbid old patients.

Ageing and its manifestation as currently understood such as frailty, functional disorders and decreasing mental abilities are not standard symptoms of ageing process but they are mostly consequences of simultaneously on-going diseases (Goldmann et al., 2000; Fauci et al., 2008). The target of new **interventional gerontology** is extension of active life period and sustaining functional abilities for maximum time.

Information about function can be used in a number of ways: as baseline information, as a measure of the patient's need for support services or placement, (Tallis & Fillit, 2003) as an indicator of possible caregiver stress, (Asplund et al., 2000) as a potential marker of specific disease activity, to determine the need for therapeutic interventions, and to indicate prognosis.

2. Comprehensive geriatric assessment (CGA) as basic tool of modern geriatry

Clinical gerontology emphasises an individual approach to old patients (Harari et al., 2007; Soriano et al., 2007). The method of operation is **comprehensive geriatric assessment - CGA** (Gupta, 2008; Gurcharan & Mulley, 2007; Williams, 2008). Apart from somatic aspects of the health status there are significant items to be underlined: self-sufficiency evaluation, knowledge and evaluation of psychic state and social conditions (see tab. 1).

Much of what has been written on evaluation of the older patient is simply attention to the details of careful clinical assessment. Contemporary emphasis on efficiency and effectiveness of clinical care requires thoughtfulness about any extension of the already lengthy evaluation of complex chronic medical problems that commonly cluster in older persons. Brief screening questions rather than elaborate instruments are appropriate for the first encounters (Stuck, 1995); more detailed assessment should be reserved for patients with demonstrated deficits (Applegate et al., 1990).

Subject of assessment	Way of evaluation
Somatic status	Somatic examination, posture, mobility, continence, nutrition, sight, hearing, geriatric syndromes, etc.
Self-sufficiency	ADL- test, ability to keep own household, IADL- test
Mental status	cognitive function - MMSE- test, Clock test; depression scale according Yesavage, etc.
Social status	social contacts, people available to summon help, bereavement, removal, dwelling and loneliness risks

Table 1. Comprehensive geriatric assessment

In its multidisciplinary context the geriatry does not substitute other clinical medical branches in care of an old person but completes them with application of **specific geriatric regimen**, which aims to reinforce the independence and improve self-sufficiency of the older patients (Williams, 2008). Following methods are based on principles of **specific geriatric regimen**.

- Considerate tailor-made diagnostics and treatment aimed at improvement of life quality
- Follow up physiotherapy
- Multi-disciplinary team active approach aimed at improvement of self-sufficiency and/or prevention of dependence

- Social work creating conditions enabling patients to return to home environment (incl. home-care)

Main target of these efforts is improvement in independence and self-sufficiency improvement in older patients (Zavazalova et al., 2007). Geriatric regimen brings benefits especially for patients aged 75+ or even 80+ who are endangered with following risks typical for this age:

- Development of immobilisation syndrome
- Self-sufficiency loss
- Atypical pathway of more diseases influencing simultaneously each other
- Occurrence of early impairment of organ function as a consequence of exhaustion of their functional reserve (lungs, kidneys etc.)
- Maladaptation towards changes
- Ageism (discrimination because of the old age).

Evaluation of the older patient can be time-consuming (Topinkova, 2005), even when it is tailored to the problem. Yet, such initial investment can reduce subsequent morbidity and resource utilization and enhance both patient's and physician's satisfaction. Additionally, the assessment can often be accomplished over several visits. Moreover, much can be gleaned from questionnaires filled out by the patient or caregiver in advance as well as from observation.

3. Geriatric patient – Particularities of health status

Geriatric patients are people of higher age (formally above 65; practically above 75 years), their involutionary and morbid changes (usually multi-morbidity) significantly influenced their functional state, adaptability, ability of regulation, toleration to stress. These patients profit from specific geriatric attitude, they need more complicated coordination of services, often active observation of health and/or functional state, they are in risk of sudden loss of self-sufficiency, danger of delay, adverse effect of remedies is more frequent, institutional care is often needed (geriatric hospitalism), also they are in danger of frequent professional mistakes for atypical symptoms in comparison to clinical picture, which is for certain disease typical in adult middle age (Friedman et al., 2006; Pathy et al., 2006; Williams, 2008).
The following principles of geriatric medicine are helpful to keep in mind while caring for older adults:

1. Diseases often present atypically.
2. Many disorders are multifactorial in origin.
3. Not all abnormalities require evaluation and treatment.
4. Polypharmacy and adverse drug events are common problems.

Comorbidities are common in older people, and the diagnostic "law of parsimony" often does not apply. A disorder in one organ system may lead to symptoms in another, especially the one that is compromised by preexisting disease. Since these organ systems are often the brain, the lower urinary tract, and the cardiovascular or musculoskeletal systems, a limited number of presenting symptoms - i.e., confusion, falling, incontinence, dizziness, and functional decline - predominate irrespectively of the underlying disease. Thus, regardless of the presenting symptoms in older people, the differential diagnosis is often similar.
Many abnormal findings in younger patients are relatively common in older people and may not be responsible for a particular symptom. Such findings may include asymptomatic

bacteriuria, premature ventricular contractions, and slowed reaction time. In addition, many older patients with multiple comorbidities may have laboratory abnormalities that, while pathologic, may not be clinically important. A complete workup for a mild anemia of chronic disease in a person with multiple other issues might be burdensome to the patient with little chance of impacting quality of life or longevity.

Ageing is associated with a decline in expectation of healthiness. Those over age 65 generally give more positive evaluations of their healthiness in the face of increasing burden of disease and disability (Kriegsman et al.., 1996; Tinetti et al., 2000). The older the person is, the more likely they are to report very good health status (Gross et al.., 1996). However, overestimating healthiness (also called normalization) often results in explaining away symptoms or problems as caused by minor illnesses or even by external events. In either case, late recognition and delayed intervention are the usual outcome. Previous neglecting of symptoms by health care professionals is also likely to teach older patients that frailty and loss of independence are normal and to be expected with ageing; again, late detection and intervention are likely, resulting in high cost and discouraging outcomes. Perhaps these attitudes explain the finding of greater pessimism in older persons compared with those middle-aged, even when health status was factored in. *Underreporting of symptoms* is a common theme in discussions of illness behavior of older persons.

The problems identified were common and usually treatable diseases; congestive heart failure, correctable hearing and vision deficits, tuberculosis, incontinence, anemia, bronchitis, claudication, cancers, malnutrition, diabetes, immobility, oral disease preventing eating, dementia, and depression were frequent. Considerable underreporting was also seen among people with chronic diseases. More than a half of chronically ill individuals, who were surveyed in one study, failed to report at least one disease. Older people tend to report inaccurately cardiac disease, arthritis, and stroke (Kriegsman et al.., 1996).

The riskiness of underreporting of symptoms by older patients is obvious; late identification of disease (inclusive of PE) leads to late initiation of treatment, usually after substantial morbidity associated with advanced pathology has already occurred and caused major functional losses. Rehabilitation to independence from these losses is difficult; permanent dependence in spite of "successful" treatment may occur.

Majority of all biological functions culminates before the age of 30 y. Some of them gradually continuously decrease afterwards (Masoro & Austad, 2006). This decay is practically of no significance in terms of current everyday activity but it can matter under stress or extended load (Humes, 2000; Hunter et al., 2002).

Seniors as such represent very heterogenous group and from the point of wiev of fitness, risk and need of help (or specific service) they can be divided to the 3 basic areas with different focus of health attention:

- **Fit seniors** - Seniors in good condition and physical efficiency. Medical attitude towards them should be the same as standards which are valid for adults in middle age. However, there can be also risk of atypical symptoms of diseases in them.
- **Independent seniors** - do not need extraordinary care and services, they can live independently in standard condition, however in stress situations (severe diseases, surgery, injuries, viral infections in epidemies, extreme variation of the weather, sudden change of social state - death of partner, loneliness, moving etc.) they fail.
- **Frail seniors** - are instable and in the risk even in standard condition. These frail seniors usually need help in common daily activities or they are limited in motion, moreover they are confined to bed (Fried et al.., 2005; Wawruch et al.., 2006). This group

of patients contains those with higher risk of falls, dementia syndrome, with very bad mobility, labile somatic disease (i.e. frail cardiac with repeated cardiac failure or electric instability), also with complicated orientation (visual disturbance and hearing loss), people in social distress and very old above 85 years old, especially when they live alone (Leng et al.., 2007; Yaffe et al.., 2007).

Health status in ageing is a result of many factors, including the chronic diseases of ageing and many other prevalent conditions that cannot be defined as classic "diseases" because they do not result from a single pathologic cause. Falls, which occur in one third of older adults, result in injuries, fractures, and high risk for disability and mortality. Severe cognitive impairment and urinary incontinence have a substantial adverse impact on an elderly person, as does sensory isolation resultnig from hearing and visual impairment; all of these conditions are frequent with aging.

Older patients differ from young or middle-aged adults with the same disease in many ways, one of which is the frequent occurrence of comorbidities and of subclinical disease.

A second way in which older adults differ from younger adults is the greater likelihood that their diseases present with nonspecific symptoms and signs. As a result, the diagnostic evaluation of geriatric patients must consider a wider spectrum of diseases than generally would be considered in middle-aged adults.

4. Biology of ageing

Ageing and advanced age is a terminal phase of ontogenetic development of every individual (Beers et al., 2006; Pathy et al., 2006). **Specific degenerative morphological** and **functional changes** occur in individual organs at all levels from the cells to whole organism (Heltweg, 2006). Important role in aging is **apoptosis.** In the cell, which may compromise the body (eg, activated leukocyt, as malignant cells), respectively a correction would be difficult to run programmed cell death.

Despite the biologic controversy, from a physiologic standpoint human ageing is characterized by progressive constriction of the homeostatic reserve of every organ system. This decline, often referred to as *homeostenosis*, is obvious by the third decade and is gradual and progressive, although the rate and extent of decline vary. The decline of each organ system appears to occur independently of changes in other organ systems and is influenced by diet, environment, and personal habits as well as by genetic factors.

Even beyond age 85, only 30% of people are impaired in any activity required for daily living and only 20% reside in a nursing home. Yet, as individuals age they are more likely to suffer from disease, disability, and the side effects of drugs, all of which, when combined with the decrease in physiologic reserve, make the older person more vulnerable to environmental, pathologic, and pharmacologic challenges.

This happens in different periods of times and in different speed. It affects any living substance from the moment of it's birth (conception). The life expectancy of an individual in nature is species specific and has important inter-individual variability. Ageing speed of an individual is genetically coded - it is presumed that this type of genetics is a multi-factorial one (Masoro & Austad, 2006). Maximum potential life expectancy of a human being attainable under ideal circumstances could be 110 - 120 y. The influence of genetic factor on the life expectancy is considered about 35 per cent. The resting 65 per cent represent an influence of a life style and external environment.

Common and **typical features of ageing** in general:

1. loss of functional parenchyma of individual organs = **involution**
2. decay of physical performance, deteriorated regeneration after load and reduced tolerance towards load
3. influence of one or more diseases
4. disintegrated ageing: big inter- and intra-individual differences (organs and systems)
5. effort to create new own homeostatic mechanisms (which accompanies growing involution) = **adaptability**.

Senile performance decline is a consequence (Beers et al.., 2006) of general weakness, impaired locomotion and balance, lower stamina. The life expectancy is significantly influenced by risk factors, contingent metabolic changes and level of resistance to stress. A choice of life style is also essential. Ageing in human population is often connected with increased occurrence of degenerative affections, tumours and Alzheimer's disease (Holmerova et al., 2007).

In fact it should be a period of life in which broad harmonic development of human personality goes on and on. Most people of advanced age should remain independent, self-sufficient and retaining their good psychic condition up to the terminal period of their life (Nemeth et al., 2007).

5. Epidemiology and demography of ageing

In the beginning of the 20th century 3 to 5 per cent of population in European industrial countries (similarly in USA) were people aged 65+ y. This percentage has grown up to 14 – 20 nowadays. Up to the fifties of previous century people died prematurely. During the last hundred years the life expectancy (LE) almost doubled which is one of the greatest achievements of mankind and science in general. Length of human life begins to approach to its biological limit. Probability of achieving advanced age is no longer exceptional, on the contrary it becomes a standard (Fauci et al., 2008; Pathy et al., 2006; Ratnaike, 2002).

Demographically, the ageing population due to changes in mortality and fertility decline – fewer children are born and more people live to old age. Crucial in this is played by more improved standard of living than in the past and progress of medicine.

Absolute and relative growth of number of the elderly both in developed and developing countries is a main feature of population development in the 21st century (Scherl, 2003). We speak about **population ageing**. There are approx. 580 mil. people aged 60+ in the today's world out of which 355 mil. live in developing countries. In 2050 there will be 2 billions of our planet inhabitants aged 60+ y. This age category will overweight children of < 14 y. The most rapid increase during the next decades is envisaged in the 80+ y. group in the industrial countries. It is the ageing of old population (Buttler, 2003). In the USA (fig.1), Canada and majority of European union countries it has been found that the most rapidly increasing group of population is the one of 85+ y.

Ageing in the industrial (developed) **countries** can be considered:

- prevailingly gradual
- connected with birth rate decrease
- a consequence of improving life conditions after the industrial revolution
- progress in medicine

In the **developing countries** on the other hand:

- ageing is more rapid
- birth rate decrease is dramatic

- life expectancy grows as a consequence of improving medical care
- ageing leads to enhanced poverty

In 2020 aged 60+ - 70 per cent of them will live in the developing countries. The highest proportion of these elderly is envisaged in Japan (31 per cent), than in Greece and Switzerland (28 per cent), USA (23 per cent), etc.

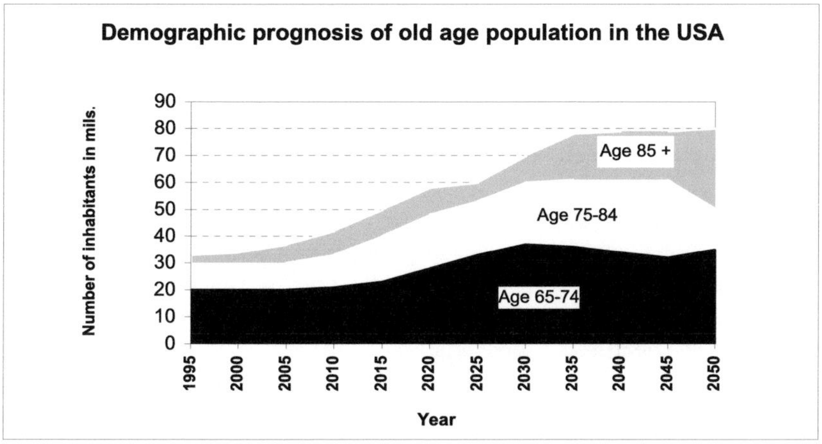

Fig. 1. Demographic prognosis of old age population in the USA

The growth of population aged 65+ in Europe and Northern America during the next 30 years is estimated to reach 24 – 35 per cent. Growing number of the elderly brings also both absolute and relative increase of occurrence of affections which are typical for the advanced age and this becomes a serious worldwide social problem (Seitz, 2003). This covers not only typically somatic diseases such as atherosclerosis, cardio- and cerebrovascular events, heart failure, peripheral vasculopathies, parkinsonism, hypo-thyreoses, diabetes, osteoporosis and osteoarthrosis, diverticulosis, anemies, etc. but also mental diseases with all manifestations and consequences of dementia, especially the Alzheimer's type (Braunwald et al.., 2001; Sinclair & Finucane, 2003).

Analogically to the population ageing in society also medical science has experienced a phenomenon of the so called "**geriatrisation of medicine**" which means a significant prevalence of the elderly among all the patients to be treated (Asplund et al.., 2000). This aspect penetrates practically all the branches of medicine to begin with the front line up to the various special fields including ophtalmology.

6. Characteristics of ageing

The elderly are highly heterogeneous group, and individuals become more dissimilar as they age. Individuals over 65 years – with or without chronic diseases – vary widely in their physical, behavioral, and cognitive functions.

The **ageing** – *is an inevitable physiological process, which is the last ontogenetic period of the human life.* People mostly achieve their old age without any enormous problems. They live to their **„successful ageing"**. in quite comfortable physical, psychical and social balance (Duthie et al., 2007; Williams, 2008). The somatic (diseases), psychical (dementia, depression) and social (loneliness) problems begin to appear apparently after 75th year (more in women) (Barba et al.., 2000)

The old age and the disease cannot be considered the same thing no matter how often it happens in both non-professional and professional community. In most cases the individual in old age is self-sufficient and fit until the last period of his/her life (many times until the last days). The dependence on care of the others comes with the disease, which can be both somatic and psychical. In between 65 and 75 years nearly 85% of people do not suffer from any significant modifying or common life restricting disease. Even in the age above 85 years 40% of the elderly can live self-sufficiently their normal life (Gammack & Morley, 2006).

Women live usually 7 - 8 years longer than men (Tallis & Fillit, 2003). The explanation can be found most likely in gender specific genetic factors and also in biological factors of the environment. The differences in surviving between genders has not changed even in contemporary era, when women smoke more often than ever before and perform originally male professions.

In gerontology we speak sometimes about the so-called **male overmortality**. The consequence of this phenomenon is increasing number of widows as the age increases. This is the base for the typical phenomenon in gerontology - the phenomenon of lonely old women. That fact indirectly increases the consumption of both institutional and non-institutional care in the health and social sphere.

The beginning of the **social old age** is usually seen in the moment of entitlement to regular retirement or the actual retirement (Blackburn & Dulmus, 2007; Woodford & George, 2007). The classification of the human age in social sphere is as follows: *the first age* (before productive age, childhood and youth, learning, preparation for profession, acquisition of social experience), *the second age* (productive age, adulthood, biological productivity - breeding, economical and social productivity), *the third age* (postproductive, the old age), eventually *the fourth age* (the period of dependance), which does not take place in every person inevitably. The calendar age is uniquely determined but does not reflect the individual differences of the real health status among the human beings.

The determination of the age zones for the old age is conventional and it is a social frame outgoing from the administrative needs of the social state. In the demographic statistics it is usually worked with the border of 60 or 65 years. Nowadays the beginnig of the old age is thought 65 years and the old age itself is considered from 75 years on. From this pattern also the most used division of the old age results:

- *65 – 74 years* old belong to group of young seniors, the main problem is the retirement, the free time, activities, self-fulfillment.
- *75 – 84 years*, the old seniors, the problem of adaptability, toleration to stress, specific ailment, loneliness. The **age above 75 years**, when the old age begins in the strict sense of the word, it seems to be breaking point of ontogenesis, when more significant changes connected with physiological ageing proceed.
- *85 and more years* very old aged seniors („oldest old") - they are segregated as an individual cathegory for the high occurrence of frail seniors and high risk of sudden rise of dependency.

7. Geriatic syndromes and frailty as golden grale of geriatric medicine

Presentation of illness in older persons less often is a single, specific symptom or sign, which in younger patients, announces the organ with pathology. Older persons often present with nonspecific problems that are in fact functional deficits (Kalvach et al., 2008). Stopping eating and drinking, or the new onset of falls, confusion, lethargy, dizziness, or incontinence in older patients may be the primary or sole manifestation of diseases with classic signs and symptoms in the young (e.g., pneumonia, myocardial infarction, pulmonary embolus, alcoholism or myxedema). These deficits have been named *geriatric syndromes;* they devastate independence without producing obvious or typical indications of disease. Geriatric syndromes may be defined as a set of lost specific functional capacities potentially caused by a multiplicity of pathologies in multiple organ systems. Comprehensive evaluation (Tinetti et al.., 2000) is usually required to identify and treat underlying causes. Although in many instances a geriatric syndrome has several contributing causes, remedying even one or a few may result in major functional improvement.

The most likely explanation for nonspecific presentation is that the additive effects of ageing restrict capacity to maintain homeostasis. Perturbation of homeostasis by disease, trauma, or drug toxicity will be manifested in the most vulnerable organ, or the weakest link, resulting from interactions of biologic ageing and chronic disease. In addition to nonspecific presentation, disease in older patients can present in other atypical ways. Blunting or absence of typical or classic symptoms and signs is well described in many conditions (Doucet et al.., 1994; Perez-Gusman et al.., 1999; Trivalle et al.., 1996).

Health status in ageing is a result of many factors, including the chronic diseases of ageing and many other prevalent conditions that cannot be defined as classic „diseases" because they do not result from a single pathologic cause. Many of the problems affecting aged individuals should be viewed as geriatric syndromes (GS), that are a collection of signs and symptoms with a number of potential causes (Hazzard, 2007). Only nowadays the causes and effective treatments of these conditions are beginning to be understood.

In spite of indisputable significance of the atypical clinical picture of diseases in the old age, the **crux of geriatric medicine** is involutionarity conditioned *decline of health potential, frailty* and *related geriatric syndromes* and *function deficiency* with their multicausal reasons. This status is connected with exhaustion of organ reservoirs - **"homeostenosis"**. Geriatric syndrome is different from the convenient meaning of the word "syndrome" in clinical medicine, where the symptoms are typical for certain disease (Inouye et al.., 2007; Pathy et al., 2006). For the geriatric syndromes numerous and various causes are typical which lead to the occurence of geriatric syndrome at the end. Geriatric syndromology is an essential component of the so-called comprehensive geriatric assessment (CGA) which is extended over the clinical examination in younger non-geriatric population (Gupta, 2008; (Gurcharan & Mulley, 2007; Williams, 2008).

Geriatric giants (Chase et al.. , 2000; Sherman, 2003;) as geriatric syndromes (GS):

- **immobility** (pressure sore etc.),
- **instability** (dizziness, posture and gait disorders, falls),
- incontinence,
- **intellectual disorders** (delirium, dementia and depression),
- **iatrogenia** (dangerous polypharmacy).

They are characterized by their:

a. Multicausality
b. Chronic course
c. Reduced independence
d. Demanding care and difficult curability

As further geriatric syndromes are respected (44,49):

- **syndrom of hypomobility, decondition and sarcopenia**
- **anorexia syndrom and malnutrition**

- **syndrom of dual combined sensoric deficiency (visual and hearing)**
- **syndrom of dehydration with subsequent manifestation of acute renal failure**
- **syndrom of thermoregulatory disturbance**
- **syndrom of elder abuse, neglect and self-neglect sy**
- **syndrom of geriatric maladaptation**
- **syndrom of terminal geriatric deterioration - FTT** („failure to thrive")

The above mentioned geriatric syndromes not always threaten patient's life but they essentially influence quality of their following life (Fauci et al., 2008; Salvedt et al.., 2002). Patients become fully dependent on other people´s assistance (family, friends, neighbours, community services). Not exceptionally they must be admitted to an institutional care (hospitals, nursing homes etc.) because of domestic care system failure or necessity to manage an acute phase of a disease. The expression of the concept of geriatric syndromes in the last decades is a very fundamental step forward in geriatric medicine. The marked part of multi-morbid disabled handicapped seniors can be better understood and earlier and effectively solved (Williams, 2008). GS are more complicated problem with inner connections very often. Their proper identification is made possible by:

- screeenig tests and observation
- optimalisation of geriatric hospital regime
- optimal coordination of community and institutional services
- influence on anorexia by adjustment of nutrition (proteins 1.3g/kg)
- psychotherapeutical support with elimination of the depression
- lasting physiotherapy (everyday walking at least for 30minutes)
- attempting to influence the disinterest and weariness by interesting daily activity
- using all of the occupational utilities, which can minimise the dependence (walker, rods, crutches, wheelchairs and other - glasses, magnifying glass, hearing aids
- recondition programs
- adjustment of the living (lightning, grab handles on toilet and corridors, the correct hight of the bed and furniture)

The involutionary loss of muscle tissue in the old age is called **sarcopenia** and it is characterized by reduction of muscle tissue, reduction of the force, tenacity, plasticity and speed of contraction (Roubenoff & Hughes, 2000a). The probable cause of sarcopenia in senium (Roubenoff, 2000b) is apart from somatopausis (lowered level of anabolic IGF-1, growth hormone and testosterone) also influence of oxidatory stress and free radicals produced by muscle mitochondrias (Masoro & Austad, 2006). The metabolic result of sarcopenia in the old age is also impaired glucose tolerance and higher risk of diabetes of 2nd type (Fauci et al., 2008; Sinclair & Finucane, 2001).

The meaningful concept which is tightly connected with ageing is **frailty** (Friedman et al., 2008; Rockwood & Hubbard, 2004; Woodhouse & O'Mahony, 1997). This belongs to key characteristics of geriatric patients, the next milestone and the keystone of geriatric medicine. Frailty is a biologic syndrome (Crome & Lally, 2011) of decreased reserves in multiple systems that results from dysregulation that can occur with ageing and is initiated by physiological changes of ageing, disease, and/or lack of activity or inadequate nutritional intake.

It is rather more multidimensional concept than just the expression of a degree of dependence in the everyday life activities. Frailty is basically connected with the grow of fatal somatic ailments and lowering of functional reserve of the old person, which is wasting away excessively without any fundamental cause disease (Juraskova et al., 2010). **Frailty** can be defined as a status of reduced physiological reserves connected with increased inclination towards invalidisation (falls, fractures, daily life restrictions, loss of independence - Leng, 2007; Walston, 2006). Apart from the clinical observations there is elevation of CRP, leukocytes (monocytes), IL-6, IL-1 and TNF. Frailty is not the synonym of multi-morbidity or disability, multi-morbidity can cause this and disability can be the consequence (Fried et al., 2005).

Frailty *is understood mainly as a risk of sudden deterioration of the status of very risky person. (above 80 years, living alone or with handicapped spouse, with serious somatic or psychical disease).* The outcome for those defined frail seniors is the long term need of help of institutions and community (nursing service). The risks of the development of frailty (Friedman et al., 2006; Szanton et al., 2010) are represented by hypomobility in pre-senium, social isolation, depression, bad subjective feeling of the own health etc.

The concept of frailty is at least coming nearer to the term risky geront, used in the past. The emphasis is put on the retrieval of these people because they can not show their frailty out. Both (the ageing and physical frailty) are conditioned by the decline of proteosynthesis in the muscles, decline of immune function, elevation of the mass of fat in the body and lowering of the amount of body water, lowering of the bone mineral density, loss of the whole body mass and strength.

The main etiological and patogenetic mechanisms (Leng et al., 2007; Walston et al., 2006) of the syndrome of frailty are:

- the inflammation or hypercoagulation
- oxidative stress
- insulin resistence
- anorexia with loosing of the weight and malnutrition
- sarcopenia
- fall of efficiency of lower hints
- loosing of spontaneous action - nutrition, hydration, movement, behavioral and social
- dysfunction of autonomic nervous system (falls, sarcopenia, decubital ulcer and healing - with the consequence like loosing the weight, incontinence, delirium, disturbance in thermoregulation etc.)
- apathy - as the consequence of lack of the dopamine in CNS (depression, dementia)
- depression, anxious status, organic psychosyndrome
- development of cognitive deficiency
- menopausis and andropausis as the consequence of hormone deficiency with the development of the syndrome ADAM and PADAM, somatopausis as the result of lack of IGF-1
- chronical pain
- hypomobility with the sedentary lifestyle
- chronic stress
- functionally important consequences of chronic diseases which limit in an activity (hemiparesis, severe diabetic neuropathy, respiratory or heart insufficiency, hard anemia of chronic diseases)
- adverse effects of the medicaments

8. Polypharmacy in the elderly

Polypharmacy is a common problem in the elderly. Particularly in those who have multiple comorbidities. Their therapy should be guided by the estimated life expectancy and the patients' values and goals. Interventions that are likely to help the elderly, who are well, may differ from those that will benefit the ones who are frail. Estimating life expectancy can help a health care provider to focus on those issues to be most likely beneficial in the given patient.

There are several reasons for the greater incidence of iatrogenic drug reactions in the elderly population, the most important of which is the high number of medications that are taken by the elderly, especially those with multiple comorbidities (Blackburn & Dulmus, 2007; Duthie et al., 2007). Older individuals often have varying responses to a given serum drug level. Thus, they are more sensitive to some drugs (eg. opioids) and less sensitive to others (eg. beta-blockers).

Following aspects should be considered in the old-age pharmacotherapy (Katzung, 2003):

1. Responses to drugs are different from preceeding age categories which is a consequence of changed pharmaco-dynamics and pharmaco-kinetics.
2. Increased occurrence of undesired effects of drugs in general
3. Increased non-compliance in the elderly
4. Increased occurrence of drug interactions

Multi-morbidity of advanced age often leads a physician in clinical practice to **polypharmacotherapy** (Nikolaus, 2000; Soriano et al., 2007), which is many times inevitable but still is sometimes hazardous because with increasing age an occurrence of undesired drug effects grows. The elderly are generally more vulnerable and the therapeutic range gets narrower. Compliance decreases inter-individual variability of an effect increases the same way as the risk of drug interactions. Basic requirement for phamacotherapy in advanced age is that it should be simple, purposeful and effective. Polypharmacy can be often risky and ineffective, many times it can be even damaging – **iatrogenia** as a syndrome. In geriatric medicine generally symptomatic treatment overweights the causal one. Its undesired effects can substantially alter the clinical picture of diseases.

The consumption of drugs in the elderly treated within the institutional care is three times higher when compared to the same number of individuals from general population and female patients need twice as many drugs as the male ones.

Distribution of drugs depends on the body composition as mentioned, bonds to plasmatic proteins and blood flow trough tissues. Poorly nourished or frail elderly persons may have a low serum albumin. A cardiac output in advanced age decreases, peripheral vessel resistance grows, liver gets smaller and blood flow trough liver and kidneys decreases. Bigger part of the cardiac output in comparison to the younger ones flows through the brains, heart and skeleton muscles. This also plays a role in the drug distribution.

9. Problems and complications of polypharmacy

Occurrence of **undesired drug effects** is generally 3 – 5 times higher in advanced age when compared to preceding age categories (Beers et al. , 2006). Higher consumption of drugs brings along higher risks (including deep venose thrombosis - DVT and PE). Side effects occur in 2 per cent of the elderly using less than 3 drugs at a time during a year. This percentage grows up to 17 in those who use 10 drugs. Combination of more drugs is preferred recently more and more frequently to mono-therapy. Except for expected and beneficial effect of synergism it can bring also adverse side effects. Number of new drugs especially in psychiatry and neurology grows dramatically during last decades. The most frequently prescribed drugs today are anxiolytics and antidepressants. They are often required also by the elderly and their usage grows also in internal medicine, geriatrics and other non-psychiatric medical branches. One third of the undesired drug effect is predictable and mere reduction of a dosage can eliminate two thirds of them.

These undesired effects are often wrongly diagnosed which leads to prescription and administration of further drugs - it is a so called prescriptive cascade. Correct medication (both with prescription drugs and commercially available medicaments) is based on the right indication appropriate dosage and forms adapted to intellectual potential and somatic skills of a patient, elimination of predictable undesired effects and drug interactions and minimisation of their impacts on patient, consideration of optimum period of drug administration and consistent monitoring of permanent administration connected with continuous evaluation of compliance (Katzung, 2003). Non-compliance occurs in 25 - 50 per cent of older patients taking drugs regularly.

When prescribing a drug the physician should ask:

- Which drug is the most convenient one regarding multi-morbidity and predictable drug interactions?
- What is the optimum dosage?
- Is a drug indication definite and undoubtful?

10. Multimorbidity in old age and its relations

Multiple pathology, or concurrence of diseases, is common among older persons. An early Scottish study of community-dwelling persons over age 65 reported 3.5 major problems per person; for those being admitted to hospitals, 6 disorders were documented per patient. Multiple pathology (Crome & Lally, 2011) poses multiple risks to older patients and their physicians. The first hazard is that active medical problems frequently interact to the detriment of the patient -*disease-disease interactions*.

Late detection of treatable problems whose neglecting and interaction have led to functional decline is common in older patients and can be one of the few discouraging features of geriatric care. Preventive dental and medical care could have avoided the sepsis, worsening of diabetes, fall, hip fracture, postoperative heart attack, stroke, and loss of independent living.

The interaction between old age and illness causes specific changes of diseases in senium (Beers et al., 2006; Pathy et al., 2006; Ratnaike, 2002).

Particularities of illness in old age include:

- Multi-morbidity - parallel occurrence of more illnesses in one person with or without causality relationship
- Mutual causality of social and health situation - each of the changes of the health state in old age influences their social status and vice versa
- Among the specialities of clinical picture of illnesses in old age we can list:

1. microsymptomathology - minimal symptoms of diseases (the iceberg phenomenon)
2. mono- or oligosyptomatology - sporadic symptoms from those, which occur usually in middle or young age
3. distant signs - to the forefront of clinical picture there are symptoms, which belong to the difficulties of other organ than the basic one ("the innocent organ complains, not the sick one")
4. tendency to chronicity - even in the diseases which are in younger and middle age acute, moreover in old age there is higher risk of death

5. tendency to complications - either of type of "chain reaction" or it is the complication, which does not have the direct relation ("crowd-out effect")
6. atypical picture of the diseases – „For the diseases in the old age it is typical that their running is atypical"

The proper symptomathology of the basic disease is usually inconspicuous. In the clinical picture manifestation of non-specific and universal symptoms dominates. These are the results of the secondary brain decompensation. Among those the universal *neurologic and psychiatric symptomathology* conditioned on hypo-perfusion (hypoxia) of the brain (TIA, delirium etc.) belong. The senior's brain is usually affected with the degenerative or vascular changes and reacts usually as the first organ.

Among the causes of the morbidity in old age the forward position (Tallis & Fillit, 2003) is being taken by the diseases of the cardiovascular system conditioned with atherosclerosis like CHD (coronary heart disease), MI (myocardial infarction), angina pectoris, stroke, transient ischemic attack, ischemic disease of the lower limbs (atherosclerosis - AS is present in 90% of the people above 75 years.). In old age we find common: the diseases of the locomotive system, sense organs, tumours, accidental injuries, the diseases of the respiratory tract, gastrointestinal tract (biliary problems etc.) and urogenital tract (the prostate in men, gynecological in women). Diabetes, mental and neurological disorders are common (Beckman et al., 2002; Sinclair & Finucane, 2003). Their coincidental and usually independent occurrence is typical for the senior's multi-morbidity. After the age of 60 there is continuous increase mainly of the cardiovascular diseases as CHD, stroke, hypertension (Ferrari, 2003; Oskvig, 1999). Similarly with the age prevalence of diabetes rises (Sinclair & Finucane, 2003).

For the quality of the senior's life crucial matter is not the presence of the disease itself (or more diseases) but the grade of the disability, it means functional disturbance, into which it is proceeding. The full self-sufficiency can be untouched even when there are more diseases present together.

The inclination of the seniors to the diseases is higher (Khaw, 1997) and the balance of the organ homeostasis is very frail (eg. homeostenosis). Similarly it is the case of "primary" mental disorders (dementia, depression, delirium) or in the geriatric social syndromes (neglect sy, elder abuse, geriatric maladaptation sy). The stressor is usually in psychosocial sphere and its clinical manifestation appears most often in cardiovascular area (heart failure, MI, stroke) or in impaired immunity (pneumonia).

As it was mentioned, the diseases and the morbid conditions in old age are marked by many extraordinarities. The diseases in old age have the tendency to cumulate and potentiate each other. In the geriatric medicine multidimensionality is typical. It is needed to comprehend the sick person in old age as the bio-psycho-social unit in more holistic way than in younger age from the viewpoint of etiopatogenesis of the disease and also in the case of everyday clinical practice.

The quoted problems from the somatic, psychic and social areas which are in the mutual interaction are hardly treatable, they are chronic with the progression of the condition and they have relatively unfavourable prognosis. They bring a lot of hardly solvable situations and problems to the ill and the surroundings. By the „old old" people ($\geq$ 80 years) the diseases proceed in the way (Crome & Lally, 2011), which differ from the progress of the diseases in middle age and they need the different approach which can improve the health condition or at least maintain the self-sufficiency and they accent the comeback home.

The most of the biological functions achieve the top before the 30th year of the life. Some of them slightly decrease afterwards linearly. For the everyday activity this decrease has not any practical importance, but can be relevant in the time of bigger stress or in the load. The physiological processes which are decreasing as the age grows are: blood flow through the kidneys, the clearance of the creatinin, the maximum heart rate and pulse volume in stress, glucose tolerance, vital capacity of the lungs, body weight, cell immunity. On the contrary the total lung capacity and the liver function do not change with increasing age, the production of the ADH is even growing.

Many of mentioned declines, which were thought as natural consequence of the ageing, are significantly influenced by the life style, behaviour, diet and environment in which the senior has been living. The most important physiological change in old age is the predisposition to the higher occurrence of severe diseases. The respiratory functions of a 70 year old healthy man are the 50% of the 30 years old man. The renal function usually goes down in 70 years by 50% and more. This decline in physiological reserve capacity does not influence the everyday life but it can influence the ability to recover from the severe disease (grave infection, life threatening internal diseases, operations, injuries etc.)

Some of the physiological changes can simulate a disease even if they are just a usual component of the ageing. Diabetes mellitus can appear and disappear in the old age. The ability of the insulin to stimulate the take up of the glucose declines with the age and is usually manifested as postprandial hyperglycaemia with normal fasting level of insulin and glucose. In the stress situations diabetes can be detected in seniors, but it can disappear when the situation gets normal. This loss of the physiological reserves contributes to the rising prevalence of diabetes with the rising age.

The age conditioned changes, which make the old age people more vulnerable in their everyday life, are usually mild. In the elderly there is an onset of hypo- or hyperthermia easier during the exposition to extreme surrounding influences, because there are a lot of changes in the coordination of the lead of the thermoregulation also in the neurological area. The loss of neurotransmitters in brain stem can cause typical senile walk, as well as it predisposes genetically determined individuals for e.g. to the progress of the Parkinson's disease. Some of the age conditioned changes cause the specific consequences. The menopausis is the physiological process connected with normal ageing but it leads to the symptoms, which predispose the organism to the loss of the bone mass and atherosclerosis.

Apart from clinically obvious forms of the diseases in the elderly the sub-clinical form is common as well. Among 6 000 individuals above 65 years which were in the Cardiovascular Health Study (Fried et al., 1991) 31% of them had clinically apparent cardiovascular disease, another 37% had sub-clinical form of the disease which was found by non-invasive methods.

The half of the people above 65 years have two or more diseases and these can mean an added risk of unfavourable consequences like mortality. In some of the seniors the cognitive disturbance can imitate symptoms of a severe disease. The therapy of one disease can act in an undesirable way on the other place - such as e.g. use of aspirin as the prevention of the ictus in the individual with the anamnesis of the gastroduodenal ulcer. The risk leading to disability or dependence on the help is getting higher with the number of co-morbidities. Certain couplets of the diseases can increase the risk of disability synergistically. The arthrosis and the diseases of the heart co-exist in 1/5 of the elderly, even though the risks of progress of disability are 3- or 4-times higher with one of them alone, the risk of both together is 14-times higher (Cassel et al., 1997).

At the end the severe and common consequence of the chronic disease in old age is physical disability, defined as the presence of difficulties or dependence on the others when doing common everyday activities, from the basic self-service (the toilet and washing up) to the tasks needed for leading the independent life (shopping, preparing food, paying the bills etc.).

On the onset and the progress of the critical conditions in old age following factors can significantly participate: the poor mobility, loneliness, bad eating habits, insufficient hydration, mental deterioration, disturbance of the sight and hearing. The mentioned ill individuals have, as it is with multi-morbidity in old age common, an atypical picture, or they can be without symptoms or the problems are seemingly moved to the other organ area. The important role is played also often by rich pharmacotherapy in old age, which can itself cause different organ symptoms (also by the mutual interactions).

The management of the critical ill persons in old age will demand very active approach from the all clinical doctors (not only intensivists) and sometimes also usage of more invasive procedures in the diagnostics and therapy of PE, which can act unfavourably in some of the cases and sometimes also iatrogenically.

11. Pulmonary embolism in the elderly – General view of a geriatritian

The entities of deep venous thrombosis (DVT) and pulmonary embolism (PE) present a continuum of venous thromboembolic disease (VTE), which is of crucial importance for elderly patients, and offer constant diagnostic and therapeutic challenges to physicians caring for patients of any age. For multiple reasons, the incidence of both DVT and PE increase with age (Hansson et al., 1997). First, there is often a decrease in the leg muscle mass, setting the stage for stasis. There are increased thrombotic tendencies in the elderly (Price et al., 1997), beginning around the age of 60, which may involve up to 20% of those over age 85; these include impaired vascular wall fibrinolysis and hypercoagulable states.

The diagnosis of venous thrombembolism (VTE) in the elderly is difficult, although the presentation is usually quite similar to that seen in younger patient groups (Matějovská-Kubešová et al., 2009). The most common presenting symptom of PE is some complaint of chest discomfort or pain, seen in approximately 35% of patients in most series, usually without hemoptysis. Dyspnea and tachypnea occur frequently. Although circulatory collapse occurs in a relatively small proportion of the elderly, these latter patients are much more likely to have sustained massive pulmonary emboli and often have evidence of neurologic deficits and findings of pulmonary hypertension. Although virtually all younger patients present with one of these syndromes, about 10% of the elderly do not, and in the setting of respiratory distress this minority may show only confusion or atypical new radiographic findings. The major diagnostic strategy (Wells, 1998) required is one of constant suspicion and concern and a consideration that, in any older hospitalized patient who is "failing to thrive," to ask whether this could be due to pulmonary embolism, because both the symptoms and standard laboratory findings are nonspecific and the diagnosis is too often made postmortem. The classic triad of hemoptysis, pleuritic chest pain, and clinically apparent thrombophlebitis is infrequently seen, in less than 10% of elderly patients with VTE.

Half of the people, who have PE, have no symptoms. With increasing age the amount of people with silent PE is growing. This is, after myocard infarction and cerebrovascular events, the third most frequent cardiovascular cause of the death. Simultaneously it is one of the least often correctly diagnosed cardiovascular diseases.

That is a medical emergency because a large embolism, or sometimes many repeated smaller ones, can be fatal in a short time. When the heart is continually overworked, it may enlarge, and it may eventually fail to perform. A large PE can cause heart or lung failure. This seems to be especially important in advanced age where CHD (heart failure too) has growing tendency. Fortunatelly chances of surviving a PE increase when a physician can diagnose and treat the patient quickly.

The acquired and genetic factors contribute to the likelihood of VTE. The acquired predispositions include generally long-haul air travel, obesity (Barba et al., 2008), cigarette smoking, oral contraceptives, pregnancy, postmenopausal hormone replacement (LaCroix et al., 2011; Sare, 2008), surgery (Einstein et al., 2008; Secin et al., 2008), trauma, and medical conditions such as antiphospholipid antibody syndrome, cancer, systemic arterial hypertension, and chronic obstructive pulmonary disease. Some patients with predisposing genetic factors will never develop clinical evidence of clotting (Reynolds et al., 2009).

PE and DVT are common problems in the elderly (Kniffin et al., 1994). They both increase with age, but the effects of race and sex are small. Current treatment patterns appear to be effective in preventing both PE after DVT and recurrence of PE. They both are associated with substantial 1-year mortality, suggesting the need to understand the role of associated conditions as well as the indications for prophylaxis and the methods of treatment. Gangireddy (Gangireddy et al., 2007) describes preoperative risk factors associated with symptomatic VTE older age, male gender, corticosteroid usage, COPD, recent weight loss, disseminated cancer, low albumin, and low haematocrit but not DM. Patients with a low probability of PE have a good prognosis in comparison to those having risk factors (Bertoletti et al., 2011). In isolation, they have limited diagnostic value and none can be used to rule in or rule out PE without further testing (West et al., 2007).

Necropsy studies in the United Kingdom (Alikhan et al., 2004) and Sweden (Hansson et al., 1997; Nordstrom et al., 1998) continued to show a high incidence of PE, which was considered the main cause of death in about 10% of necropsies. Since the inpatient mortality in general hospitals is about 10%, it is estimated that about 1% of patients admitted to hospital die from PE. However, for every patient who dies of PE in a surgical ward, three die in nonsurgical wards. This is not only a common problem but a serious one: the in-hospital mortality of elderly patients over the age of 65 with documented pulmonary embolism was 21% in the Prospective Investigation of Pulmonary Embolism Diagnosis (PIOPED, 1990) Study, and the 1-year mortality was 39% (Stein, 2008).Recent data suggest these numbers may be even higher (Heit et al., 1998).

The clinical non-recognition of venous thrombembolism prior to fatal PE implies that its detection and treatment cannot have a major impact on its mortality; hence, identificaton and primary prophylaxis of hospitalized in-patients (medical and surgical) at high absolute risk of DVT is required for its prevention.

The high occurrence of PE (particularly its silent form) has crucial importance in the elderly mortality. Our recommendations would like to emphasize the need of no underestimation of this fact and to carry out preventive measures in all age groups (including "oldest old" and frail persons.

Immobilization in medical ward is due to illness (e.g. infection, malignancy, heart failure, myocardial infarction and stroke). The cumulative risk of DVT and PE increases with the duration of immobility, suggesting a role for venous stasis in the inactive leg in the pathogenesis of DVT.

Prophylaxis against PE is of paramount importance because venous thromboembolism is difficult to detect and poses an excessive medical and economic burden (Kakkar et al., 2010).

Mechanical and pharmacologic measures often succeed in preventing this complication. Patients who have undergone total hip replacement, total knee replacement, or cancer surgery will benefit from extended pharmacologic prophylaxis for a total of 4 to 6 weeks, especially with LMWH or UFH about 2 in 3 cases (Bottaro et al., 2008; Reynolds et al., 2009).
Thromboembolic complications are prevalent in the perioperative period. It has been estimated that between 20% and 30% of patients undergoing general surgery develop deep venous thrombosis, and the incidence is as high as 40% in hip and knee surgery, gynecological cancer operations, open prostatectomies, and major neurosurgical procedures. Although fatal pulmonary embolism occurs in 1% to 5% of all surgical patients, it accounts for a larger proportion of operative deaths in middle-aged and older individuals. Because venous thrombosis and pulmonary emboli can be difficult to diagnose and treat, considerable effort has been focused on prophylaxis.
Patients at high risk can receive a combination of mechanical and pharmacologic modalities. Graduated compression stockings and pneumatic compression devices may complement mini-dose unfractionated heparin (5000 units subcutaneously twice or preferably three times daily), low-molecular-weight heparin, a pentasaccharide or warfarin administration.
Overall the literature suggests that any association of age with risk of bleeding on heparin or warfarin is weak, and contrasts with the strong, consistent finding of an exponential increase in thrombembolic risk with age (Kanaan et al., 2007; Kakkar et al., 2010). However, geriatritians should consider several practical considerations when prescribing oral anticoagulants to the elderly (Beers et al., 2006; Cassel et al., 2003).

1. Sensitivity to the anticoagulant effect of a given dose increases with age (e.g. decrease of daily dose of warfarin)
2. Polypharmacy (including self-medication) increases the risk of drug interactions which alter oral anticoagulant effect, or which increase the risk of bleeding (e.g. aspirin and other NSAD)
3. Increased prevalence of concurrent or intercurrent illness also increases the risk of bleeding (e.g. severe anemia, renal failure, gastrointestinal bleeding, hemorrhagic stroke, bleeding disorder)
4. Decreased compliance or decreased access to monitoring - whether performed by the general practitioner or hospital anticoagulant clinic - also increases risk of bleeding.

12. DVT and PE in the elderly – Two sides of the same coin VTE

The continuum of DVT and PE in the elderly is quite similar to that of the younger patient. Constant consideration of the diagnosis and application of standard diagnostic and therapeutic strategies will be a benefit for the patients and also enhance the mental equanimity and professional satisfaction of physicians caring for the elderly.

12.1 Deep vein thrombosis

The incidence of deep vein thrombosis increases with age.

12.1.1 Etiology

Immobilization, prolonged sitting (as it may occur during long drives or air travel), or even a relatively sedentary existence can lead to venous stasis and predisposes to thrombosis, because the emptying of veins in the extremities depends entirely on skeletal muscles that pump blood and on one-way venous valves that inhibit retrograde flow. Since incompetent

venous valves lead to deep vein thrombosis, which damages the valves, deep vein thrombosis tends to recur.
Deep vein thrombosis occurs in 20 to 25% of patients > 40 after routine surgery and in almost 50% after hip surgery when no prophylaxis is given.

12.1.2 Symptoms and signs

DVT usually occurs in the leg, regardless of the cause. The hallmark symptom is rapid onset of unilateral leg swelling with dependent edema - in advanced age predominantly asymptomatic. Generally, patients first note swelling when they awaken. In ambulatory patients, swelling is maximal at the ankle and lower leg, usually developing over 1 or 2 days.
Calf vein thrombosis may produce no symptoms or mild tenderness and mild edema. Calf vein thrombosis without swelling is common only among sedentary or bedridden patients.
Complications of DVT include venous thromboembolism, particularly pulmonary embolism (which can lead to death within 30 minutes of onset).

12.1.3 Diagnosis

Risk factors (eg, dehydration, estrogen use (LaCrox et al., 2011; Sare et al., 2008), heart failure, hip fracture, hypercoagulable states, immobilization or decreased physical activity, malignancy, obesity (Barba et al., 2008), polycythemia, thrombocytosis, trauma, venous damage) should be sought unless the cause is clear.

12.1.4 Prophylaxis

Orthopedic procedures: DVT is common among the elderly because they commonly undergo high-risk orthopedic procedures, particularly semi-elective or urgent procedures (eg, after a traumatic fracture). If the procedure involves the extremities, the value of low-dose heparin is limited; full-dose heparin or warfarin is effective, but each has a significant risk of bleeding.
After elective total hip replacement, the incidence of proximal deep vein thrombosis (without prophylaxis after surgery) approaches 25%, and the incidence of fatal pulmonary embolism is 3 to 4%. Prophylaxis reduces the occurrence of venous thromboembolism by 30 to 50%.
Low-dose heparin or low-molecular-weight heparin reduces the occurrence of deep vein thrombosis by at least 50%.

12.1.5 Treatment

The objective is to prevent pulmonary embolism and chronic venous insufficiency. Patients > 70 (especially women) receiving warfarin therapy are at high risk of hemorrhage. Since many elderly persons with arthritic or neurologic disorders fall frequently, warfarin is often contraindicated in patients > 80 and frail patients > 70.

12.2 Pulmonary embolism

Since the symptoms and signs are nonspecific, pulmonary embolism may be overdiagnosed or underdiagnosed, especially in the elderly. Patients with cardiac and respiratory disorders are especially at risk of misdiagnosis.
The first step in making the diagnosis is a careful physical examination to evaluate alternative diagnoses, for example, congestive heart failure, coronary artery disease,

malignancy, and infections that are all frequent in the elderly and may on occasion be confused with pulmonary embolism.
The most common and serious major error is one of omissions, when the diagnosis simply is not considered clinically and is confirmed only at autopsy. Pleural changes and possibly some local asymmetric changes in vascularity may be detected if the film is keenly studied; however, the most common finding is that of an essentially normal chest roentgenogram in a very sick patient.

12.2.1 Etiology

Bed rest and inactivity pose the greatest risk for developing of deep vein thrombosis. Certain medical conditions common among the elderly (eg, trauma to leg vessels, obesity (Barba et al., 2008), heart failure, malignancy, hip fracture, myeloproliferative disorders) predispose them to venous thrombosis, as do smoking, estrogen usage (LaCroix et al., 2011; Sare et al., 2008), tamoxifen therapy, the presence of a femoral venous catheter, and surgery (Barba et al., 2008). Risk factors for venous thrombosis are vessel wall injury, stasis, and conditions that increase the tendency of the blood to clot, including rare deficiencies of antithrombin III, protein C, and protein S as well as disseminated intravascular coagulation, polycythemia vera, or the presence of a lupus anticoagulant or antiphospholipid antibodies. Ageing is also associated with increased coagulation and products of fibrinolysis, resulting in an overall prethrombotic state.
About 90% of blood clots that cause pulmonary embolism originate in the legs. The risk that a clot will embolize and lodge in the lungs is greater if the clot is in the popliteal or iliofemoral vein (about 50%) than if it is confined to the calf veins (< 5%). Less common sites of thrombosis that may lead to pulmonary embolism are the right atrium, the right ventricle, and the pelvic, renal, hepatic, subclavian, and jugular veins.

12.2.2 Symptoms and signs

In elderly patients, the most common symptoms are tachypnea (respiratory rate > 16 breaths/minute), shortness of breath, chest pain that may be pleuritic, anxiety, leg pain or swelling, hemoptysis, and syncope. Patients who have small thromboemboli may be asymptomatic or have atypical symptoms. Nonspecific symptoms suggestive of pulmonary emboli in the elderly include persistent low-grade fever, change in mental status, or a clinical picture that mimics airway infection.
Patients with pulmonary embolism (West, 2007) usually present with one of the following symptom patterns: (1) diagnostically confusing syndromes (confusion, unexplained fever, wheezing, resistant heart failure, unexplained arrhythmias); (2) transient shortness of breath and tachypnea; (3) pulmonary infarction (pleuritic pain, cough, hemoptysis, pleural effusion, pulmonary infiltrate); (4) right-sided heart failure along with shortness of breath and tachypnea secondary to pulmonary embolism; or (5) cardiovascular collapse with hypotension and syncope. Fewer than 20% of elderly patients have the classic triad of dyspnea, chest pain, and hemoptysis. If tachypnea is absent, pulmonary embolism is unlikely to occur.
The most common physical findings are tachypnea, tachycardia, fever, leg edema or tenderness, cyanosis, and a pleural friction rub. Although most elderly patients with pulmonary embolism have deep vein thrombosis as the initial source of the embolus, only 33% have clinical signs of leg thrombosis.

About 33% of elderly patients with pulmonary embolism have pleural effusions, which are usually unilateral. About 67% of these effusions are bloody. Bloody pleural effusions generally have a pulmonary infiltrate on chest x-ray that suggests hemorrhagic consolidation of the lung parenchyma. The infiltrate usually resolves over several days. About 10% of patients with pulmonary emboli, especially those with severe heart failure, develop pulmonary infarction.

Syncope, a systolic blood pressure < 100 mm Hg, or a markedly decreased systolic blood pressure in a hypertensive patient suggests the possibility of a massive pulmonary embolism or, in a patient with marginal cardiopulmonary function, a significant embolus.

A patient who is hypotensive because of pulmonary embolism has elevated right atrial and ventricular pressures (as measured by a pulmonary arterial catheter). Thus, a normal right atrial or ventricular pressure in a patient with hypotension argues against pulmonary embolism as the cause.

12.2.3 Diagnosis

The most important consideration for determining the extent of testing is the clinical assessment of pretest probability (Bertoletti et al., 2011). The clinical probability (Wells or Geneva score) of pulmonary embolism pretest places patients into low-, moderate-, or high-probability groups. This grouping is combined with the results of ventilation-perfusion scans or of spiral chest CT scans to determine whether further testing is needed.

Very useful and easy for diagnosis of PE in daily clinical practice in elderly patients seems to be the combination of clinical pretest probability (PTP) and D-dimer result (Pasha et al., 2010). In VIDAS study the combination of a negative D-dimer result and non-high PTP effectively and safely excludes PE in an important proportion of outpatients with suspected PE (Carrier et al., 2009).

12.2.4 Laboratory findings

A chest x-ray, an ECG, and arterial blood gas values should be obtained. If pulmonary embolism is still considered to be likely, the next step is usually to obtain a ventilation-perfusion lung scan. If the lung scan is likely to be indeterminate (because of underlying lung disease), spiral chest CT scans may be useful. Finding deep vein thrombosis with ultrasonography indicates the need for anticoagulation and usually eliminates the need for further testing for pulmonary emboli. The gold standard for diagnosing pulmonary embolism is pulmonary angiography.

Chest x-rays: Results of chest x-rays may be normal or may show nonspecific abnormalities, eg, atelectasis, an elevated hemidiaphragm, pleural effusion, or an infiltrate.

ECG: ECG findings are usually nonspecific; 33% of patients with pulmonary embolism have a normal ECG.

BNP (brain natriuretic peptid) and echocardiography may be also useful determinants of the short-term outcome for patiens with PE (Sanchez et al., 2010).

d-Dimer: Levels of d-dimer, a fibrin-specific product, are increased in patients with acute thrombosis (Douma et al., 2010; Kabrhel et al. 2010). About 60% of patients < 50 who are suspected of having a pulmonary embolus have an abnormal d-dimer result. In contrast, 92% of patients > 70 have abnormal d-dimer levels, probably due to comorbid conditions (Douketis et al., 2010). Therefore, if d-dimer test results are negative, deep vein thrombosis or pulmonary embolism is unlikely to be present, but positive test results are not useful in patients > 70.

The use of d-dimers as a secondary strategy to exclude the diagnosis of VTE has been recommended because the test has a high sensitivity, although a low specificity. False positives may occur in patients with recent trauma or surgery, malignancy, pregnancy, severe infections, and liver disease.

12.2.5 Prognosis

The mortality rate for hospitalized patients > 65 with pulmonary embolism is 21%. If pulmonary embolism is the primary diagnosis, the mortality rate is 13%; if it is a secondary diagnosis, the rate is 31%. Thus, many diseases and medical conditions--including heart failure, chronic obstructive pulmonary disease, cancer, myocardial infarction, stroke, and hip fracture--greatly increase the risk of death among hospitalized patients > 65 with pulmonary embolism. Prognosis is poorest for patients with severe underlying cardiac or pulmonary disease.

In patients > 65 with a pulmonary embolus, the recurrence rate in the first year is 8%, and the 1-year mortality rate is 39% (21% inpatient mortality and an additional 18% mortality during the first year). Elderly patients with deep vein thrombosis but without pulmonary emboli have a 21% mortality rate in the first year.

12.2.6 Treatment

Pulmonary embolectomy is not recommended in the elderly because it has a very low success rate and medical therapy is generally quite effective. These procedures should regularly be found in the armamentarium of geriatritians.

Heparin prevents clot formation and extension. As the risk of death from pulmonary embolism is the greatest in the first few hours of development of a clot and since diagnostic test results often are not available for 8 to 12 hours, heparin should be given to patients with a moderate to high clinical probability of pulmonary embolism or deep vein thrombosis until all diagnostic results are available. Low-molecular-weight heparin (LMWH) is preferred to unfractionated heparin. **LMWH** can be given subcutaneously once or twice a day, and laboratory monitoring may not be necessary.

Long-term anticoagulation is begun in the hospital with heparin and is continued after discharge, usually with **warfarin**.

Thrombolytic (fibrinolytic) therapy should be considered for patients with deep vein thrombosis involving the iliofemoral system. It is also useful for patients with massive pulmonary embolism who have significant pulmonary hypertension, obstruction of multiple segments of the pulmonary circulation, right ventricular dysfunction, or systemic hypotension.

12.2.7 Prophylaxis

Prophylaxis reduces the incidence of fatal pulmonary emboli by two thirds in hospitalized patients at risk of developing venous clots. LMWH (eg, enoxaparin 40 mg sc once daily) is as effective and safe as prophylaxis with subcutaneous heparin (5000 IU sc bid or tid) and may reduce drug-induced adverse effects. Postoperative prophylaxis with LMWH (eg, sc q 12 h for up to 14 days) also dramatically reduces the incidence of venous thrombosis after knee or hip replacement and in abdominal surgery (Bottaro et al., 2008). For total hip replacement, some investigators find that 4 to 6 weeks of LMWH postoperatively may be more effective (Kanaan et al., 2007).

13. Conclusion

The approach to older patients should be consistently individualised. New diagnostic methods and therapeutic algorithms used in acute geriatric wards together enable us to treat successfully also multi-morbid patients in advanced age admitted by hospital's doctors. Modern iatrotechniques make possible also the treatment (including recovery) and protect self-sufficiency and preserve quality of life in the elderly being acutely ill.

Physicians committed to the care of elderly patients, are challenged with the diagnosis of venous thrombembolism due to a higher incidence, co-morbidities masking signs and symptoms and burdening referrals (Siccama et al., 2011).

We would like to emphasize the need to permanently think of the possibility of PE in elderly persons with present risk factors and in suspected cases the use of pretest probability scale as Wells or Geneva score as soon as possible (Carrier et al., 2009` Pasha et al., 2010). The requirement of correctly assessed diagnosis and starting of therapeutic procedures is crucial and essential proceeding for giving the hope to patient and generally, from the professional viewpoint, improvement of the prognosis.

14. References

Alikhan R, Peters F, Wilmott R, Cohen AT. (2006). *Fatal pulmonary embolism in hospitalised patients: a necropsy review,* J Clin Pathol, Vol.57, No.12, pp.1254-7, ISSN 0021-9746

Applegate WB, Blass JP, Williams TF. (1990). *Instruments for the functional assessment of older patients,* N Engl J Med, Vol.322, pp.1207-14, ISSN 0028-4793.

Asplund K, Gustafson Y, Jacobsson C. (2000). *Geriatric- Based Versus General Wards for Older Acute Medical Patients: A Randomized Comparison of Outcomes and Use of Resources,* JAGS, Vol.48, pp.1381-88, ISSN 0002-8614

Barba R, Martinez-Espinosa S, Rodriguez-Garcia E. (2000). *Poststroke dementia: clinical features and risk factors,*. Stroke, Vol. 31, pp. 1494-501, ISSN 00392499

Barba R, Zapatero A, Losa JE, Valdaos V, Todola JA, Di Micco P, Monreal M, Riete Investigators (2008) *Body mass index and mortality in patients with acute venous thromboembolism: findings from the RIETE registry,* J Thromb Haemost, Vol.6, No.4, pp. 595-600, ISSN: 1538-7933

Beckman JA, Creager MA, Libby P. (2002). *Diabetes and Atherosclerosis. Epidemiology, Pathophysiology, and Management,*. JAMA, Vol. 287, pp. 2570-81, ISSN: 00987484

Beers MH, Thomas VJ & Jones TV (eds.) (2006) *The Merck Manual of Geriatrics- 7th edition,* Merck & Co, ISBN-13: 978-0911910667, New York, USA

Bertoletti L, Le Gal G, Aujesky D, Roy PM, Sanchez O, Verschuren F, Bounameaux H, Perrier A, Righini M. (2011). *Prognostic value of the Geneva prediction rule in patients in whom pulmonary embolism is ruled out.* J Intern Med, 2011 Vol. 269, No. 4, pp. 433-40, ISSN: 0954-6820

Blackburn JA & Dulmus CN. (eds.). (2007). *Handbook of gerontology : evidence-based approaches to theory, practice, and policy,* Hoboken, N.J. Wiley, ISBN-13: 978-0471771708, New York, USA

Bongard FS & Sue DY. (eds.). (2003). *Current Critical Care Diagnosis & Treatment, Second Edition,* Lange Medical Books/McGraw-Hill Medical Publishing Division, ISBN: 0-07-121206-X, New York, USA

Bottaro FJ, Elizondo MC, Doti C, Bruetman JE, Perez Moreno PD, Bullorsky EO, Ceresetto JM. (2008). *Efficacy of extended thrombo-prophylaxis in major abdominal surgery: what does the evidence show? A meta-analysis.* Thromb Haemost, Vol.99, No.6, pp.1104-11, ISSN: 1538-7933

Braunwald E, Zipes DP, Libby P. (eds.). (2001). *Heart Disease, 6th edition – a Textbook of Cardiovascular Medicine,* W.B.Saunders Comp., ISBN-13: 978-0721685618, Philadelphia, USA

Brunner-Ziegler S, Heinze G, Ryffel M, Kompatscher M, Slany J, Valentin A. (2007) *"Oldest old" patients in intensive care: prognosis and therapeutic activity.* Wien Klin Wochenschr, Vol. 119, pp. 14-19, ISSN 0043-5325

Buttler G. (2003). *Increasing life expectancy - what are the promises of demography?* Z Gerontol Geriat, Vol.36, pp. 90-94, ISSN (printed): 0948-6704

Campbell AJ, Cook JA, Adey G, Cuthbertson BH. (2008). *Predicting death and readmission after intensive care discharge.* Br J Anaesth, Vol. 100, pp. 556-562, ISSN 1471-6771

Carrier M, Righini M, Djurabi RK, Huisman MV, Perrier A, Wells PS, Rodger M, Wuillemin WA, Le Gal G. (2009). *VIDAS D-dimer in combination with clinical pre-test probability to rule out pulmonary embolism. A systematic review of management outcome studies.* Thromb Haemost, Vol.101, No.5, pp. 886-92, ISSN: 1538-7933

Cassel ChK, Cohen HJ, Larson EB et al. (eds.). (2003). *Geriatric medicine: an evidence-based approach,* Springer, ISBN-13: 978-0387955148, New York, USA

Chase P, Mitchell K, Morley JE. (2000) *In the steps of giants: the early geriatrics texts.* J Am Geriatr Soc, Vol. 48, No.1, pp. 89-94

Crome P & Lally F. (2011). *Frailty: joining the giants.* CMAJ, Vol.183, No.8, pp. 889-90, ISSN 0820-3946

Doucet J, Trivalle CH, Chassagne PH. (1994). *Does age lay a role in clinical presentation of hypothyroidism?* J Am Geriatr Soc, Vol.42, pp.984-986, ISSN: 0002-8614

Douketis J, Tosetto A, Marcucci M, Baglin T, Cushman M, Eichinger S, Palareti G, Poli D, Tait RC, Iorio A. (2010) *Patient-level meta-analysis: effect of measurement timing, threshold, and patient age on ability of D-dimer testing to assess recurrence risk after unprovoked venous thromboembolism.* Ann Intern Med, Vol.153, No.8, pp.523-31, ISSN: 0003-4819

Douma RA, le Gal G, Sauhne M, Righini M, Kamphuisen PW, Perrier A, Kruip MJ, Bounameaux H, Baller HR, Roy PM. (2010). *Potential of an age adjusted D-dimer cut-off value to improve the exclusion of pulmonary embolism in older patients: a retrospective analysis of three large cohorts.* BMJ, Vol.340, c 1475, ISSN: 0959 8138

Duthie EH, Katz PR & Malone ML. (eds.). (2007). *The practice of geriatrics 4th ed.,* Saunders Elsevier, ISBN-13: 978-1416022619, Philadelphia, USA

Einstein MH, Kushner DM, Connor JP, Bohl AA, Best TJ, Evans MD, Chappell RJ, Hartenbach EM. (2008). *A protocol of dual prophylaxis for venous thromboembolism prevention in gynecologic cancer patients,* Obstet Gynecol, Vol.112, No.5, pp.1091-7, ISSN: 0300-8835

Fauci AS, Braunwald E, Kasper DL, Longo DL, Jameson JL, Loscalzo L. (eds.). (2008). *Harrison's Principles of Internal Medicine 17th Edition,* McGraw-Hill Medical Publishing Division, ISBN-13: 978-0071466332, New York, USA

Ferrari AU, Radaelli A, Centolla M. (2003). *Aging and the cardiovascular system,*. J Appl Physiol, Vol. 95, pp. 2591-97, ISSN: 8750-7587

Fried LP, Borhani NO, Enright P, Furberg CD, Gardin JM, Kronmal RA, Kuller LH, Manolio TA, Mittelmark MB, Newman A. (1991). *The Cardiovascular Health Study: design and rationale,* Ann Epidemiol, Vol.1, pp. 263-276, ISSN: 1047-2797

Fried LP, Hadley EC, Walston JD, Newman AB, Guralnik JM, Studenski S, Harris TB, Ershler WB, Ferrucci L. (2005). *From bedside to bench: research agenda for frailty,* Sci Aging Knowledge Environ, Vol. 31: pp.24, ISSN 1539-6150

Friedman SM, Mendelson DA, Kates SL, McCann RM (2008). *Geriatric co-management of proximal femur fractures: total quality management and protocol-driven care result in better outcomes for a frail patient population.* J Am Geriatr Soc, Vol. 56, pp. 1349-56, ISSN: 0002-8614

Friedman SM, Steinwachs DM, Temkin-Greener H, Mukamel DB. (2006). *Informal caregivers and the risk of nursing home admission among individuals enrolled in the program of all-inclusive care for the elderly,* Gerontologist, Vol. 46, pp. 456-463, ISSN: 0016-9013

Gammack JK & Morley JE. (eds.). (2006). *Geriatric medicine,* Saunders, ISBN-13: 9780801635267, Philadelphia, USA

Gangireddy C, Rectenwald JR, Upchurch GR, Wakefield TW, Khuri S, Henderson WG, Henke PK. (2007). *Risk factors and clinical impact of postoperative symptomatic venous thromboembolism,* J Vasc Surg, Vol. 45, No.2, pp.335-41

Goldmann L, Ausiello DA, Arend W. et al. (eds.). (2007). *Cecil Medicine: Expert Consult - Online and Print,* W. B. Saunders Comp., ISBN-13: 978-1416028055, Philadelphia, USA

Gross R, Bentur N, Einayany A. (1996). *The validity of self-reports on chronic disease: characteristics of underreporters and implications for the planning of services,* Public Health Rev, Vol.24, No.2, pp. 167-82, ISSN (printed): 0301-0422

Gupta A. (2008). *Measurement scales used in elderly care,* Radcliffe Publishing, OBE, ISBN-13: 978-1846192661, Oxford, UK

Gurcharan RS & Mulley GP. (eds.). (2007). *Elderly medicine : a training guide, 2nd ed.,* Churchill Livingstone Elsevier, ISBN 9058232344, 9789058232342, Edinburgh, UK

Hall JB, Schmidt GA, Wood LDH et al.(eds). (2005). *Principles of Critical Care. care.3. ed.,* McGraw-Hill, Medical Publishing Division , ISBN 0-07-141640-4, New York, USA

Hansson PO, Welin L, Tibblin G, Eriksson H. (1997). *Deep vein thrombosis and pulmonary embolism in the general population. 'The Study of Men Born in 1913,* Arch Intern Med, Vol.157, No.15, pp.1665-70, ISSN 0003-9926

Harari D, Martin FC, Buttery A, O'Neill S, Hopper A. (2007). *The older persons' assessment and liaison team 'OPAL': evaluation of comprehensive geriatric assessment in acute medical inpatients,* Age Ageing, Vol. 36, No. 6, pp. 670-5, ISSN: 0002-0729

Hazzard WR. (2007) *Scientific progress in geriatric syndromes: earning an "A" on the 2007 report card on academic geriatrics,* J Am Geriatr Soc, Vol. 55, pp. 794-96, ISSN: 0002-8614

Heit JA, Silverstein MD, Mohr DN. (1999). *Predictors of survival after deep vein thrombosis and pulmonary embolism: a population-based cohort study,* Arch Intern Med, Vol. 159, pp. 445-56, ISSN 0003-9926

Heltweg B. (2006). *Antitumor Activity of a Small-Molecule Inhibitor of Human Silent Information Regulator 2 Enzymes,* Cancer Research, Vol. 66, pp. 4368-77, ISSN: 0008-5472

Holmerová I, Jurasková B, Kalvach Z, Rohanová E, Rokosová M, Vanková H. (2007). Dignity and palliative care in dementi, J Nutr Health Aging, Vol. 11, No. 6, pp. 489-94, ISSN (printed): 1279-7707

Humes D. (ed. in chief). (2002). *Kelley's Textbook of Internal Medicine,* Lippincott Williams & Wilkins, ISBN-13: 978-0781717878, Philadelphia, USA

Hunter JA, Haslett C, Chilver AR, Boon NA, et al.(eds.). (2002).: *Davidson's Principle and Practice of Medicine.* Churchill Livingstone, 2002, ISBN-13: 978-0781717878, Edinburgh, UK

Inouye SK, Studenski S, Tinetti ME, Kuchel GA. (2007). *Geriatric syndromes: clinical, research, and policy implications of a core geriatric koncept,* J Am Geriatr Soc, Vol. 55, pp. 780-91, ISSN: 0002-8614

Juraskova B, Andrys C, Holmerova I, Solichova D, Hrnciarikova D, Vankova H, Vasatko T, Krejsek J. (2010). *Transforming growth factor beta and soluble endoglin in the healthy senior and in Alzheimer's disease patiens,* J Nutr Health Aging, Vol. 14, No. 9, pp. 758-61, ISSN (printed): 1279-7707

Kabrhel C, Mark Courtney D, Camargo CA Jr, Plewa MC, Nordenholz KE, Moore CL, Richman PB, Smithline HA, Beam DM, Kline JA. 2010). *Factors associated with positive D-dimer results in patients evaluated for pulmonary emboliím,* Acad Emerg Med, Vol.17, No.6, pp.589-97, ISSN 1069-6563

Kakkar VV, Balibrea JL, Martanez-Gonzalez J, Prandoni P. (2010). *CANBESURE Study Group: Extended prophylaxis with bemiparin for the prevention of venous thromboembolism after abdominal or pelvic surgery for cancer: the CANBESURE randomized study,* J Thromb Haemost, Vol. 8, No.6, pp. 1223-9, ISSN: 1538-7933

Kalvach Z,. Zadák Z, Jirák R., Zavázalová H., Holmerová I., Weber P. a kolektiv (2008). *Geriatrické syndromy a geriatrický pacient.* Galén, ISBN 978-80-247-2490-4, Praha, Czech Republic

Kalvach Z., Zadák Z, Jirák R, Zavázalová H.,Sucharda P. a kol. (eds.- in czech). (2004). *Geriatrie a gerontologie,* Grada Publishing a.s., ISBN 80-247-0548-6, Praha, Czech republic

Kanaan AO, Silva MA, Donovan JL, Roy T, Al-Homsi AS. (2007). *Meta-analysis of venous thromboembolism prophylaxis in medically Ill patients,* Clin Ther, Vol.29, No.11, pp. 2395-405, ISSN: 0149-2918

Katzung BG. (ed.). (2007). : *Basic and Clinical Pharmacology.* McGraw- Hill Professional Publishing, ISBN 0071451536, 9780071451536, San Francisco, USA

Khaw KT. (1997). *How many, how old, how soon.* BMJ, Vol. 319, pp. 1350-52, ISSN: 0959 8138.

Kniffin WD Jr, Baron JA, Barrett J, Birkmeyer JD, Anderson FA Jr. (1994). *The epidemiology of diagnosed pulmonary embolism and deep venous thrombosis in the elderly,* Arch Intern Med. Vol.154, No.8, pp. 861, ISSN 0003-9926

Kriegsman DM, Penninx BW, van Eijk JT. (1996). *Self-reports and general practitioner information on the presence of chronic diseases in community-dwelling elderly. A study on the accuracy of patients' self-reports and on determinants of inaccuracy,* J Clin Epidemiol, Vol. 49, No.12, pp. 1407-17, ISSN: 0895-4356.

LaCroix AZ, Chlebowski RT, Manson JE, Aragaki AK, Johnson KC, Martin L, Margolis KL, Stefanick ML, Brzyski R, Curb JD, Howard BV, Lewis CE, Wactawski-Wende J; WHI Investigators. (2011). *Health outcomes after stopping conjugated equine estrogens among postmenopausal women with prior hysterectomy: a randomized controlled trial,* JAMA, Vol.305, No.13, pp. 1305-14, ISSN: 00987484

Leng SX, Xue QL, Tian J, Walston JD, Fried LP. (2007). *Inflammation and frailty in older women,* J Am Geriatr Soc, Vol. 55, 864-71, ISSN: 0002-8614

Masoro EJ & Austad SN (editors). (2011). *Handbook of the biology of aging, 7th ed.,* Elsevier Academic Press, Burlington, MA, ISBN: 978-0-12-378638-8, London, UK

Matějovská- Kubešová H et al. (2009). *Akutní stavy v geriatrii,* Galén, ISBN 978-80-7262-620-5, Praha, Czech Republic.

Moody HR. (2009). *Aging : concepts and controversies, 6th ed.,* Pine Forge, ISBN 1412969662, 9781412969666, London, UK

Nemeth F, Koval S, Zavazalova H, Banik M. (2007). End of life, Bratisl Lek Listy, Vol. 108, No. 6, pp. 239-45, ISSN 0006-9248

Nikolaus T. (Hrsg.). (2000). *Klinische Geriatrie,* Springer, Springer, ISBN-13: 978-3540665687, Berlin, Germany

Nordstrom M & Lindblad B. (1998). *Autopsy-verified venous thromboembolism within a defined urban population – the city of Malmo, Sweden,* APMIS, Vol. 106, No.3, pp. 378-84, ISSN (printed): 0903-4641

Oskvig RM. (1999). *Special problems in the elderly,* Chest,, Vol. 115, pp. 158-64, ISSN: 0012-3692

Pasha SM, Klok FA, Snoep JD, Mos IC, Goekoop RJ, Rodger MA, Huisman MV. (2010). *Safety of excluding acute pulmonary embolism based on an unlikely clinical probability by the Wells rule and normal D-dimer concentration: a meta-analysis,* Thromb Res, Vol.125, No.4, e123-7, ISSN: 0049-3848

Pathy MSJ, Sinclair AJ, Morley JE. (eds.) (2006). *Principles and practice of geriatric medicine, 4th ed.,* Wiley, ISBN: 0-470-09055-3, Chichester, UK

Perez-Guzman C, Vargas MH, Torres-Cruz A. (1999). *Does aging modify pulmonary tuberculosis? a mentaanalytical review,* Chest, Vol.116, No.4, pp. 961-7, ISSN: 0012-3692

PIOPED Investigators. (1990). *Valve of the ventilation/perfusion scan in acute pulmonary embolism: results of the prospective investigation of pulmonary embolism diagnosis (PIOPED),* JAMA, Vol. 263, pp. 2753-59, ISSN: 00987484

Price DT & Ridken PM. (1997). *Factor V Leiden mutation and the risks for thromboembolic disease: a clinical perspective*, Ann Intern Med, Vol. 127, pp. 895-903. ISSN: 0003-4819

Ratnaike RN (ed.). (2002). *Practical Guide to Geriatric Medicine*. Mc Graw Hill Comp., Inc., ISBN-13: 978-0074708019, New York, USA

Reynolds MW, Shibata A, Zhao S, Jones N, Fahrbach K, Goodnough LT. (2008). *Impact of clinical trial design and execution-related factors on incidence of thromboembolic events in cancer patients: a systematic review and meta-analysis,* Curr Med Res Opin, Vol.24, No.2, pp.497-505, ISSN (printed): 0300-7995

Roberts JR & Hedges JR. (eds.). (2009). *Clinical Procedures in Emergency Medicine, 5th ed.,* Saunders, An Imprint of Elsevier, ISBN: 978-1-4160-3623-4, New York, USA

Rockwood K & Hubbard R. (2004). *Frailty and the geriatrician,* Age Ageing, Vol.33, No.5, pp.429-30, ISSN (printed): 0002-0729

Roubenoff R, Hughes VA. (2000). *Sarcopenia: Current Concepts,* J Gerontology, Vol. 55, pp. 716-24, ISSN 0022-1422

Roubenoff R. (2000). *Sarcopenia and its implications for the elderly,* European J of Clinical Nutrition, Vol. 54, pp. 40-47, ISSN: 0954-3007

Salvedt I, Ophdal Mo E-S, Fayers P. (2002). *Reduced Mortality in Treating Acutely Sick, Frail Older Patients in a Geriatric Evaluation and Management Unit, A Prospective Randomized Trial,* JAGS, Vol.50, No.5: pp. 792-8, ISSN: 0002-8614

Sanchez O, Trinquart L, Caille V, Couturaud F, Pacouret G, Meneveau N, Verschuren F, Roy PM, Parent F, Righini M, Perrier A, Lorut C, Tardy B, Benoit MO, Chatellier G, Meyer G. (2010). *Prognostic factors for pulmonary embolism: the prep study, a prospective multicenter cohort study,* Am J Respir Crit Care Med, Vol.181, No.2, pp.168-73, ISSN: 1073-449X

Sare GM, Gray LJ, Bath PM. (2008). *Association between hormone replacement therapy and subsequent arterial and venous vascular events: a meta-analysis,* Eur Heart J, Vol.29, No.16, pp.2031-41, ISSN 0195-668x

Scherl H. (2003). *Increasing life expectancy – the big social issue of the 21st century?* Z Gerontol Geriat, Vol.36, pp.95-103, ISSN (printed): 0948-6704

Secin FP, Jiborn T, Bjartell AS, Fournier G, Salomon L, Abbou CC, Haber GP, Gill IS, Crocitto LE, Nelson RA, Cansino Alcaide JR, MartĂnez-PiĂ±eiro L, Cohen MS, Tuerk I, Schulman C, Gianduzzo T, Eden C, Baumgartner R, Smith JA, Entezari K, van Velthoven R, Janetschek G, Serio AM, Vickers AJ, Touijer K, Guillonneau B. (2008). *Multi-institutional study of symptomatic deep venous thrombosis and pulmonary embolism in prostate cancer patients undergoing laparoscopic or robot-assisted laparoscopic radical prostatectomy,* Eur Urol., Vol.53, No.1, pp.134-45, ISSN: 0302-2838

Seitz M. (2003). *A long life – a wish and its limits. Aging with dignity and meaning,* Z Gerontol Geriat, Vol.36, pp. 104- 9, ISSN (printed): 0948-6704

Sherman FT. (2003). *The geriatric giants. Don't miss their footprints!* Geriatrics, Vol.58, No.4, pp.8, ISSN: 0016-867X

Siccama RN, Janssen KJ, Verheijden NA, Oudega R, Bax L, van Delden JJ, Moons KG. (2011). *Systematic review: diagnostic accuracy of clinical decision rules for venous thromboembolism in elderly,* Ageing Res Rev, Vol.10, No.2, pp.304-13, ISSN (printed): 1568-1637

Sinclair AJ & Finucane P (eds.). (2002). *Diabetes in Old Age. second edition.* John Wiley & Sons, Chichester, U.K.

Soriano RP, Fernandez HM, Cassel ChK, Leipzig R (eds.). (2007). *Fundamentals of geriatric medicine : a case-based approach,* Springer, ISBN 0-387-32326-8, New York, USA

Stein PD, Gottschalk A, Sostman HD, Chenevert TL, Fowler SE, Goodman LR, Hales CA, Hull RD, Kanal E, Leeper KV Jr, Nadich DP, Sak DJ, Tapson VF, Wakefield TW, Weg JG, Woodard PK. (2008). *Methods of Prospective Investigation of Pulmonary Embolism Diagnosis III (PIOPED III),* Semin Nucl Med, Vol.38, No.6, pp.462-70, ISSN: 0001-2998

Stone CK & Humphries R (eds.). (2007). *Current Emergency Diagnosis & Treatment 6th Edition,* McGraw-Hill Companies, Inc., ISBN-13: 978-0071443197, New York, USA

Stuck AE. (1995). *A trial of annual in-home comprehensive geriatric assessments for elderly people living in the community,* N Engl J Med, Vol.333, pp.1184-9, ISSN 0028-4793

Szanton SL, Seplaki CL, Thorpe RJ Jr, Allen JK, Fried LP. (2010). *Socioeconomic status is associated with frailty: the Women's Health and Aging Studies,* J Epidemiol Community Health, Vol. 64 pp. 63-7, ISSN: 0141-7681

Tallis R & Fillit H (eds.). (2003). *Brocklehurst's Textbook of Geriatric Medicine and Gerontology 6th ed.,* Churchill Livingstone, ISBN-13: 978-0443070877, London, U.K.

Tallis R. & Fillit H. (eds.). (2003). Effects of aging on the heart, In: *Brocklehurst's Textbook of Geriatric Medicine and Gerontology 6th ed.,* Churchill Livingstone, ISBN-13: 978-0443070877 , London, UK

Tinetti ME, Williams CS, Gill TM. (2000). *Dizziness among older adults: a possible geriatric syndrome,* Ann Intern Med, Vol.132, pp.337-44, ISSN: 0003-4819

Topinková E. (2005). *Geriatrie pro praxi.* Galén, ISBN 8072623656, 9788072623655, Praha, Czech Republic

Trivalle C, Doucet J, Chassagne P, (1996). *Differences in the signs and symptoms of hyperthyroidism in older and younger patients,* J Am Geriatr Soc, Vol.44, pp. 50-3, ISSN: 0002-8614

Walston J, Hadley EC, Ferrucci L, Guralnik JM, Newman AB, Studenski SA, Ershler WB, Harris T, Fried LP. (2006). *Research agenda for frailty in older adults: toward a better understanding of physiology and etiology: summary from the American Geriatrics Society/National Institute on Aging Research Conference on Frailty in Older Adults,* J Am Geriatr Soc, Vol. 54 pp. 991-1001, ISSN: 0002-8614

Wawruch M, Zikavska M, Wsolova L, Jezova D, Fialova D, Kunzo M, Kuzelova M, Lassanova M, Kruty P, Kriska M. (2006). *Perception of potentially inappropriate medication in elderly patients by Slovak physicians,* Pharmacoepidemiol Drug Saf, Vol. 15, pp. 829-34, ISSN: 1099-1557

Wells PS, Ginsberg JS, Andersen DR. (1998). *Use of a clinical model for safe management of patients with pulmonary embolism,* Ann Intern Med, Vol.129, pp.997-1005, ISSN: 0003-4819

West J, Goodacre S, Sampson F. (2007). *The value of clinical features in the diagnosis of acute pulmonary embolism: systematic review and meta-analysis,* QJM, Vol.100, No.12, pp.763-9, ISSN 1460-2725

Williams ME. (2008). *Geriatric physical diagnosis : a guide to observation and assessment,* McFarland & Co. Inc. ISBN-13: 978-0-7864-3009-3, Jefferson, N.C. , USA

Woodford H & George J. (eds.) (2007). *Essential geriatrics,* Radcliffe Publishing, 184619170X, 9781846191701, Abingdon, USA

Woodhouse KW & O'Mahony MS. (1997). *Frailty and ageing,* Age Ageing, Vol. 26, pp. 245-6, ISSN (printed): 0002-0729

Yaffe K, Haan M, Blackwell T, Cherkasova E, Whitmer RA, West N. (2007). *Metabolic syndrome and cognitive decline in elderly Latinos: findings from the Sacramento Area Latino Study of Aging study,* J Am Geriatr Soc, Vol. 55, pp. 758-62, ISSN: 0002-8614

Zavazalova H, Nemeth F, Zikmundova K, Zaremba V, Rais V. (2007). Some indicators of quality of life in senior age in two regions international comparative study--the Czech Republic and the Slovak Republic, Bratisl Lek Listy. Vol. 108, No. 4-5, pp. 212-7, ISSN 0006-9248

4

Venous Thromboembolism in Bariatric Surgery

Eleni Zachari, Eleni Sioka, George Tzovaras and Dimitris Zacharoulis
Department of Surgery, University Hospital of Larissa
Greece

1. Introduction

Deep venous thrombosis (DVT) and pulmonary embolism (PE) constitute clinical presentations of the same vascular disease, known as venous thromboembolism (VTE). VTE is responsible for hospitalization of >250000 Americans annually. It is associated with high morbidity and mortality and represents a primary cause of preventable death. There is strong evidence that obesity is an independent risk factor for DVT and PE. Bariatric surgery is proven to be an effective means in the therapy of morbid obesity and its related co-morbidities, thus its prevalence is rapidly increasing. Well established and widely performed procedures include laparoscopic adjustable gastric band (LAGB), Roux-en-Y gastric bypass (RYGBP), biliopancreatic diversion (BPD, with or without duodenal switch) and sleeve gastrectomy (SG). LAGB is a purely restrictive method, while RYGBP and BPD are considered as mainly malabsorbptive procedures. SG was performed as a bridge to further by-pass surgery, however nowadays is performed as a single stage procedure. The risk of VTE in patients undergoing elective bariatric surgery is high, attributable to obesity, intraoperating factors and the lack of an established guidance describing optimal VTE prophylaxis. Overall incidence of VTE in this population is reported to be 1-3%. Diagnosis of PE postoperatively in obese patients can be difficult due to physical limitations and consequently may be underdiagnosed. Furthermore, although VTE is usually diagnosed as immediate postoperative complication, PE can occur in nonhospitalized patients, within the first month after surgery, despite pharmacologic prophylaxis.

2. Obesity

The most widely applied tool to diagnose obesity is body mass index (BMI). BMI is defined as weight in kilograms divided by the square of height in meters. World health Organization defines obesity as a BMI≥ 30. This cutoff was selected because according to epidemiological studies mortality curve increases at this value. Moreover, morbid obesity is defined as BMI≥40.

The prevalence of obesity increases rapidly in both developed and developing countries and is considered as one of the most serious public health problems.

Recent scientific data from long-term studies support the strong association between obesity and type 2 diabetes, hypertension, cardiovascural disease, dyslipidemia, arthritis, gallbladder disease, sleep apnea syndrome and many types of cancer. Furthermore, obesity deteriorates quality of life and induces severe psychological disorders.

3. Bariatric surgery

Bariatric surgery holds an important and well established role in the management of obese and morbid obese patients. Furthermore, it is proved to be the most efficient mode of treatment that provides sustained weight loss in morbidly obese patients.

International medical and surgical societies (International Federation for the Surgery of Obesity (IFSO), European Association for Study of Obesity (EASO), European Childhood Obesity Group (ECOG)) created guidelines in order to assure safe and effective clinical practice in the field of bariatric surgery.

3.1 Indications of bariatric surgery

a. Patients from 18-60 years

- with BMI≥40 kg/m^2
- with BMI 35-40 kg/m^2 and with co-morbidity which weight loss is expected to improve (metabolic disorders, cardio-respiratory disease, severe joint disease, obesity-induced severe psychological problems)

To be candidates for surgical management, patients must have failed to lose weight or to maintain a substantial weight-loss following conservative treatment.

Bariatric surgery is indicated in patients who managed to lose weight prior to scheduled surgery and have reach a BMI below the required for surgery.

b. Patients aged above 60

In these patients the primary objective is to improve quality of life. Benefits should be contemplated with potential risks, thus indications for surgery should be individualized.

3.2 Contraindications of bariatric surgery

- Absence of effort to lose weight following an appropriate non-surgical medical program.
- Psychotic disorders, severe depression, personality disorders.
- Alcohol abuse and/or drug dependencies.
- Life-threatening diseases (in a short term).
- Patients who are unable to care for themselves or to participate and conform to the required long-term medical follow-up.
- Patients in very high or unacceptable anaesthetic risk.

3.3 Bariatric surgery techniques

Nowadays a variety of surgical procedures is available for the surgical treatment of obesity. Furthermore, although primary objective of bariatric surgery is the weight loss, significant long-term amelioration or total remission of co-morbidities has been established. Bariatric surgery procedures modify the gastrointestinal track in order to reduce its volume and/or its absorptive function.

Restrictive procedures induce volume limitation and include laparoscopic adjustable gastric band (LAGB), vertical banded gastroplasty (VBG), laparoscopic sleeve gastrectomy (LSG), gastric bypass (GBP).

Malabsorptive procedures induce limited absorption of nutrients and include biliopancreatic diversion with (BPD-DS) or without duodenal switch (BPD).

Roux-en-Y gastric bypass (RYGBP), open or laparoscopic, encompasses characteristics of both types of procedures, as it provides restriction and mild- malabsorption.

4. Venous thromboembolism

4.1 Predisposing factors to venous thromboembolism in bariatric surgery

Morbid (BMI>50) and truncal obesity are identified as major predisposing factors for VTE. Sedentary lifestyle, increased abdominal pressure and excessive weight resting on the inferior vena cava drainage attribute to the increased risk. Additional risk factors include advanced age, history of previous VTE, immobilization, venous insufficiency and stasis, smoking, estrogen- containing oral contraceptives and hormone replacement therapy, hypercoaguable state, hypoventilation syndrome and anastomotic leakage. According to current literature, obesity interferes in intrinsic and extrinsic coagulation pathways, as well as in the anticoagulant mechanism, leading to a hypercoagulating state. Plasma concentration of fibrogen, von Willebrand, t-PA, PAI-1 and factor VII are significantly elevated in obese patients, while platelet aggregation is promoted due to leptin. There is evidence that treatment of morbid obesity can reverse partially some of the above abnormalities, as weight loss is associated with significant reduction in fibrogen, t-PA, PAI-1 and improvement of deficiency of antithrombin III.

Perioperative factors contributing to VTE include extend of surgical trauma, operative duration, length of postoperative immobilization and the use of general versus regional anesthesia. The risk of developing VTE depends on the type of major abdominal surgical procedure. Mukherjee et al. reported lower incidence of VTE among bariatric surgery patients (0.35%), while VTE rates were higher in patients undergoing nephrectomy, hepatectomy, colorectal resection, splenectomy, gastrectomy, pancreatectomy and esophagectomy. This lower rate may reflect strict adherence of bariatric surgeons to VTE prophylaxis guidelines relative to other surgical specialties.

More specifically, in laparoscopic bariatric surgery, reverse Trendelenburg position and pneumoperitoneum are associated with venous stasis of lower extremity and impaired venous return due to the compression of iliac veins and inferior vena cava. Furthermore several studies show the development of a hypercoagulable state during laparoscopy. Conversely, the risk of VTE during laparoscopy could be compensated by lower degree of surgical injury, early mobilization and reduced postoperative acute-phase response. Podnos et al. in a review of 3464 cases of GBP demonstrated that although the difference was not statistically significant, the incidence of PE was lower in laparoscopic group rather than the open group. In absence of randomized controlled studies, the evidence remains inconclusive as to the relative risk of VTE after laparoscopic bariatric surgery.

4.2 Prophylaxis of venous thromboembolism in bariatric surgery

4.2.1 Mechanical prophylaxis

Mechanical modalities include graduated compression stockings, intermittent pneumatic compression devices (IPC) and venous foot pump. Perioperative use of the above devices and early mobilization of patients reduce the risk of VTE by increasing venous outflow and preventing venous stasis. Remarkable advantage of mechanical prophylaxis is lack of interference in the coagulation path, which renders it safe for patients in high risk for bleeding. Limitations of the use of mechanical devices are skin irritation and poor compliance.

4.2.2 Pharmacological prophylaxis

Unfractionated heparin (UFH) and low molecular weight heparins (LMWH) are effective in the prophylaxis of VTE in surgical patients. An initial dose of 5000 units UFH is administrated subcutaneous preoperatively and repeated doses every 8 or 12 hours are required. On the contrary, LMWH shows improved pharmacological characteristics, as it requires a single dose per day, has lower degree of plasma protein binding, longer half-life and an enhanced bioavailability. Contraindications in anticoagulation agents are allergy, heparin-induced thrombocytopenia, coagulation disorders, active bleeding or patient at high risk of bleeding.

There is no consensus in literature considering the optimal regimen, dosage, and duration or application mode for VTE preventions in bariatric surgery patients. Furthermore, there is a paucity of data confirming the scaling of dosage according to body weight and renal function. Several authors support low rate of VTE when weight-adapted dosages are administrated, while others suggest that there is no significant difference. American College of Chest Physicians recommend the administration of LMWH, UFH 3 times daily, fontaparinux or the combination of one of these pharmacologic method with optimally used IPC (Grade 1C). Although according to recommendations administrated doses should be higher than those for nonobese patients (Grade 2C), adjusting doses according to BMI remain debatable. Current statement of American Society for Metabolic and Bariatric Surgery suggests the use of both mechanical and pharmacological prophylaxis in bariatric patients, without providing further adaptation guidance. Data on compliance of bariatric surgeons with the above guidelines are inconsistent, however treating high-risk bariatric patients seems to have a positive effect in adherence. Wu et al reported that 95% of bariatric surgeon comply with guidelines, while ENDORSE trial proved that only 58,5% of all surgical patients in risk for VTE receive prophylaxis.

4.2.3 The role of inferior vena cava filters

The prophylactic use of inferior vena cava filters (IVCF) remains controversial. Although recent studies report lower incidence of DVT and PE, other suggest that IVCF may reduce the rate of PE, but increase the incidence of DVT. Risk and complications deriving from the implantation of such a device should not be underestimated. Inferior Vena Cava, filter breakage, caval perforation, insertion site hematoma and infection have been reported. Based on the above, American Society of Hematology stated that the evidence to support the efficacy of IVCF in bariatric surgery is insufficient (Grade 2C recommendation against their use).

4.3 Diagnosis of venous thromboembolism

4.3.1 Clinical findings

Presenting symptoms of VTE are rather non-specific (dyspnea, chest pain, tachypnea), rendering the clinical diagnosis difficult. The key to early detection of VTE in bariatric patients is the high degree of vigilance for clinical features of DVT or PE. Physical examination may reveal increased respiratory rate, rales, wheeze, pleural friction rub, cyanosis, tachycardia, loud second heart sound, sings of DVT (oedema, redness, Homan's sign- pain on passive dorsiflexion of the ankle) and temperature above 38,5°C. Syncope and severe hypotension when present should be considered as signs of hemodynamic compromise.

In obese patients typical clinical findings of DVT or PE can be underestimated, as some of them (edema of lower extremity, tachycardia, dyspnea, tachypnea) pre-exist, due to obesity related co-morbidities, such as cardiac or respiratory failure, varicose veins, obesity related hypoventilation syndrome.

Clinical prediction rules were established in order to overcome the above limitations and provide effective risk stratification of VTE. Wells Score and Revised Geneva Score assess the clinical probability of VTE based on patient's risk factors and clinical findings.

4.3.2 Laboratory findings

The role of arterial blood gas (ABG) in the diagnosis of VTE is rather limited. Respiratory alkalosis and hypoxemia constitute common but non-specific findings and although their presence should raise suspicion, cannot be used solely for the confirmation of the diagnosis.
D-dimers blood test detects a fibrin degradation product and has a high negative predictive value. In bariatric patients has limited value only to exclude VTE, as recent surgery, inflammation and trauma can induce false positive readings.

4.3.3 Imaging studies

Several diagnostic imaging studies can be performed in bariatric population, although limitations occur.
Electrocardiogram (ECG) in acute pulmonary embolism can reveal sinus tachycardia, ST segment depression and signs of right ventricular strain (more commonly incomplete right bundle branch block). Echocardiogram may detect right ventricular dysfunction. The high prevalence of cardiovascular diseases (coronary heart disease, left ventricular hypertrophy, atrial fibrillation, arrhythmias) in obese patients renders ECG and echocardiogram diagnostic tools of limited value.
Chest radiograph in acute pulmonary embolism may appear normal, while rarely, infiltrates, pleural effusion, atelectasis may be present. Consequently, chest radiograph is more useful in the exclusion of other pathological entities (pneumonia, pneumothorax) that may present with the same clinical picture with pulmonary embolism.
In the detection of DVT, Duplex Doppler Ultrasound remains the standard noninvasive examination for the visualization of thrombus, although when performed in obese patients may have reduced accuracy.
Chest Spiral CT has recently replaced pulmonary angiography and is now considered as the gold standard in the diagnosis of PE. However, special equipment must be available for morbidly obese patient, given the weight limitation of the conventional ones.

5. Differential diagnosis

Pathological entities that present with the same clinical features and sings as venous thromboembolism and should be part of the differential diagnosis are: pneumonia, pleural effusion, pneumothorax, congestive heart failure, and cardiac ischemia, exacerbation of chronic obstructive pulmonary disease, asthma and pulmonary edema.
Furthermore, differential diagnosis of PE after bariatric surgery should include anastomotic leakage, which may also present with tachycardia, fever, chest pain and respiratory insuffiency. An upper gastrointestinal study or surgical intervesion may be necessary in order to exclude such a complication.

6. Treatment of venous thromboembolism

European Society of Cardiology guidelines and American Heart Association statement provide evidence-based therapeutic strategies of VTE. Hemodynamic and respiratory support is vital in patients presenting with PE and right ventricle dysfunction. Standard treatment remains the administration of UFH, LMWH and fontaparinux with the considerations mentioned in the prophylactic use of these agents. Data confirming the safety of weight-based dosage of LMWH are insufficient. Performance of thrombolysis, surgical pulmonary embolectomy, percutaneous catheter embolectomy and IVCF should be guided by evidence-based indications. In the absence of nationwide established guidelines standardized to this special surgical population, potential risk of all the above pharmacological and mechanical means should be taken into account when treating bariatric patients.

7. References

Bonanomi G, Hamad GG, Bontempo F. Venous thrombosis and pulmonary embolism. In Schauer PR and Schirmer BD (Eds). Minimally Invasive Bariatric Surgery - Springe Verlag - New York 2007. Pp. 407-411

Buchwald H, Avidor Y, Braunwald E, et al. Bariatric surgery: a systematic review and meta-analysis. JAMA. 2004;292:1724.

Clinical Issues Committee of the American Society for Metabolic and Bariatric Surgery.Prophylactic measures to reduce the risk of venous thromboembolism in bariatric surgery patients.Surg Obes Relat Dis. 2007 Sep-Oct;3(5):494-5.

Cohen AT, Tapson VF, Bergmann JF et al. Venous thromboembolismrisk and prophylaxis in the acute hospital care setting (ENDORSE study): a multinational cross-sectional study. Lancet 2008;371:387–394

Eppsteiner RW, Shin JJ, Johnson J, van Dam RM. Mechanical compression versus subcutaneous heparin therapy in postoperative and posttrauma patients: a systematic review and meta-analysis.World J Surg. 2010 Jan;34(1):10-9.

Fried M, Hainer V, Basdevant A, Buchwald H, Deitel M, Finer N, Greve JW, Horber F, Mathus-Vliegen E, Scopinaro N, Steffen R, Tsigos C, Weiner R, Widhalm K; Bariatric Scientific Collaborative Group Expert Panel. Interdisciplinary European guidelines for surgery for severe (morbid) obesity. Obes Surg. 2007 Feb;17(2):260-70

Geerts WH, Bergqvist D, Pineo GF, Heit JA, Samama CM, Lassen MR, Colwell CW Prevention of venous thromboembolism: American College of Chest Physicians Evidence-Based Clinical Practice Guidelines (8th Edition). American College of Chest Physicians. Chest. 2008 Jun;133(6 Suppl):381S-453S.

Goldhaber SZ, Savage DD, Garrison RJ, et al. Risk factors for pulmonary embolism. The Framingham study. Am J Med 1983;74:1023–1028.

Hamad CG, Choban PS. Enoxaparin for thromboprophylaxis in morbidly obese patients undergoing bariatric surgery; findings of the prophylaxis against VTE outcomes in bariatric surgery patients receiving enoxaparin (PROBE) study. Obes Surg. 2005;15:1368-1374.

Hamad GG, Bergqvist D. Venous thromboembolism in bariatric surgery patients: an update of risk and prevention. Surg Obes Relat Dis. 2007;3(1):97–102.

Jaff MR, McMurtry MS, Archer SL, Cushman M, Goldenberg N, Goldhaber SZ, Jenkins JS, Kline JA, Michaels AD, Thistlethwaite P, Vedantham S, White RJ, Zierler BK; on behalf of the American Heart Association Council on Cardiopulmonary, Critical Care, Perioperative and Resuscitation, Council on Peripheral Vascular Disease, and Council on Arteriosclerosis, Thrombosis and Vascular Biology.Management of

Massive and Submassive Pulmonary Embolism, Iliofemoral Deep Vein Thrombosis, and Chronic Thromboembolic Pulmonary Hypertension: A Scientific Statement From the American Heart Association.Circulation. 2011 Mar 21.

Kalfarentzos F, Stavropoulou F, Yarmenitis S, et al. Prophylaxis of venous thromboembolism using two different doses of lowmolecular- weight heparin (nadroparin) in bariatric surgery: a prospective randomized trial. Obes Surg. 2001;11:670–6.

Le Gal G, Righini M, Roy PM, Sanchez O, Aujesky D, Bounameaux H et al. Prediction of pulmonary embolism in the emergency department: the revised Geneva score. Ann Intern Med 2006;144:165–171.

López-Jiménez F, Cortés-Bergoderi M. Update: systemic diseases and the cardiovascular system: obesity and the heart. Rev Esp Cardiol. 2011 Feb;64(2):140-9. Review

Maggard MA, Shugarman LR, Suttorp M, et al. Meta-analysis:surgical treatment of obesity. Ann Intern Med. 2005;142:547.

Manganelli D, Palla A, Donnamaria V, Giuntini C. Clinical features of pulmonary embolism. Doubts and certainties.Chest. 1995 Jan;107(1 Suppl):25S-32S. Review.

Mukherjee D, Lidor AO, Chu KM, Gearhart SL, Haut ER, Chang DC. Postoperative venous thromboembolism rates vary significantly after different types of major abdominal operations. J Gastrointest Surg. 2008 Nov;12(11):2015-22.

Nguyen NT, Owings JT, Gosselin R, Pevec WC, Lee SJ, Goldman C, Wolfe BM. Systemic coagulation and fibrinolysis after laparoscopic and open gastric bypass. Arch Surg. 2001 Aug;136(8):909-16.

Podnos YD, Jimenez JC, Wilson SE, Stevens CM, Nguyen NT. Complications after laparoscopic gastric bypass: a review of 3464 cases. Arch Surg. 2003 Sep;138(9):957-61

Rajasekhar A, Crowther MA. ASH evidence-based guidelines: what is the role of inferior vena cava filters in the perioperative prevention of venous thromboembolism in bariatric surgery patients? Hematology Am Soc Hematol Educ Program. 2009:302-4. Review

Rocha AT, de Vasconcellos AG, da Luz Neto ER, Araújo DM, Alves ES, Lopes AA. Risk of venous thromboembolism and efficacy of thromboprophylaxis in hospitalized obese medical patients and in obese patients undergoing bariatric surgery. Obes Surg. 2006 Dec;16(12):1645-55

Roger VL et al. Heart disease and stroke statistics--2011 update: a report from the American Heart Association. Circulation. 2011 Feb 1;123(4):e18-e209.

Sapala JA, Wood MH, Schuhknecht MP, et al. Fatal pulmonaryembolism after bariatric operations for morbid obesity: a 24-year retrospective analysis. Obes Surg. 2004;14:738.

Scholten DJ, Hoedema RM, Scholten SE. A comparison of two different prophylactic dose regimens of low molecular weight heparin in bariatric surgery. Obes Surg. 2002;12:19–24.

Singh K, Podolsky ER, Um S, Saba S, Saeed I, Aggarwal L, Zaya M, Castellanos A. Evaluating the Safety and Efficacy of BMI-Based Preoperative Administration of Low-Molecular-Weight Heparin in Morbidly Obese Patients Undergoing Roux-en-Y Gastric Bypass Surgery. Obes Surg. 2011 Apr 9

Sjostrom L, Narbro K, Sjostrom CD, et al. Effects of bariatric surgery on mortality in Swedish obese subjects. N Engl J Med.2007;357:741–52.

Stroh C, Birk D, Flade-Kuthe R, Frenken M, Herbig B, Höhne S, Köhler H, Lange V, Ludwig K, Matkowitz R, Meyer G, Pick P, Horbach T, Krause S, Schäfer L, Schlensak M, Shang E, Sonnenberg T, Susewind M, Voigt H, Weiner R, Wolff S, Wolf AM, Schmidt U, Meyer F, Lippert H, Manger T; Study Group Obesity Surgery.Evidence of thromboembolism prophylaxis in bariatric surgery-results of a quality assurance trial in bariatric surgery in Germany from 2005 to 2007 and review of the literature. Obes Surg. 2009 Jul;19(7):928-36.

Torbicki A, Perrier A, Konstantinides S, Agnelli G, Galiè N, Pruszczyk P, Bengel F, Brady AJ, Ferreira D, Janssens U, Klepetko W, Mayer E, Remy-Jardin M, Bassand JP; ESC Committee for Practice Guidelines (CPG). Guidelines on the diagnosis and management of acute pulmonary embolism: the Task Force for the Diagnosis and Management of Acute Pulmonary Embolism of the European Society of Cardiology (ESC).Eur Heart J. 2008 Sep; 29(18):2276-315.

Vaziri K, Bhanot P, Hungness ES, Morasch MD, Prystowsky JB, Nagle AP. Retrievable inferior vena cava filters in high-risk patients undergoing bariatric surgery. Surg Endosc. 2009 Oct;23(10):2203-7.

Vaziri K, Devin Watson J, Harper AP, Lee J, Brody FJ, Sarin S, Ignacio EA, Chun A, Venbrux AC, Lin PP. Prophylactic Inferior Vena Cava Filters in High-Risk Bariatric Surgery. Obes Surg. 2010

Wells PS, Anderson DR, Rodger M, Ginsberg JS, Kearon C, Gent M et al. Derivation of a simple clinical model to categorize patients probability of pulmonary embolism: increasing the models utility with the SimpliRED D-dimer. Thromb Haemost 2000;83:416–420.

Wu EC, Barba CA. Current practices in the prophylaxis of venous thromboembolism in bariatric surgery. Obes Surg 2000;10:7–13.

5

Non-Thrombotic Pulmonary Embolism

Vijay Balasubramanian, Malaygiri Aparnath and Jagrati Mathur
University of California, San Francisco, Fresno (UCSF Fresno)
USA

1. Introduction

Pulmonary thrombo-embolism (PTE) remains a common cause of morbidity and mortality worldwide. Annually, as many as 300,000 people in the United States die from acute pulmonary embolism and the diagnosis is often not made until autopsy (Tapson, 2008). Obstruction of the pulmonary artery or one of its branches by material other than thrombi is commonly referred to as Non-thrombotic Pulmonary Embolism (NTPE). The lungs are a prominent target for the embolization of any material larger than approximately 10 microns that gains access to the venous circulation. This includes thrombi, air, amniotic fluid, fat, injected foreign material, and tumor (Fig 1). In comparison with pulmonary thrombo-embolism, NTPE is a less common condition (M. B. King & Harmon, 1994). Its complex and diverse etiologies renders it more difficult to accurate diagnosis and characterization. Therefore, there is a gross scarcity of epidemiologic data pertaining to this group. We speculate that it is often underestimated (both due to under-recognition and under-diagnosis). In contrast to pulmonary thrombo-embolism, the complex and diverse pathogenesis of different subtypes of emboli is subject to continuing speculation and extends beyond "simple" mechanical obstruction of pulmonary vasculature. Non-thrombotic emboli may also be associated with a severe inflammatory response both in the systemic and pulmonary circulation, unlike pulmonary thrombo-emboli.

The diagnosis of NTPE is even more challenging given lack of specific clinical features, heterogeneity of radiographic findings as well as lack of specific laboratory blood tests. Nonetheless, NTPE can be associated with some specific radiographic findings and familiarity with these features should aid in prompt diagnosis (Han et al.,2003). High index of clinical suspicion in the appropriate clinical setting often paves the way to prompt diagnosis. It is important that the correct type of pulmonary emboli be identified, since treatment and prognosis vary considerably. In this chapter, we have summarized the current concepts of various types of NTPE.

2. Fat embolism

Fat Embolism (FE) is by far the most frequent NTPE observed outside the clinical setting of Obstetrics-Gynecology. The term FE refers to the presence of fat globules within the

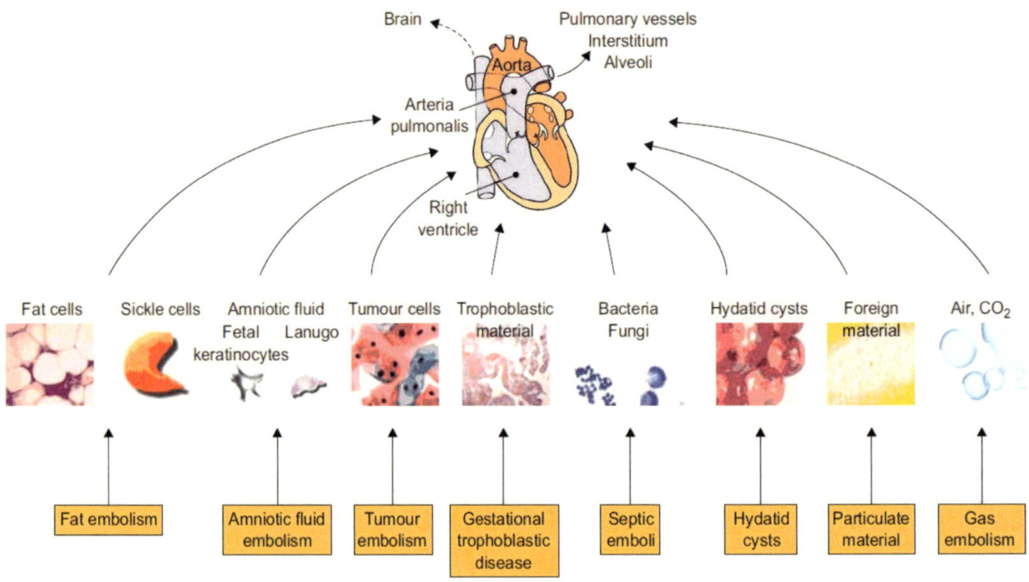

Fig. 1. Different sub-types of NTPE (Reproduced with permission - Jorens et al, ERJ 2009)

peripheral and pulmonary circulation. It can range from being asymptomatic to life threatening respiratory failure with or without neurological and other systemic manifestations often described as Fat Embolism Syndrome (FES).

3. Epidemiology

The reported incidence of FE & FES varies widely in literature. FE occurs in great majority of patients who sustain pelvic or long-bone fractures, endo-medullary nailing of long-bone fractures or placement of knee and hip prosthesis. Embolic showers of circulating fat globules have been demonstrated in up to 41% of patients following surgical nailing of long bone fractures (Talbot & Schemitsch, 2006). However, only a small percentage of these patients develop FES (406th Medical General Laboratory, Professional Section, 1951; Deland, 1956; Gossling & Pellegrini, 1982; Gurd & Wilson, 1974; Koessler et al., 2001; Levy, 1990; Lozman et al., 1986; Palmovic & McCarroll, 1965; Peltier, 1969; Shier & Wilson, 1980; Talbot & Schemitsch, 2006). The incidence of posttraumatic FES can range from 0.25% (Peltier, 1969) to 35% (Gurd & Wilson, 1974; Lindeque et al., 1987; Riska & Myllynen, 1982). The timing of the fracture fixation also appears to impact the incidence of FES. Delayed surgery predisposes to a higher incidence. Non-traumatic FE or FES is rare.

4. Risk factors

Trauma, orthopedic procedures and soft tissue injuries including severe burns are by far the most common causes of FE and FES. FES is more likely to develop after pelvic or lower extremity fractures; it is seldom observed in patients with isolated upper extremity fractures.

Characteristics	Comments
Age: 10-40 years - peak incidence Sex : M > F	• Physically most active age group - higher risk of trauma • Children <10 yrs old: lower fat and olein content of the bone marrow (hence, less likely to develop FES) • Elderly : low impact fractures, mostly single fracture, mainly involving the neck of the femur thus less intramedullary pressure and less marrow is available for embolization.
Location of fracture(s) in order of incidence: • Lower extremity and/or pelvic • Upper extremity • Rib & vertebrae	Femur (excluding neck) is the single most common site
Number of fracture(s) Multiple > single	More marrow is available for embolization
Type of fracture Closed > open	Higher pressure is more likely to develop in closed than open (Dedhia & Mushambi, 2007; ten Duis et al., 1988; Thomas & Ayyar, 1972).

Table 1. Traumatic Fat Embolism - Factors predisposing to FES among Trauma patients

5. Non-traumatic fat embolism

Non traumatic Fat embolism or FES is rare and overall incidence is extremely low (Stein et al., 2008). It can be divided into three categories.

- Procedures related (Table-2)
- Diseases related (Table-3)
- Drugs related (Table-4)

6. Non orthopedic procedures associated with fat embolization (Table-2)

Soft tissue filling	(Coronado-Malagon et al., 2010)
Bone marrow transplantation	(Bulger et al., 1997; Hasan et al., 2001; Jenkins et al., 2002; Lipton et al., 1987; Robert et al., 1993)
Renal transplantation	(Jones et al., 1965; Lipton et al., 1987)
Lipectomy	(Laub & Laub, 1990)
Autologous fat harvesting	(Currie et al., 1997)
Periurethral injection	(Currie et al., 1997)
Lymphangiography	(Francis et al., 1983)
Mineral oil enemas	(Rabah et al., 1987)
Injection of rice bran oil into breasts	(Kiyokawa et al., 1995)
Cardiopulmonary resuscitation	(Buchanan & Mason, 1982; Bulger et al., 1997; Jackson & Greendyke, 1965; Jenkins et al., 2002; Robert et al., 1993)
Liposuction	Bulger et al., 1997; Guardia et al., 1989; Jenkins et al., 2002; M. B. King & Harmon, 1994; Laub & Laub, 1990; Platt et al., 2002; Richards, 1997; Robert et al., 1993; R. M. Ross & Johnson, 1988)
Intraosseous fluid and drug administration	(Hasan et al., 2001; Vichinsky et al., 2000)
Extracorporeal circulation such as extracorporeal membrane oxygenation or cardiopulmonary bypass	(Akhtar, 2009; Bulger et al., 1997; Gravante et al., 2008; Jenkins et al., 2002; M. B. King & Harmon, 1994; Richards, 1997; Robert et al., 1993; ten Duis, 1997)

Table 2. Procedures related

7. Conditions associated with fat embolization (Table-3)

Pancreatitis	(Bulger et al., 1997; Godeau et al., 1996; Goldhaber, 2004; Guardia et al., 1989; Jenkins et al., 2002; M. B. King & Harmon, 1994; Lynch, 1954; Richards, 1997; Robert et al., 1993)
Panniculitis	(Goldhaber, 2004)
Osteomyelitis	(Broder & Ruzumna, 1967; Goldhaber, 2004; M. B. King & Harmon, 1994; Richards, 1997; Wagner, 1865)
Sickle cell crisis	(Bulger et al., 1997; Goldhaber, 2004; Hutchinson et al., 1973; Jenkins et al., 2002; M. B. King & Harmon, 1994; Richards, 1997; Robert et al., 1993)
Alcoholic fatty liver	(Goldhaber, 2004)
Liquefying subcutaneous hematoma	(Jorens et al., 2009)
Viral hepatitis in pre-existing fatty liver	(Schulz et al., 1996)
Bone tumor lysis	(Weinhouse, January 2011)
Burns	(Bulger et al., 1997; Jenkins et al., 2002; M. B. King & Harmon, 1994; Levy, 1990; Patil & Wakankar, 2008; Richards, 1997; Robert et al., 1993; Weisz, 1974)
Decompression sickness	(Bulger et al., 1997; Haymaker & Davison, 1950; Jenkins et al., 2002; M. B. King & Harmon, 1994; Ober et al., 1959; Richards, 1997; Robert et al., 1993)
Diabetes mellitus	(Cuppage, 1963; M. B. King & Harmon, 1994; Richards, 1997; Weinhouse, January 2011)

Table 3. Diseases related

8. Drugs associated with fat embolization (Table-4)

Cyclosporine A solvent	(Weinhouse, January 2011)
Carbon tetrachloride poisoning	(Macmahon & Weiss, 1929; Taviloglu & Yanar, 2007)
Infusion of lipids at a rate greater than normal clearing capacity, i.e. 3.8 gm/kg/day,	(Bulger et al., 1997; Haber et al., 1988; Jenkins et al., 2002; Kitchell & Balogh, 1986; Rayburg et al., 2010; Ritter et al., 1997; Robert et al., 1993)
Intraosseous fluid and drug administration	(Hasan et al., 2001; Vichinsky et al., 2000)
Corticosteroids	(Bulger et al., 1997; Jenkins et al., 2002; Robert et al., 1993; Weinhouse, January 2011)

Table 4. Drugs related

In view of the large number of patients who are treated with liposome-embedded drugs, reports of fatal FE caused by intravenous liposome drug delivery or intra-venous hyperalimentation are debatable (Kitchell & Balogh, 1986; Tolentino et al., 2004).
Pathophysiology of FES remains unknown. Two main theories, namely mechanical and biochemical, dominate the literature and have gained acceptance (Bulger et al., 1997; Choi et al., 2002; Mellor & Soni, 2001; Parisi et al., 2002).

9. Mechanical hypothesis

Gauss first proposed the mechanical theory of fat embolization which requires that large fat cells in the bone marrow rupture into the venous circulation through torn venules at the fracture site in the setting of a favorable pressure gradient (increased intra-medullary pressure). These fat globules subsequently embolize to the lungs and obstruct the pulmonary capillaries (Gauss, 1924). Systemic embolization takes place via intra-cardiac shunts or PFO. Small fat droplets (7-10 micrometers) can pass through pulmonary capillaries (Parisi et al., 2002) causing systemic embolization in the absence of anatomic shunt. The clinical picture is dictated by the extent of the organ(s) involved. However, mechanical theory does not explain the following observations:

- Not all patients who have fat emboli develop FES (Aoki et al., 1998)
- "Latent period": from the time of onset of injury to the onset of symptoms and signs of FES
- Non-Traumatic causes of FES

Therefore factors other than mechanical obstruction must be playing a role which led to the biochemical hypothesis.

10. Biochemical hypothesis

In 1927, Lehman and Moore first postulated that a substance exists that causes destabilization of the emulsion of chylomicrons in the bloodstream with coalescence of fat stores in response to stress and catecholamine release (Lehman & Moore, 1927). Currently the most widely held view is that there is physiochemical alteration leading to degradation of embolized fat and production of toxic intermediates—mainly Free Fatty Acids (FFAs). Circulating FFAs originating from triglycerides at the fracture site may become concentrated as a result of systemic lipolysis induced by catecholamines. Alternatively, fat emboli trapped in pulmonary vessels may be metabolized to FFAs and glycerol by lipase secreted by lung parenchymal cells (P. L. Baker et al., 1971). However the exact source of FFAs remains unknown. Regardless of the source of the FFAs, circulating FFAs level is elevated in patients with fractures and in animal models of nontraumatic fat embolism. It has been postulated that decreased hepatic clearance as in shock, sepsis, or decreased plasma concentration of albumin also increase the risk of FES (Mays, 1970; Moylan et al., 1976). FFAs have been shown in both animal and human studies to have the following systemic effects

- Toxicity to lung parenchyma:
  - capillary leak
  - curtailed surfactant production
  - interstitial hemorrhage and pulmonary edema (Herndon, 1975; Parker et al., 1974; Szabo et al., 1977)
- Cerebral cortical cell damage (Parisi et al., 2002)
- Cardiac contractile dysfunction (Dedhia & Mushambi, 2007; Hulman, 1988b)
- C-reactive protein which is elevated in these patients appears to interact with circulating chylomicrons to form fat globules **de novo,** which can explain non traumatic fat embolism (Hulman, 1988a).

Coagulation cascade activation, disseminated intravascular coagulation (DIC), and antifibrinolytic pathways may further contribute to lung injury (E. G. King et al., 1971; Saldeen, 1970).The biochemical theory, could explain "latent period" and nontraumatic forms of FES (Schnaid et al., 1987). It must be emphasized that evidence is largely circumstantial and the exact pathophysiologic mechanism responsible for FES remains unknown.

11. Clinical features

FES usually presents as multisystem disorder in the setting of long bone fracture(s) or major trauma. The most commonly affected organs are brain and lung. The presentation is heterogeneous given diverse causes as well as multi-organ involvement. Latent period is typically 12 to 72 hours although rarely it can be as short as few hours in the setting of major trauma or as long as 2 weeks (Gary, 2004; Johnson & Lucas, 1996; M. B. King & Harmon, 1994; Mellor & Soni, 2001; Moreau, 1974; Parisi et al., 2002; Peltier, 1984; Schonfeld et al., 1983; Shier & Wilson, 1980). 85% of patients will develop signs and symptoms within 48 hours of injury (Sevitt, 1962). The classic triad of hypoxemia, neurological dysfunction and petechial rash is seen in only about 50% of the patients.

12. Pulmonary

It is uncommon to develop FES in the absence of respiratory manifestations. A great majority of patients present with varying degrees of respiratory insufficiency that can range from nearly asymptomatic hypoxemia to severe hypoxemia and ARDS requiring mechanical ventilation (Bernard et al., 1994). The most "fulminant" form of FES presents as "acute cor pulmonale" with respiratory failure causing death within a matter of few hours, usually after a major trauma (Mellor & Soni, 2001; Parisi et al., 2002; Peltier, 1984; Schonfeld et al., 1983). Although frequently clinically inapparent, hypoxemia is nearly universal (Peltier et al., 1974; A. P. Ross, 1970).

13. Central nervous system

Neurological findings are nonspecific and usually completely reversible. They can range from anxiety and restlessness to comatose state requiring mechanical ventilation. The early signs and symptoms are delirium, restlessness, confusion or anxiety. Diffuse encephalopathy and coma can ensue (Jacobson et al., 1986). Focal neurological deficits are common. These findings are frequently not responsive to correction of hypoxemia (Metting et al., 2009) and have infrequently been observed in absence of pulmonary involvement.

14. Skin

The characteristic petechial rash has been reported to be in present in about 50% to 60% of patients with FES. Upper anterior torso, axillae, neck, upper arm, conjunctivae and oral mucosa are usual sites. The rash is NOT due to thrombocytopenia but from fat emboli obstructing capillaries and causing capillary damage and subsequent hemorrhages. The petechial rash may be the only physical sign.

15. Eye

Retinopathy has been reported in up to 50% of patients (Adams, 1971). Fundoscopic findings (Kearns, 1956) include macular edema, cotton-wool spots, retinal hemorrhages and occasional fat droplets. The findings are attributed to microvascular injury in the form of microinfarcts of retina which usually disappear with possible residual scotomas.

16. Cardiovascular

Tachycardia is invariably present. Hemodynamic changes include: (Aebli et al., 2005; Krebs et al., 2007; Murphy et al., 1997)

- Increase in pulmonary arterial pressure due to not only mechanical obstruction from fat embolism but also from pulmonary vasoconstriction.
- Reduction in systemic arterial pressure
- Reduction in cardiac output
- Arrythmias

Cardiovascular deterioration is often transient but can be fulminant resulting in severe cardiac failure, cardiac arrest and even death.

Other findings: Rarely severe hypocalcemia leading to tetany has been reported (Gurd & Wilson, 1974). Jaundice/icterus can be present. Hematological findings include anemia, thrombocytopenia and DIC (Dines et al., 1972; Herndon, 1975; Hulman, 1988b; McCarthy et al., 1973; Peltier, 1984; Peltier, 1988). Elevation of ESR & CRP, presence of fat globules in the urine, sputum or blood, elevation of serum lipase and phospholipase A2 have been described.

17. Role of bronchial alveolar lavage (BAL)

Presence of lipid inclusions in alveolar macrophages in the BAL has been associated with various traumatic and nontraumatic conditions, especially aspiration pneumonia and lipid infusion. Quantification of cells containing fat droplets in bronchial alveolar lavage (BAL) fluid within the first 24 hours after trauma have also been shown to correlate with clinical fat embolism in some studies) (Al-Khuwaitir et al., 2002; Chastre et al., 1990; Mellor & Soni, 2001; Mimoz et al., 1995). In the absence of an exogenous source of fat, BAL fluid that contains more than 30% macrophages laden with lipid inclusions is highly suggestive of FES.

18. Imaging

The findings are nonspecific and appear after a variable lag period as related to clinical symptoms. Chest roentgenogram may reveal diffuse evenly distributed alveolar and interstitial densities suggestive of pulmonary edema or acute lung injury. Computed tomography (CT) of the chest may rarely show fat in the pulmonary artery. Multiple sub-centimeter, ill-defined centrilobular and subpleural nodules can be seen in the acute phase of FES. Diffuse lung calcifications located in the branches of the pulmonary arteries have been described in the late course of FES (Hamrick-Turner et al., 1994). Ventilation perfusion scan (V/Q scan) may reveal subsegmental perfusion defects (H. M. Park et al., 1986).

Computed tomography (CT) of the brain may show nonspecific signs of cerebral edema and hemorrhagic infarcts in multiple areas (Meeke et al., 1987). Magnetic resonance imaging (MRI) of the brain and MR spectroscopy seem to be the most sensitive method in detection of cerebral emboli, but nonspecific (J. J. Chen et al., 2008; Eguia et al., 2007; Guillevin et al., 2005; Sasano et al., 2004; Satoh et al., 1997; Stoeger et al., 1998). Diffusion-weighted imaging may reveal bright spots on a dark background, a finding known as the "Starfield pattern" (Parizel et al., 2001). Cerebral micro-emboli can be detected in vivo after long bone fracture by transcranial Doppler (Barak et al., 2008; Forteza et al., 1999).

Transesophageal Echo (TEE) is most useful for diagnosing intra-operative FES. TEE has sensitivity of 80% and specificity of 100% in patients with fat embolism large enough to cause hemodynamic instability (Pruszczyk et al., 1997). TEE cannot reliably distinguish fat emboli from tumor emboli.

19. Diagnosis

Given the extremely heterogeneous pattern of presentation, precise diagnosis of FES remains elusive. Various diagnostic criteria have been proposed. However given the lack of gold standard diagnostic tests and lack of pathognomic signs, it is difficult to determine validity of these criteria. Therefore the diagnosis of FES is based on a constellation of clinical and laboratory findings and exclusion of other potential diagnoses (Taviloglu & Yanar, 2007).

The following diagnostic criteria are widely used.

Major	Minor
• Respiratory insufficiency • Cerebral involvement • Petechial rash	• Pyrexia • Tachycardia • Retinal changes • Jaundice • Renal changes (anuria or oliguria) • Thrombocytopenia (a drop of >50% of the admission platelet count) • High erythrocyte sedimentation rate • Fat macroglobulinemia

Table 5. Gurd and Wilson: FES = 1 major + 4 minor + Fat microglobulinemia

Criterion	Points
Diffuse petechiae	5
Alveolar infiltrates	4
Hypoxemia <70 mm Hg	3
Confusion	1
Fever 38 C	1
Heart rate >120/min	1
Respiratory rate >30/min	1

Table 6. Schonfeld's criteria - FES = 5 or more points

20. Management

There is no definitive therapy for FES. The treatment is mainly supportive. Maintenance of adequate oxygenation, ensuring hemodynamic stability, prophylaxis of venous thrombosis and stress related gastrointestinal bleeding and nutrition are key aspects. Therefore clinical management strategies should be geared towards prophylactic measures in trauma victims. Early stabilization of the fractures as well as early operative intervention reduces the incidence and severity of FES (Al-Khuwaitir et al., 2002; A. B. Baker, 1976; Bone et al., 1989; Jenkins et al., 2002; Johnson & Lucas, 1996; Parisi et al., 2002; Riska et al., 1976; Riska & Myllynen, 1982; Svenningsen et al., 1987; Tachakra et al., 1990; Talucci et al., 1983). Early (< 24 hours) fixation of the fracture of the femur was associated with an improved outcome even in patients with concomitant head and chest trauma (Brundage et al., 2002). When fracture stabilization was delayed in patients with multiple injuries, the incidence of ARDS, FE and pneumonia, the costs of hospital care and the number of days in the intensive care unit (ICU) were increased (Behrman et al., 1990; Bone et al., 1989). Intraosseous pressure limitation during orthopedic procedures reduces the intravasation of intramedullary fat and other debris and therefore may reduce the incidence and severity of FES (Y. H. Kim et al., 2002; Kropfl et al., 1999; Pitto et al., 1999; Pitto et al., 2002; Pitto, Schramm et al., 1999).

Incidence and severity of FES are decreased when corticosteroids are given prophylactically, although no mortality benefit has been demonstrated (Alho et al., 1978; Bederman et al.,

2009; Kallenbach et al., 1987; Lindeque et al., 1987; Schonfeld et al., 1983). Nonetheless, prophylactic use of corticosteroids remains controversial mainly because of lack of large scale studies. The results of treatment with drugs, including clofibrate, dextran-40, ethyl alcohol, heparin, and aspirin are inconclusive (K. M. Chan et al., 1984; Gossling & Pellegrini, 1982; Peltier, 1984; Shier et al., 1977; Stoltenberg & Gustilo, 1979).

21. Prognosis

With timely supportive care and hemodynamic support, most patients with FES recover completely. Mortality rate has been variably reported to be 10 to 20% (Fabian et al., 1990; Moreau, 1974; Peltier, 1965; Peltier et al., 1974).

22. Septic pulmonary embolism

Septic pulmonary embolism (SPE) is an uncommon but serious disorder that is often difficult to diagnose. SPE are thrombi containing microorganisms in a fibrin matrix that are mobilized via the bloodstream from an infectious nidus to get implanted into the vascular system of the lungs. The organisms can be bacteria, fungi or parasites.

23. Epidemiology

In 1978, MacMillan et al. (MacMillan et al., 1978) studied 60 patients with SPE over a 5-year period and reported that most of SPE cases occurred in drug users. Intravenous drug abuse (IVDA-78%) and tricuspid endocarditis were identified as the embolic source in 53% of these IVDA cases (fig 2b) (MacMillan et al., 1978). However, the epidemiology and outcome of patients with SPE have changed over the past 30 years with the increased use of long term indwelling catheters and devices (pacemakers, prosthetic vascular devices) and also increase in the number of immune-compromised patients. The predominant cause of SPE in the current era is infections related to intravascular devices/catheters or soft-tissue infections. Its incidence is declining among IVDA presumably due to greater needle hygiene (Fig 2a) (Cook et al., 2005). Intravascular devices are a common cause of local site infection and cause up to 50% of the nosocomial bacteremias. Central venous catheters account for 80-90% of these infections.

In a large series of postmortem examinations in Japan, a total of 11,367 PE cases were identified from 396,982 postmortem examinations. In this study, the incidence of septic PE was found to be 2.2% (Sakuma et al., 2007).

24. Risk factors

A prerequisite for the development of SPE appears to be a heavily infected source such as long-term indwelling vascular devices, bacterial endocarditis of the right heart valves or peripheral thrombophlebitis (head and neck or pelvic infections) leading to showers of septic emboli to the lung. In the above-mentioned recent Japanese study with 247 SPE patients, fungal emboli were more common than bacterial emboli. Among the fungi, Aspergillus was the most common pathogen (20.8%) encountered preceding Mucor or Candida. Cancer was the most common predisposing factor associated with fungal SPE (63%) - Leukemia (43.2%), followed by adenocarcinoma and lymphoma. The top three infectious sources showering septic emboli were pneumonia, sepsis and infective endocarditis.

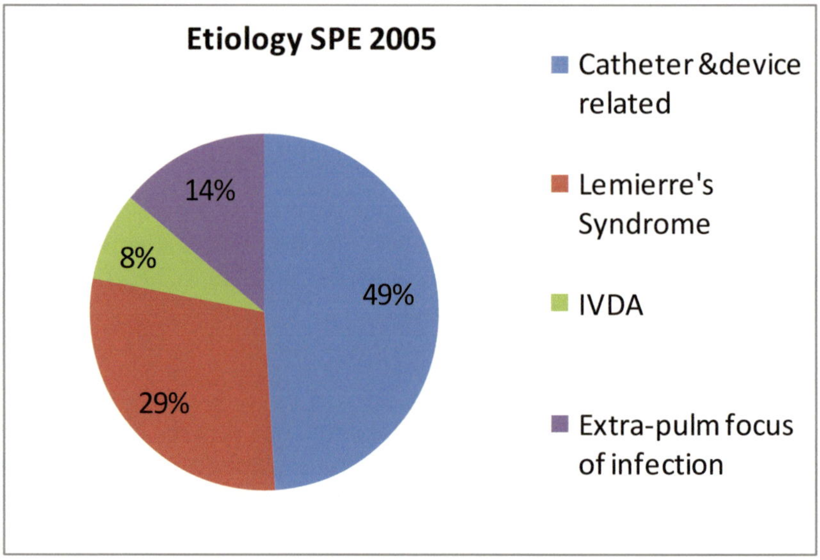

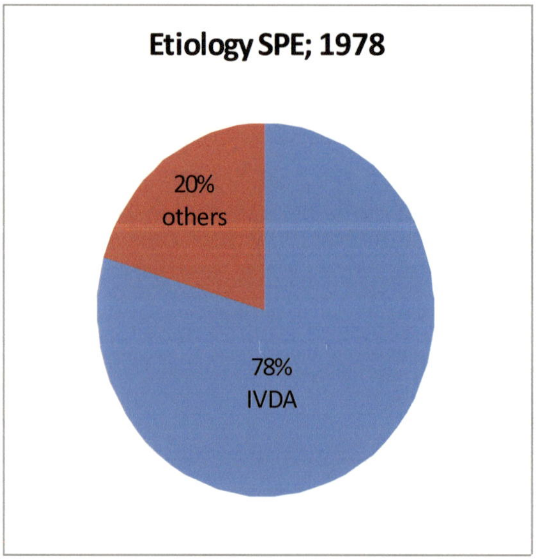

Fig. 2. (a & b): Causes of Septic Pulmonary Embolism
(Cook et al., 2005; MacMillan et al., 1978)

25. Pathophysiology

Septic emboli are transported to the lung via the hematogenous route from various sources of infection. These emboli cause occlusion of the small, peripheral pulmonary arteries leading to pulmonary infarction which could further complicate to microabscesses. Extravasation from the bronchial arteries – "pulmonary hemorrhages", may cause peripheral consolidation. (Fig 3- Flow chart).

A peculiar subtype is Lemierre's syndrome (postanginal sepsis), a severe illness caused by the anaerobic bacterium, Fusobacterium necrophorum which typically occurs in healthy teenagers and young adults. The infection originates in the throat as tonsillo-pharyngitis, odontogenic infection, mastoiditis or sinusitis and spreads via a septic thrombophlebitis of the tonsillar vein and internal jugular vein. The ensuing bacteremia is complicated by septic emboli to a range of sites such as lung, joints, and bones. Pulmonary involvement in Lemierre's syndrome has been reported in up to 97% with SPE, lung abscesses and empyema (Golpe et al., 1999; Riordan & Wilson, 2004; Sinave et al., 1989). The causative organisms of Lemierre's syndrome include the anaerobic gram-negative Fusobacterium species, and also Eikenella, Porphyromonas, Streptococci and Bacteroides. Recently, methicillin-resistant Staphylococcus aureus has been identified as a new causative agent (Riordan & Wilson, 2004).

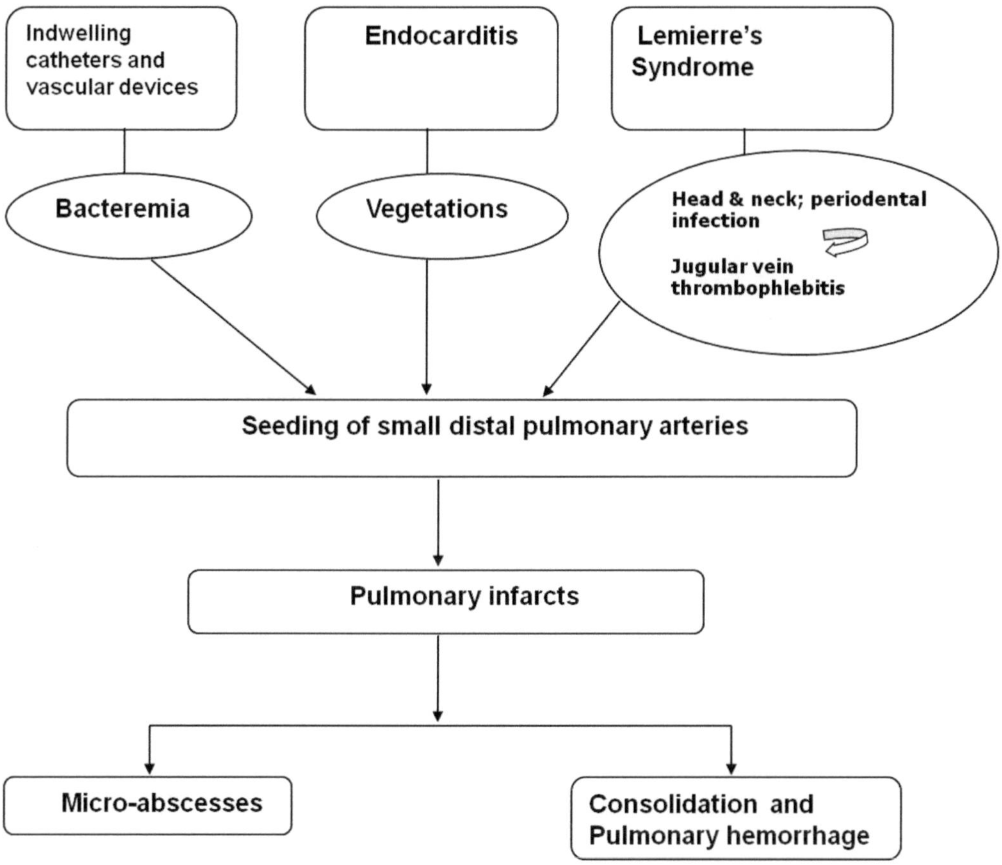

Fig. 3.

26. Clinical features

The clinical features of SPE are non-specific and patients generally present with a febrile illness, cough, hemoptysis, dyspnea and pleuritic chest pain. Diffuse cavitary lung nodules and infiltrates associated with an active focus of extra-pulmonary infection should clue the clinician into thinking about a diagnosis of SPE. Other pulmonary complications of SPE include pleural effusion, empyema, and rupture of subpleural lesions leading to spontaneous pneumothorax.

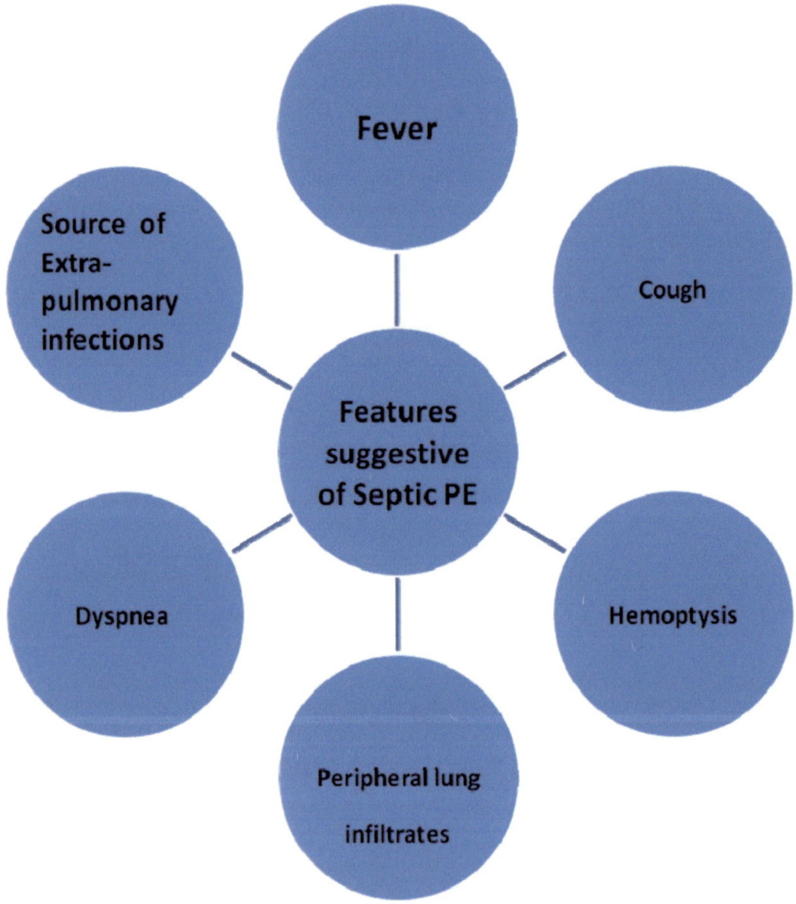

Fig. 4. Clinical manifestations of SPE

Lemierre's syndrome usually occurs in previously healthy adolescent or young adults, generally presenting with high grade fever (39-41°C) and rigors. History is usually significant for sore throat, tooth ache, odynophagia, dysphagia and chest pain in the week preceding the presentation. On examination the patient appears ill, may have signs of periodontal disease, the tonsils are usually inflamed with exudates and peritonsillar abscesses releasing foul-smelling pus. "The diagnosis of this infection may be suggested by the peculiar odour—like Limburger or overripe Camembert cheese—of pus produced by it."(Alston, 1955). Signs of internal jugular vein thrombosis may be present in 26–45% of cases. Features suggestive of the development of internal jugular vein thrombophlebitis include neck pain and stiffness, cervical lymphadenopathy often in the anterior triangle and more characteristically a tender (normally unilateral) swelling at the angle of the jaw-anterior to, and parallel with, the sternomastoid muscle (Riordan & Wilson, 2004).

27. Diagnosis

Clinical and radiological features at presentation are usually nonspecific and the diagnosis is frequently delayed (Huang et al., 1989). Radiographic findings, predisposing background or illness, and clinical evidence of infection usually are clues to the diagnosis. Blood cultures, chest CT and echocardiography are valuable when evaluating a patient with suspected SPE. Basic laboratory testing provides some clues to diagnosis. Patients typically have a neutrophil predominant leucocytosis. Liver function tests are abnormal in approximately 50% of patients. C-reactive protein is invariably raised.

Microbiology: The diagnosis of bacteremia or fungemia is confirmed by recovery of the same species of micro-organisms from the peripheral blood cultures and from quantitative cultures obtained from the source of SPE. Pus drained from any site should be sent for culture, including catheter tip, localized abscesses in the neck, empyema, septic arthritis, bone, and soft tissue abscesses.

Chest radiograph findings are usually nonspecific with a spectrum of radiological abnormalities. The usual findings include patchy air space opacities simulating nonspecific broncho-pneumonia, multiple ill-defined nodules (usually 1-3 cm) in various stages of cavitation with irregular thick walls or wedge-shaped densities of varying sizes located peripherally abutting the pleura. Other x-ray features also include blunting of the costophrenic angle, indicating small pleural effusions or empyema.

Computed tomography (CT) of the chest: Common findings are patchy consolidation with air bronchograms, nodules in various stages of cavitation (predominant in the lower lobes), wedge-shaped peripheral lesions abutting the pleura with or without extension into the pleural space - pleural effusion/empyema, and hilar or mediastinal lymphadenopathy. The *"feeding vessel sign"* has been considered highly suggestive (although not pathognomonic) of septic PE and consists of a distinct vessel leading directly into the center of a nodule (Fig 5). This sign may represent hematogenous spread to the lungs and may also be seen in metastasis. The prevalence of this sign varies from 67–100% in various series and the heterogeneous sub pleural wedge-shaped opacities are seen in 70–75% of patients (Kwon et al., 2007). Multi-detector CT is faster and superior to the classical CT technology for detection of this sign (Dodd et al., 2006).

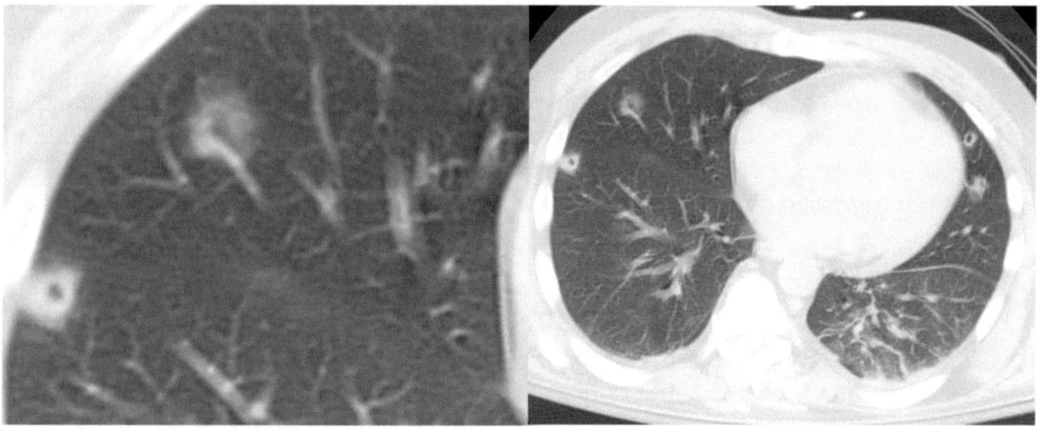

Fig. 5. The "Feeding vessel" sign and multiple peripheral cavitating lesions suggestive of SPE

Features	Gram Positive SPE	Gram negative SPE
1) Size of emboli	Larger	Smaller
2) Radiographic Characteristics	1) Cavitation 2) Air bronchograms in nodules 3) Peripheral wedge shaped opacities	1) 'Halo sign': Central area of soft tissue attenuation surrounded by a halo of ground-glass attenuation. 2) Hemorrhagic nodules and infarcts 3) "Feeding vessel" sign

Table 7. Characteristics of SPE

Echocardiography is an important tool in evaluating patients for endocarditis. Trans-esophageal echocardiography (TEE) increases the sensitivity of detecting vegetations from 75 to 95 percent while maintaining the specificity of 85 to 98 percent and is thus, superior to the transthoracic technique (TTE) in delineating vegetations, abscesses and leaflet perforations in the heart (Dodd et al., 2006).

28. Treatment

Recent studies demonstrate improved outcomes for patients with SPE with virtually all patients recovering from their illness. This may be attributable to earlier diagnosis, prompt administration of broad-spectrum antibiotics and improvements in surgical and supportive care. Discontinuation of vascular catheters/devices is recommended. In Lemierre's syndrome, vigorous antibiotic treatment for 4-6 weeks, targeting the organism and drainage of accessible abscesses are indicated. Internal jugular vein ligation/excision is rarely indicated as is the use of anticoagulation (Armstrong et al., 2000; Lustig et al., 1995). Consensus recommendation(American Heart Association (AHA), British Society for Antimicrobial Chemotherapy (BSAC), and the European Society for Cardiology (ESC)) is that, prompt use of antibiotics in treatment of endocarditis may result in reduction of incidence of SPE (Baddour et al., 2005; Elliott et al., 2004). The recommended duration of antibiotics is 4 to 6 weeks. The 2008 American College of Chest Physicians (ACCP) guidelines recommend against the use of routine antithrombotic therapy unless a separate indication exists.

29. Amniotic fluid embolism

AFE is an exceedingly rare and one of the most catastrophic complications of pregnancy. It remains an enigma to this date, more than half a century after the first published autopsy series. AFE is responsible for significant proportion of maternal mortality (Lang & King, 2008; Lewis, 2007). The presence of fetal debris in the pulmonary circulation of a mother who died suddenly during labor was first reported by Meyer in 1926 (Meyer, 1926) and subsequently by Steiner and Lushbaugh in 1941 as an autopsy series (Steiner & Lushbaugh, 1941).

30. Epidemiology and risk factors

The true incidence of AFE remains unknown and is variably reported in literature. The incidence of AFE has been estimated to be in 1 in 8000 to 80000 deliveries with reported mortality rates in older reports as high as 60%. However, more recent data suggest lower mortality rates ranging between 27-37% (Clark et al., 1995; Morgan, 1979; Tuffnell, 2005). For unknown reasons, the incidence of AFE is much higher in North America, around 1 in 15000 deliveries, Australia -1 in 30000 deliveries (C. L. Roberts et al., 2010), United Kingdom - 1 in 50000 (Abenhaim et al., 2008; Knight et al., 2010; Kramer et al., 2006).
AFE usually occurs during immediate postpartum period. Data from a national registry revealed that AFE occurred during labor but before delivery in 70% of cases and during caesarean section in 19% (Clark et al., 1995). Although, reported as early as second trimester, the diagnosis in cases occurring as late as 36 h postpartum has been described (Devriendt et al., 1995). AFE following trans-abdominal amniocentesis is very rare (Hasaart & Essed, 1983). It has been estimated that AFE accounted for 12% of all maternal deaths related to legally induced abortion since 1972 (Grimes & Schulz, 1985; Guidotti et al., 1981). It is seldom associated with (surgical) manipulation during caesarean section (Laforga, 1997), curettage (Grimes & Cates, 1977), cervical suture removal (Margan et al., 1984) or repair of an incompetent cervix (Margan et al., 1984), or after car or motor vehicle accidents (Olcott et al., 1973). Large fetal size, use of oxytocics and vaginal prostaglandins, advanced gestational age, amnio-infusion or complicated labor have all been implicated (Maher et al., 1994; Morgan, 1979). In reality, specific risk factors have not been conclusively identified. Logistic regression identified advanced maternal age, placental pathologies and caesarean deliveries in a large population-based cohort study (Abenhaim et al., 2008). Maternal age below 20 years and dystocia has been associated with lower incidence of AFE.
Pathophysiology: The pathogenesis of AFE remains poorly understood. The detection of fetal tissue in maternal pulmonary artery is not pathognomonic. In fact, there is no clear temporal relationship between entry of amniotic fluid in to maternal circulation and symptom onset. The "antigenic" nature of AF along with pulmonary eosinophilic infiltrates, elevated antitryptase activity suggestive of mast cell degranulation has resulted in some authors to propose "Anaphylactoid syndrome of Pregnancy" as an alternative name to AFE. Autopsy findings frequently reveal disseminated intravascular coagulation (DIC). Isolated DIC may herald AFE. Amniotic fluid accelerates clot initiation and propagation.
Hemodynamic Effects: A biphasic pattern of hemodynamic changes have been favored in most recent descriptions. The "acute phase" comprising of acute elevation of pulmonary arterial pressure ("acute Cor Pulmonale"), followed by left ventricular dysfunction/failure.

31. Clinical features

AFE is a diagnosis of exclusion. It typically occurs during labor and delivery or in the immediate postpartum period, although it can occur as late as 48 hours postpartum. About 70% of cases occur before delivery (range, 63–76%). The symptoms are often sudden and protean. AFE is typified by maternal collapse associated with breathlessness, cyanosis, cardiac dysrhythymia, hypotension and then haemorrhage associated with DIC. Clark et al,

Adjusted odds ratio (95% confidence interval)		
Characteristics	Kramer et al (Canadian Cohort) (Kramer et al., 2006)	Abenhaim et al (American Cohort) (Abenhaim et al., 2008)
Maternal age 35 years	1.9 (1. -2.7)	2.2 (1.5-2.)
Cesarean delivery	12.5 (7.9 -19.9) - cephalic presentation 8.6 (4.3–17.4) – non-cephalic presentation	5.7 (3.7–8.7)
Forcep delivery	5.9 (3.4–10.3)	4.3 (1.9–6.6)
Vacuum delivery	2.9 (1.6–5.3)	1.9 (1 -3.7)
Abr ptio placen a	---	8.0 (4.0–15.9)
Placenta previa	----	30.4 (15.4–60.1)
Abruptio placenta or placenta previa	3.5 (2.3–5.5)	
Eclampsia	11.5 (2.8–46.9)	29.1 (7.1–119.3)
Fetal distress	1.7 (1.2–2.5)	1.5 (1.0–2.2)

Table 8. Risk factors associated with an increased risk of AFE in two large registries.

found the most common presenting signs and symptoms were hypotension and signs of non-reassuring fetal status (100%), pulmonary edema or respiratory symptoms (93%), cardiac arrest (87%), cyanosis (83%), and coagulopathy (83%). A majority develop seizures, encephalopathy and permanent neurological sequelae [85], due to cerebral ischemia and anoxia. The clinical course seems to have phases that are likely temporally related to pathophysiologic changes (Clark, 1990).

Induced abortion	(Grimes & Schulz, 1985; Guidotti et al., 1981; Lawson et al., 1990)
foeticide	(Edwards & Davies, 2000; Shojai et al., 2003)
Intrapartum amnioinfusion	(Dorairajan & Soundararaghavan, 2005; Maher et al., 1994)
Transabdominal amniocentesis	(Hasaart & Essed, 1983; Paterson et al., 1977)
Blunt abdominal trauma	(Judich et al., 1998; Olcott et al., 1973)
Surgical trauma	(Pluymakers et al., 2007)
Removal of cervical sutures	(Haines & Wilkes, 2003; Margan et al., 1984)
Manual removal of placenta	(Manchanda & Sriemevan, 2005)

Table 9. Procedures associated with AFE.

32. Diagnosis

The diagnosis of AFE is "clinical" and one of exclusion. AFE should be suspected if a woman experiences one or more of the following during late pregnancy or within 48 hours of delivery: acute or sudden onset of hypotension and/or cardiac arrest, hypoxemia, seizures or coma, DIC and in absence of potential alternative explanation for these manifestations (Table 2). Demonstration of fetal squamous cells in pulmonary arterial circulation is not pathognomonic. Presence of AF cells in BAL may be supportive. There are no specific laboratory tests for diagnosing AFE. Diagnostic markers for AFE have been developed which rely on detection of fetal or amniotic fluid constituents in maternal circulation, such as Serum Sialyl Tn Antigen, (Benson et al., 2001; Kobayashi et al., 1993; Oi et al., 1998) and plasma zinc coproporphyrin (a component of meconium) (Kanayama et al., 1992). Serum Tryptase, a marker of mast cell degranulation may be elevated but unreliable (Dorne et al., 2002; Farrar & Gherman, 2001; Marcus et al., 2005; Nishio et al., 2002).

33. Management

There is no specific treatment for AFE. The condition can be neither predicted nor prevented. The principles of management of AFE are mainly supportive, ie, to restore and maintain hemodynamic stability, to correct hypoxia and maintain adequate oxygenation, correction of coagulopathy with blood products as necessary and to deliver the fetus promptly at the earliest sign of maternal or fetal distress. Given sudden or hyperacute manner of presentation, prompt and aggressive response from the treating clinician is a must. As the diagnosis is not always clear from the onset of collapse, the role of diagnostic tests is to exclude conditions that can be treated specifically such as, Thrombotic PE which is more common compared to AFE. Hypoxia must be corrected promptly as significant proportions of survivors have residual neurological impairment due to cerebral anoxia (Moore & Baldisseri, 2005). Hypotension and shock should be aggressively treated with intravenous fluids, vasopressors and ionotropes as necessary. Since clinical manifestations are biphasic and complex, invasive hemodynamic monitoring is essential. Additional data from trans-thoracic or trans-esophageal echocardiography may be useful (James et al., 2004; Koegler et al., 1994; Stanten et al., 2003; van Haeften et al., 1989; Verroust et al., 2007). Administration of blood component is considered the first line treatment for coagulopathy associated with AFE. DIC is frequently associated with severe hemorrhage, so transfusion of packed red blood cells is a priority to maintain adequate tissue oxygenation. Uterine atony with DIC is a dangerous complication that might require immediate surgical intervention such as, hysterectomy.

As AFE occurred during labor in a predominant number of cases, immediate delivery of fetus by means of caesarian section is mandatory to prevent fetal hypoxic damage and to facilitate resuscitation (Davies & Harrison, 1992; Prasad & Howell, September 2001). Advanced cardiac life support (ACLS) protocol should be followed in case of cardiac arrest. The goal of drug therapy is to restore normal maternal hemodynamics in conjunction with the delivery of the fetus as soon as possible after the onset of asystole or malignant arrhythmia. During resuscitation, the uterus should be displaced to the left to avoid compression of the large vessels and improve venous return.

34. Prognosis

AFE accounts for approximately 10% of all maternal death within the USA (Atrash et al., 1990). Case fatality rate has declined significantly in recent years due to the prompt and aggressive resuscitation measures. (Abenhaim et al., 2008; Benson, 1993; Clark et al., 1995; Morgan, 1979). There is higher likelihood of survival if the women survive long enough to be transferred to intensive care unit. AFE still carries significant morbidity which includes neurological deficit in significant proportions of mothers as well as newborn. Neonatal survival is reported to be at 70%.

Either In the absence of any other clear cause Acute maternal collapse with one or more of the following features: • Acute fetal compromise • Cardiac arrhythmias or arrest • Coagulopathy • Convulsion • Hypotension • Maternal haemorrhage • Premonitory symptoms, e.g. restlessness, numbness, agitation, tingling • Shortness of breath Excluding women with maternal haemorrhage as the first presenting feature in whom there was no evidence of early coagulopathy or cardiorespiratory compromise ***Or*** Women in whom the diagnosis was made at post-mortem examination by finding fetal squames or hair in the lungs

Table 10. UK Obstetric Surveillance System (UKOSS) criteria for defining cases of AFE

35. Tumor embolism

Pulmonary tumor emboli are defined as clumps of malignant cells within the lumina of pulmonary arteries and arterioles (Kane et al., 1975). Microscopic pulmonary tumor emboli involve the small pulmonary arteries, arterioles and alveolar septal capillaries which are occluded by aggregates of tumor cells accompanied by platelet-fibrin thrombosis.
Types:

1. "Acute" tumor emboli - "massive" tumor emboli that can result in symptoms over "days"
2. "Sub-acute" tumor emboli - multiple small emboli resulting in "symptoms" over weeks to months

36. History and epidemiology

In 1897, Schmidt (M. B. Schmidt, 1903) first described pulmonary tumor embolization in a patient with gastric carcinoma. Autopsy showed the pulmonary bed was massively occluded by tumor emboli and pathology was similar to gastric tumor cells. It was not until 1937 that Brill and Robertson (Brill & Robertson, 1937) described the clinical syndrome of sub acute cor-pulmonale due to multiple tumor emboli to the pulmonary microvasculature. This syndrome is rare and exceedingly difficult to recognize before death. Since then pulmonary tumor embolism has been described in a variety of malignancies.
The estimated incidence of pulmonary tumor embolism is 3-26% among patients with solid tumors as reported by autopsy series (Bast et al., 2000; Kane et al., 1975; Shields & Edwards,

1992). Despite the relative prevalence at autopsy, the diagnosis is infrequently made ante mortem and thus the incidence of clinically significant tumor embolism is unclear (C. K. Chan et al., 1987). Retrospective chart reviews demonstrate that only 8% of patients with pathological evidence of tumor emboli have documented morbidity and mortality (Kane et al., 1975; Shields & Edwards, 1992).

37. Etiology

The risk appears to be greatest with mucin secreting adenocarcinomas of the breast, lung, stomach and colon. However, PTE has also been reported in hepatocellular, prostate, renal cell and choriocarcinomas. Other rare associations are listed below (K. E. Roberts et al., 2003).

Breast
Stomach
Lung
Liver
Prostate
Pancreas
Bone
Undifferentiated carcinoma
Ovary
Bladder
Cervix
Colorectal
Kidney
Mesothelioma
Wilms' tumor
Esophageal
Parotid
Melanoma
Myxoma
Thyroid
Trophoblastic
Vulva
Neurogenic sarcoma

Table 11. Primary Tumors associated with Tumor Embolism

38. Pathology

Histological studies of tumor emboli in humans and animals have provided some insights into the fate of pulmonary tumor emboli. Schimdt noted that tumor emboli are usually associated with intravascular platelet-fibrin rich thrombi. As a result, cancer cells become fewer and degenerative in appearance during the organization of these thrombi. The tumor emboli have no tendency to invade the arterial wall (Winterbauer et al., 1968). Necropsy studies and animal model studies suggest that tumor emboli are destroyed or remain latent and are not truly metastases. Soares et al (Soares et al., 1993) studied 222 consecutive autopsies of cancer cases and detected pulmonary hypertensive arteriopathy with proliferative endarteritis. Thus, PTE may be pathologically indistinguishable from other forms of pulmonary arterial hypertension, except for the notable absence of plexiform lesions. Some investigators describe tumor emboli as possessing an unusual level of resistance to recannulation (as compared to thromboembolism) and therefore likely lead to progressive and irreversible obstruction of the pulmonary vascular bed (Winterbauer et al., 1968).

Pathophysiology: Pulmonary vasculature provides the first capillary bed to the circulating tumor cells. The process of pulmonary metastasis consists of sequential steps that includes intravascular and/or lymphatic invasion of the lung by the neoplastic cells. Large scale autopsy studies suggest that tumor cells spread to the pulmonary vasculature in basically 4 ways (Kane et al., 1975; Winterbauer et al., 1968):

1. Large tumor emboli to the main pulmonary artery or large lobar branches producing the syndrome of acute pulmonary hypertension.
2. Microscopic tumor embolization involving small arteries and arterioles accounting for progressive dyspnea and subacute pulmonary hypertension.
3. Generalized lymphatic dissemination leading to pulmonary microvascular involvement (lymphatic carcinomatosis) causing diffuse interstitial infiltrates.
4. A combination of the above three mechanisms.

Clinical features: In most patients, primary malignancy was established when tumor emboli were noted. The signs and symptoms are non-specific. Patients with large proximal emboli have rapid onset of symptoms due to acute right heart failure indistinguishable from the presentation of a massive thromboembolism. Lymphangitic carcinomatosis and microvascular disease involving small pulmonary arteries, follow a more deliberate and progressive course resulting in subacute cor pulmonale.

Physical examination shows evidence of pulmonary hypertension and signs of right heart dysfunction. Common findings included: tachypnea, tachycardia, cyanosis, hypotension, elevated Jugular venous distension (JVD), audible pulmonic sound (P2), ascites and peripheral edema. Although considered "classic", signs of right heart failure are only reported in 15% to 20% of patients with this syndrome (Veinot et al., 1992).

Diagnosis: Ante-mortem diagnosis of pulmonary tumor embolism can be very difficult due to lack of distinctive features compared to thrombo-embolism which is more common. Diagnosis often made via tissue specimens from open lung biopsy or autopsy. Pulmonary arterial sampling (in a wedge position) has resulted in diagnosis in a few cases (Masson & Ruggieri, 1985; K. E. Roberts et al., 2003).

39. Management

Treatment of the pulmonary tumor embolism is directed at the primary tumor. Complete surgical resection of the primary tumor results in gradual resolution of the tumor emboli and reversal of the respiratory symptoms in patients with renal cell carcinoma, atrial myxoma and choriocarcinoma (C. K. Chan et al., 1987). The curative surgical resection in these cases may be due to early recognition or related to the less aggressive nature of the underlying malignancies. Embolectomy and IVC filter placement have been employed in the rare patients suffering from large, central pulmonary tumor emboli arising from infra-diaphramatic tumors. Chemotherapy generally does not affect the prognosis unless the primary tumor is very chemo-sensitive i.e. Wilm's tumor or trophoblastic tumors.

40. Pulmonary cement embolism

Pulmonary Cement Embolism (PCE) is a complication of Percutaneous Vertebroplasy (PVP) and Balloon Kyphoplasty which are minimally invasive procedures used to treat osteoporotic and other vertebral fractures (Galibert et al., 1987; Garfin et al., 2001;Gigante & Pierangeli, 2008; McDonald et al., 2008; Oner et al., 2006; Stoffel et al., 2007; Wu & Fourney, 2005). Polymethylmethacrylate (PMMA, "cement") leakage is a frequent occurrence during these procedures and the source of PCE (Gangi et al., 1999; Garfin et al., 2001; Hauck et al., 2005; Hodler et al., 2003; R. Schmidt et al., 2005; Vasconcelos et al., 2002; Yeom et al., 2003). The risk of pulmonary cement embolism (PCE) ranges from 3.5% to 23% for osteoporotic fractures (Anselmetti et al., 2005; Choe et al., 2004; Duran et al., 2007; Y. J. Kim et al., 2009). A recent report suggested a prevalence of 8.8% (Gill et al., 2010). Exact incidence is difficult to estimate as many are asymptomatic and escape detection. Patients with malignant lesions of the vertebrae might be at a higher risk of developing PCE due to damaged cortical substance and increased vascularity, while technical factors such as inappropriate viscosity of the cement at the time of injection, lack of visual guidance and higher cement volume injected during the procedure increase the risk of PCE (Baroud et al., 2006; Bohner et al., 2003; Choe et al., 2004; Deramond et al., 1998).The clinical spectrum following PMMA leakage is broad: asymptomatic extravasation into surrounding tissues, features of nerve root compression (Kelekis et al., 2003; Laredo & Hamze, 2005; Ratliff et al., 2001), asymptomatic and symptomatic pulmonary cement embolism (Anselmetti et al., 2005; Choe et al., 2004; Duran et al., 2007; Y. J. Kim et al., 2009), even cardiac perforation (S. Y. Kim et al., 2005; Lim et al., 2008; Schoenes et al., 2008; Son et al., 2008) and death (H. L. Chen et al., 2002; Monticelli et al., 2005; Stricker et al., 2004; Yoo et al., 2004) have been reported. Fat embolism occurring simultaneously with cement embolism may also contribute to the clinical picture (Aebli et al., 2002; Rauschmann et al., 2004). Clinically PCE cannot be distinguished from thrombotic pulmonary embolism (Bernhard et al., 2003; Jang et al., 2002; Padovani et al., 1999; Tozzi et al., 2002). Diagnosis is based on history and imaging which shows presence of radio-opaque densities (Figs 6 a&b). There is not enough evidence to underlay treatment guidelines. Since cement is regarded as "thrombogenic", (Francois et al., 2003; Perrin et al., 1999; Righini et al., 2006; Tozzi et al., 2002) anticoagulation for 6 months is recommended for symptomatic patients or patients with central PCE. Asymptomatic patients with peripheral PCE should have close clinical follow up with no anticoagulation. Surgical embolectomy may be considered for exceptional cases of central embolism. Routine chest roentogenogram should be obtained after PVP and BKP regardless of the symptoms as many patients are asymptomatic.

41. Gas embolism

Gas embolism (GE) is mainly ambient "air" embolism (AE) but also includes other gases such as carbon dioxide, nitrous oxide, nitrogen and helium. It is a rare and potentially fatal condition. There are 2 main types of GE, i.e, venous and arterial. They are distinguished by the mechanism of entry. Venous GE (VGE) occurs usually as a complication of iatrogenic procedures such as vascular catheter placement, mechanical ventilation and rarely surgical procedures (pulmonary lung biopsy, open heart surgeries, craniotomy). Arterial GE causes ischemia. As little as 0.5ml of air can result in coronary ischemia, cardiac arrhythmias, serious brain damage and even death.

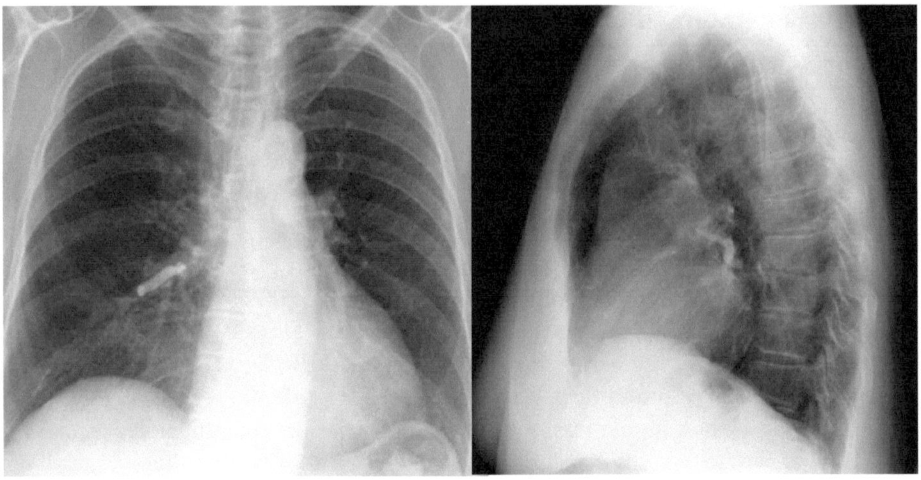

Fig. 6. a: Chest radiograph showing radio-opaque density in right main pulmonary artery

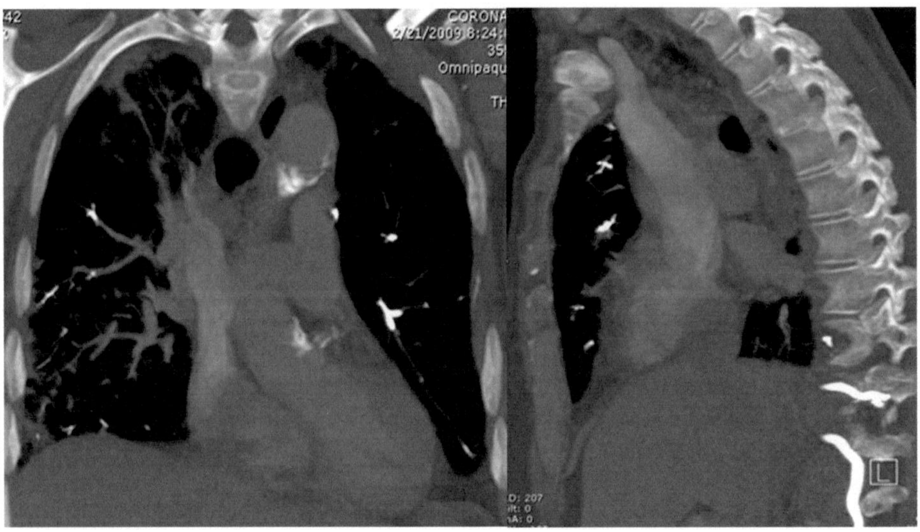

Fig. 6. b: CT Chest revealing bright intravascular densities in segmental and subsegmental pulmonary arteries

In venous GE, manifestations include cough, dyspnea, tachypnea and a hypoxemic "gasp" reflex when 10% or more of the pulmonary vessels are occluded (Souders, 2000; Sviri et al., 2004). Arterial embolization into the coronary arteries induces a specific drum-like or "mill-wheel" murmur along with electrocardiographic changes of ischemia (Rossi et al., 2000).

The key to controlling air embolism lies in prevention. First line of treatment includes administration of 100% oxygen, placing the patient in left lateral decubitus position to prevent right ventricular outflow obstruction by airlock. Hyperbaric Oxygen (HBO) may be used. 100% oxygen decreases the size of the gas bubbles by increasing the ambient pressure and by establishing a diffusion gradient that favors the elimination of gas from the bubbles and by increasing the gradient for the egress of nitrogen from the bubbles (Muth & Shank, 2000; Van Liew et al., 1993). Adjunctive treatment, includes fluid administration and prophylaxis against venous thromboembolism in paralyzed patients. Treatment is effective in most cases, although residual deficits can remain in serious cases.

42. Foreign body embolism

42.1 Silicone embolism

Silicone is thought to be an immunological inert substance and a component of many implantable medical devices. Silicone emboli (SIE) were first reported in trans-sexual males in 1970's and then later in young healthy women seeking low cost enhancements. Silicone implants are approved and widely used for breast augmentation, however liquid silicone used for aesthetic purposes cause significant morbidity when injected in the hips and buttocks, face, breasts, and vagina and is illegal in the US (Bartsich & Wu, 2010). Clinical features are similar to fat embolism with majority of patients meeting Schonfeld criteria (Schmid et al., 2005). The most common presentation is hypoxemia (92%) (Bartsich & Wu, 2010). Silicone embolic syndrome (SES) is a constellation of mainly pulmonary symptoms including dyspnea, fever, cough, hemoptysis, chest pain, hypoxia, alveolar hemorrhage, and altered consciousness presenting in patients shortly after silicone injection (within the first few hours) (Schmid et al., 2005). Later sequelae may occur within a few days and the possibility of delayed-onset pneumonitis or local inflammation at injection sites can occur up to years after administration (Chastre et al., 1987). Several factors have been implicated in leading to silicone emboli, including large volume injections, high-pressure infiltration, particle migration, and intravascular injection (Villa & Sparacio, 2000). It is thought that alveolar macrophages ingest silicone and fat to provoke an inflammatory response by increasing vascular permeability, activating endothelial cells, inducing the accumulation of activated neutrophils and modulating immunoregulatory responses in the lung. Imaging is usually suggestive of an embolic, congestive, pneumonitis or diffuse alveolar damage pattern. Treatment is supportive, consisting mainly of supplemental oxygen and steroid therapy.

43. Hyaluronic acid embolism

Hyaluronic acid (HA) is an approved dermal filler used for correction of facial wrinkles and folds (H. J. Park et al., 2010). All other uses are considered off label and illegal. HA associated pulmonary emboli (HAAPE) have been described in few case reports (Famularo et al., 2001; H.J. Park et al., 2010). Typical presentation of HAAPE is acute respiratory failure within hours after the HA injection in the anterior wall of the vagina, G-Spot amplification or for lip amplification by an unlicensed medical practitioner. Due to the extensive venous plexus, procedures involving injections in and around the injection site can cause NTPE. Although HA is thought to be non-immunogenic, it can cause localized granulomatous foreign body reactions with multinucleated giant cells around amorphous basophilic materials in the pulmonary vessels and lung parenchyma, as seen on video-assisted lung biopsy (Fernandez-Acenero et al., 2003; Honig et al., 2003; Raulin et al., 2000). Treatment is mainly supportive.

44. Others

Any material that is injected intravenously can potentially enter the pulmonary circulation leading to pulmonary embolism. Foreign materials such as talc, starch, cotton, and cellulose used as insoluble binding agents in oral tablets, are first pulverized, then dissolved in water and injected by intravenous drug users, and may be carried by the bloodstream until they lodge in the pulmonary capillary bed to cause NTPE (Farber et al., 1989; Ferrer et al., 2002; Low & Nicol, 2006; Pare et al., 1989).

The advent of modern percutaneous interventional procedures has led to a rise in catheter or fragment related pulmonary embolism. Catheter embolism usually takes place when the catheter is withdrawn from the introducing needle causing the distal portion of the catheter be sheared off (Propp et al., 1988). Spontaneous catheter breakage accounts for 25% of the catheter emboli. Retained catheter fragments have high rate of complications such as arrhythmias, perforations and thrombus formation (Fisher & Ferreyro, 1978; Richardson et al., 1974).

Prostate brachytherapy can also lead to embolization of radioactive seeds. On imaging the radioactive seeds appear as small (Iodine-125 measures 4.8 mm in length and 0.8 mm in diameter) metallic densities, usually detected incidentally. Clinical implications of these embolized radioactive seed implants remain unclear. Patients with arteriovenous malformations undergo therapeutic cerebral embolization with different materials such as cyano-acrylate agents, polyvinyl alcohol foam particles, micro-coils, silk or dacron thread and balloons. Cyano-acrylate has been reported to cause symptomatic pulmonary embolism (Kjellin et al., 2000; Pelz et al., 1995). Intravenous injection of elemental mercury is rare and has typically been reported in relation to psychiatric or suicidal incidents (Givica-Perez et al., 2001). Systemic embolization of mercury has been reported as well (Shareeff et al., 2000; Vas et al., 1980). On imaging, multiple metallic densities are seen. Mercury may remain in the body for a long time and metallic densities may remain visible for years after the injection (Ambre et al., 1977).

45. Conclusion

NTPE continues to pose a diagnostic challenge in clinical medicine despite much advancement in laboratory testing and imaging. Improved awareness along with techniques to allow for more accurate ante-mortem diagnosis may faciltitate early and prompt recognition of these syndromes which may in turn pave the way for better treatment modalities.

46. Acknowledgement

We wish thank Ms. Judy Kammerer (Librarian, UCSF Fresno) for her invaluable contribution in preparation of this chapter.

47. References

406th Medical General Laboratory, Professional Section. (1951). *Fat embolism: Annual publication, historical report,* Tokyo

Abenhaim, H. A., Azoulay, L., Kramer, M. S. & Leduc, L. (2008). Incidence and risk factors of amniotic fluid embolisms: A population-based study on 3 million births in the united states. *American Journal of Obstetrics and Gynecology,* Vol.199, No.1, pp. 49.e1-49.e8, 1097-6868; 0002-9378

Adams, C. B. (1971). The retinal manifestations of fat embolism. *Injury,* Vol.2, No.3, pp. 221-224, 0020-1383

Aebli, N., Krebs, J., Davis, G., Walton, M., Williams, M. J. & Theis, J. C. (2002). Fat embolism and acute hypotension during vertebroplasty: An experimental study in sheep. *Spine,* Vol.27, No.5, pp. 460-466, 1528-1159; 0362-2436

Aebli, N., Schwenke, D., Davis, G., Hii, T., Theis, J. C. & Krebs, J. (2005). Polymethylmethacrylate causes prolonged pulmonary hypertension during fat embolism: A study in sheep. *Acta Orthopaedica,* Vol.76, No.6, pp. 904-911, 1745-3674

Akhtar, S. (2009). Fat embolism. *Anesthesiology Clinics,* Vol.27, No.3, pp. 533-50, table of contents, 1932-2275

Alho, A., Saikku, K., Eerola, P., Koskinen, M. & Hamalainen, M. (1978). Corticosteroids in patients with a high risk of fat embolism syndrome. *Surgery, Gynecology & Obstetrics,* Vol.147, No.3, pp. 358-362, 0039-6087

Al-Khuwaitir, T. S., Al-Moghairi, A. M., Sherbeeni, S. M. & Subh, H. M. (2002). Traumatic fat embolism syndrome. *Saudi Medical Journal,* Vol.23, No.12, pp. 1532-1536, 0379-5284

Alston, J. M. (1955). Necrobacillosis in great britain. *British Medical Journal,* Vol.2, No.4955, pp. 1524-1528, 0007-1447

Ambre, J. J., Welsh, M. J. & Svare, C. W. (1977). Intravenous elemental mercury injection: Blood levels and excretion of mercury. *Annals of Internal Medicine,* Vol.87, No.4, pp. 451-453, 0003-4819

Anselmetti, G. C., Corgnier, A., Debernardi, F. & Regge, D. (2005). Treatment of painful compression vertebral fractures with vertebroplasty: Results and complications. *La Radiologia Medica,* Vol.110, No.3, pp. 262-272, 0033-8362

Aoki, N., Soma, K., Shindo, M., Kurosawa, T. & Ohwada, T. (1998). Evaluation of potential fat emboli during placement of intramedullary nails after orthopedic fractures. *Chest,* Vol.113, No.1, pp. 178-181, 0012-3692

Armstrong, A. W., Spooner, K. & Sanders, J. W. (2000). Lemierre's syndrome. *Current Infectious Disease Reports,* Vol.2, No.2, pp. 168-173, 1534-3146; 1523-3847

Atrash, H. K., Koonin, L. M., Lawson, H. W., Franks, A. L. & Smith, J. C. (1990). Maternal mortality in the united states, 1979-1986. *Obstetrics and Gynecology,* Vol.76, No.6, pp. 1055-1060, 0029-7844

Baddour, L. M., Wilson, W. R., Bayer, A. S., Fowler, V. G.,Jr, Bolger, A. F., Levison, M. E., . . . Infectious Diseases Society of America. (2005). Infective endocarditis: Diagnosis, antimicrobial therapy, and management of complications: A statement for healthcare professionals from the committee on rheumatic fever, endocarditis, and kawasaki disease, council on cardiovascular disease in the young, and the councils on clinical cardiology, stroke, and cardiovascular surgery and anesthesia, american heart association: Endorsed by the infectious diseases society of america. *Circulation,* Vol.111, No.23, pp. e394-434, 1524-4539; 0009-7322

Baker, A. B. (1976). The fat embolism syndrome, results of a therapeutic regime. *Anaesthesia and Intensive Care,* Vol.4, No.1, pp. 53-55, 0310-057X

Baker, P. L., Pazell, J. A. & Peltier, L. F. (1971). Free fatty acids, catecholamines, and arterial hypoxia in patients with fat embolism. *The Journal of Trauma,* Vol.11, No.12, pp. 1026-1030, 0022-5282

Barak, M., Kabha, M., Norman, D., Soudry, M., Kats, Y. & Milo, S. (2008). Cerebral microemboli during hip fracture fixation: A prospective study. *Anesthesia and Analgesia,* Vol.107, No.1, pp. 221-225, 1526-7598; 0003-2999

Baroud, G., Crookshank, M. & Bohner, M. (2006). High-viscosity cement significantly enhances uniformity of cement filling in vertebroplasty: An experimental model and study on cement leakage. *Spine,* Vol.31, No.22, pp. 2562-2568, 1528-1159; 0362-2436

Bartsich, S. & Wu, J. K. (2010). Silicon emboli syndrome: A sequela of clandestine liquid silicone injections. A case report and review of the literature. *Journal of Plastic, Reconstructive & Aesthetic Surgery : JPRAS,* Vol.63, No.1, pp. e1-3, 1878-0539; 1748-6815

Bast, R. C., Kufe, D. W., Pollock, R. E. & Weichselbaum, R. R. (2000). *Cancer medicine* (5th ed.), B.C. Decker, 9781550091137, Ontario

Bederman, S. S., Bhandari, M., McKee, M. D. & Schemitsch, E. H. (2009). Do corticosteroids reduce the risk of fat embolism syndrome in patients with long-bone fractures? A meta-analysis. *Canadian Journal of Surgery.Journal Canadien De Chirurgie,* Vol.52, No.5, pp. 386-393, 1488-2310; 0008-428X

Behrman, S. W., Fabian, T. C., Kudsk, K. A. & Taylor, J. C. (1990). Improved outcome with femur fractures: Early vs. delayed fixation. *The Journal of Trauma,* Vol.30, No.7, pp. 792-7; discussion 797-8, 0022-5282

Benson, M. D. (1993). Nonfatal amniotic fluid embolism. three possible cases and a new clinical definition. *Archives of Family Medicine,* Vol.2, No.9, pp. 989-994, 1063-3987

Benson, M. D., Kobayashi, H., Silver, R. K., Oi, H., Greenberger, P. A. & Terao, T. (2001). Immunologic studies in presumed amniotic fluid embolism. *Obstetrics and Gynecology,* Vol.97, No.4, pp. 510-514, 0029-7844

Bernard, G. R., Artigas, A., Brigham, K. L., Carlet, J., Falke, K., Hudson, L., Spragg, R. (1994). The american-european consensus conference on ARDS. definitions, mechanisms, relevant outcomes, and clinical trial coordination. *American Journal of Respiratory and Critical Care Medicine,* Vol.149, No.3 Pt 1, pp. 818-824, 1073-449X

Bernhard, J., Heini, P. F. & Villiger, P. M. (2003). Asymptomatic diffuse pulmonary embolism caused by acrylic cement: An unusual complication of percutaneous vertebroplasty. *Annals of the Rheumatic Diseases,* Vol.62, No.1, pp. 85-86, 0003-4967

Bohner, M., Gasser, B., Baroud, G. & Heini, P. (2003). Theoretical and experimental model to describe the injection of a polymethylmethacrylate cement into a porous structure. *Biomaterials,* Vol.24, No.16, pp. 2721-2730, 0142-9612

Bone, L. B., Johnson, K. D., Weigelt, J. & Scheinberg, R. (1989). Early versus delayed stabilization of femoral fractures. A prospective randomized study. *The Journal of Bone and Joint Surgery.American Volume,* Vol.71, No.3, pp. 336-340, 0021-9355

Brill, I. C. & Robertson, T. D. (1937). Subacute cor pulmonale. *Archives of Internal Medicine,* Vol.60, pp. 1043-1057, 0003-9926

Broder, G. & Ruzumna, L. (1967). Systemic fat embolism following acute primary osteomyelitis. *JAMA : The Journal of the American Medical Association,* Vol.199, No.13, pp. 150-152, 0098-7484

Brundage, S. I., McGhan, R., Jurkovich, G. J., Mack, C. D. & Maier, R. V. (2002). Timing of femur fracture fixation: Effect on outcome in patients with thoracic and head injuries. *The Journal of Trauma,* Vol.52, No.2, pp. 299-307, 0022-5282

Buchanan, D. & Mason, J. K. (1982). Occurrence of pulmonary fat and bone marrow embolism. *The American Journal of Forensic Medicine and Pathology,* Vol.3, No.1, pp. 73-78, 0195-7910

Bulger, E. M., Smith, D. G., Maier, R. V. & Jurkovich, G. J. (1997). Fat embolism syndrome. A 10-year review. *Archives of Surgery (Chicago, Ill.: 1960),* Vol.132, No.4, pp. 435-439, 0004-0010

Chan, C. K., Hutcheon, M. A., Hyland, R. H., Smith, G. J., Patterson, B. J. & Matthay, R. A. (1987). Pulmonary tumor embolism: A critical review of clinical, imaging, and hemodynamic features. *Journal of Thoracic Imaging,* Vol.2, No.4, pp. 4-14, 0883-5993

Chan, K. M., Tham, K. T., Chiu, H. S., Chow, Y. N. & Leung, P. C. (1984). Post-traumatic fat embolism--its clinical and subclinical presentations. *The Journal of Trauma,* Vol.24, No.1, pp. 45-49, 0022-5282

Chastre, J., Brun, P., Soler, P., Basset, F., Trouillet, J. L., Fagon, J. Y., . . . Hance, A. J. (1987). Acute and latent pneumonitis after subcutaneous injections of silicone in transsexual men. *The American Review of Respiratory Disease,* Vol.135, No.1, pp. 236-240, 0003-0805

Chastre, J., Fagon, J. Y., Soler, P., Fichelle, A., Dombret, M. C., Huten, D., . . . Gibert, C. (1990). Bronchoalveolar lavage for rapid diagnosis of the fat embolism syndrome in trauma patients. *Annals of Internal Medicine,* Vol.113, No.8, pp. 583-588, 0003-4819

Chen, H. L., Wong, C. S., Ho, S. T., Chang, F. L., Hsu, C. H. & Wu, C. T. (2002). A lethal pulmonary embolism during percutaneous vertebroplasty. *Anesthesia and Analgesia,* Vol.95, No.4, pp. 1060-2, table of contents, 0003-2999

Chen, J. J., Ha, J. C. & Mirvis, S. E. (2008). MR imaging of the brain in fat embolism syndrome. *Emergency Radiology,* Vol.15, No.3, pp. 187-192, 1070-3004

Choe, D. H., Marom, E. M., Ahrar, K., Truong, M. T. & Madewell, J. E. (2004). Pulmonary embolism of polymethyl methacrylate during percutaneous vertebroplasty and kyphoplasty. *AJR.American Journal of Roentgenology,* Vol.183, No.4, pp. 1097-1102, 0361-803X

Choi, J. A., Oh, Y. W., Kim, H. K., Kang, K. H., Choi, Y. H. & Kang, E. Y. (2002). Nontraumatic pulmonary fat embolism syndrome: Radiologic and pathologic correlations. *Journal of Thoracic Imaging,* Vol.17, No.2, pp. 167-169, 0883-5993

Clark, S. L. (1990). New concepts of amniotic fluid embolism: A review. *Obstetrical & Gynecological Survey,* Vol.45, No.6, pp. 360-368, 0029-7828

Clark, S. L., Hankins, G. D., Dudley, D. A., Dildy, G. A. & Porter, T. F. (1995). Amniotic fluid embolism: Analysis of the national registry. *American Journal of Obstetrics and Gynecology,* Vol.172, No.4 Pt 1, pp. 1158-67; discussion 1167-9, 0002-9378

Cook, R. J., Ashton, R. W., Aughenbaugh, G. L. & Ryu, J. H. (2005). Septic pulmonary embolism: Presenting features and clinical course of 14 patients. *Chest,* Vol.128, No.1, pp. 162-166, 0012-3692

Coronado-Malagon, M., Visoso-Palacios, P. & Arce-Salinas, C. A. (2010). Fat embolism syndrome secondary to injection of large amounts of soft tissue filler in the gluteal area. *Aesthetic Surgery Journal / the American Society for Aesthetic Plastic Surgery,* Vol.30, No.3, pp. 448-450, 1527-330X; 1090-820X

Cuppage, F. E. (1963). Fat embolism in diabetes mellitus. *American Journal of Clinical Pathology,* Vol.40, pp. 270-275, 0002-9173

Currie, I., Drutz, H. P., Deck, J. & Oxorn, D. (1997). Adipose tissue and lipid droplet embolism following periurethral injection of autologous fat: Case report and review of the literature. *International Urogynecology Journal and Pelvic Floor Dysfunction,* Vol.8, No.6, pp. 377-380,

Davies, M. G. & Harrison, J. C. (1992). Amniotic fluid embolism: Maternal mortality revisited. *British Journal of Hospital Medicine,* Vol.47, No.10, pp. 775-776, 0007-1064

de Falco, R., Scarano, E., Di Celmo, D., Grasso, U. & Guarnieri, L. (2005). Balloon kyphoplasty in traumatic fractures of the thoracolumbar junction. preliminary experience in 12 cases. *Journal of Neurosurgical Sciences,* Vol.49, No.4, pp. 147-153, 0390-5616

Dedhia, J. D. & Mushambi, M. C. (2007). Amniotic fluid embolism. *Continuing Education in Anaesthesia, Critical Care & Pain,* Vol.7, No.5, pp. 152-156, 1743-1816; 1743-1824

Deland, F. H. (1956). *Bone marrow embolism and associated fat embolism to the lungs.* Thesis, Graduate School, University of Minnesota).

Deramond, H., Depriester, C., Galibert, P. & Le Gars, D. (1998). Percutaneous vertebroplasty with polymethylmethacrylate. technique, indications, and results. *Radiologic Clinics of North America,* Vol.36, No.3, pp. 533-546, 0033-8389

Devriendt, J., Machayekhi, S. & Staroukine, M. (1995). Amniotic fluid embolism: Another case with non-cardiogenic pulmonary edema. *Intensive Care Medicine,* Vol.21, No.8, pp. 698-699, 0342-4642

Dines, D. E., Linscheid, R. L. & Didier, E. P. (1972). Fat embolism syndrome. *Mayo Clinic Proceedings.Mayo Clinic,* Vol.47, No.4, pp. 237-240, 0025-6196

Dodd, J. D., Souza, C. A. & Muller, N. L. (2006). High-resolution MDCT of pulmonary septic embolism: Evaluation of the feeding vessel sign. *AJR.American Journal of Roentgenology,* Vol.187, No.3, pp. 623-629, 1546-3141; 0361-803X

Dorairajan, G. & Soundararaghavan, S. (2005). Maternal death after intrapartum saline amnioinfusion--report of two cases. *BJOG : An International Journal of Obstetrics and Gynaecology,* Vol.112, No.9, pp. 1331-1333, 1470-0328

Dorne, R., Pommier, C., Emery, J. C., Dieudonne, F. & Bongiovanni, J. P. (2002). Amniotic fluid embolism: Successful evolution course after uterine arteries embolization. [Embolie de liquide amniotique: evolution favorable apres embolisation therapeutique des arteres uterines] *Annales Francaises d'Anesthesie Et De Reanimation,* Vol.21, No.5, pp. 431-435, 0750-7658

Duran, C., Sirvanci, M., Aydogan, M., Ozturk, E., Ozturk, C. & Akman, C. (2007). Pulmonary cement embolism: A complication of percutaneous vertebroplasty. *Acta Radiologica (Stockholm, Sweden : 1987),* Vol.48, No.8, pp. 854-859, 1600-0455; 0284-1851

Edwards, G. J. & Davies, N. J. (2000). Amniotic fluid embolus following feticide - a cautionary tale. *Journal of Obstetrics and Gynaecology : The Journal of the Institute of Obstetrics and Gynaecology,* Vol.20, No.2, pp. 191, 0144-3615

Eguia, P., Medina, A., Garcia-Monco, J. C., Martin, V. & Monton, F. I. (2007). The value of diffusion-weighted MRI in the diagnosis of cerebral fat embolism. *Journal of Neuroimaging : Official Journal of the American Society of Neuroimaging,* Vol.17, No.1, pp. 78-80, 1051-2284

Elliott, T. S., Foweraker, J., Gould, F. K., Perry, J. D., Sandoe, J. A. & Working Party of the British Society for Antimicrobial Chemotherapy. (2004). Guidelines for the antibiotic treatment of endocarditis in adults: Report of the working party of the british society for antimicrobial chemotherapy. *The Journal of Antimicrobial Chemotherapy,* Vol.54, No.6, pp. 971-981, 0305-7453

Fabian, T. C., Hoots, A. V., Stanford, D. S., Patterson, C. R. & Mangiante, E. C. (1990). Fat embolism syndrome: Prospective evaluation in 92 fracture patients. *Critical Care Medicine,* Vol.18, No.1, pp. 42-46, 0090-3493

Famularo, G., Liberati, C., Sebastiani, G. D. & Polchi, S. (2001). Pulmonary embolism after intra-articular injection of methylprednisolone and hyaluronate. *Clinical and Experimental Rheumatology,* Vol.19, No.3, pp. 355, 0392-856X

Farber, H. W., Fairman, R. P., Millan, J. E., Rounds, S. & Glauser, F. L. (1989). Pulmonary response to foreign body microemboli in dogs: Release of neutrophil chemoattractant activity by vascular endothelial cells. *American Journal of Respiratory Cell and Molecular Biology,* Vol.1, No.1, pp. 27-35, 1044-1549

Farrar, S. C. & Gherman, R. B. (2001). Serum tryptase analysis in a woman with amniotic fluid embolism. A case report. *The Journal of Reproductive Medicine,* Vol.46, No.10, pp. 926-928, 0024-7758

Fernandez-Acenero, M. J., Zamora, E. & Borbujo, J. (2003). Granulomatous foreign body reaction against hyaluronic acid: Report of a case after lip augmentation. *Dermatologic Surgery : Official Publication for American Society for Dermatologic Surgery [Et Al.],* Vol.29, No.12, pp. 1225-1226, 1076-0512

Ferrer, J., Montes, J. F., Villarino, M. A., Light, R. W. & Garcia-Valero, J. (2002). Influence of particle size on extrapleural talc dissemination after talc slurry pleurodesis. *Chest,* Vol.122, No.3, pp. 1018-1027, 0012-3692

Fisher, R. G. & Ferreyro, R. (1978). Evaluation of current techniques for nonsurgical removal of intravascular iatrogenic foreign bodies. *AJR.American Journal of Roentgenology,* Vol.130, No.3, pp. 541-548, 0361-803X

Forteza, A. M., Koch, S., Romano, J. G., Zych, G., Bustillo, I. C., Duncan, R. C. & Babikian, V. L. (1999). Transcranial doppler detection of fat emboli. *Stroke; a Journal of Cerebral Circulation,* Vol.30, No.12, pp. 2687-2691, 0039-2499

Francis, R. A., Barnes, P. A. & Libshitz, H. I. (1983). Pulmonary oil embolism after lymphangiography. *Journal of Computer Assisted Tomography,* Vol.7, No.1, pp. 170-171, 0363-8715

Francois, K., Taeymans, Y., Poffyn, B. & Van Nooten, G. (2003). Successful management of a large pulmonary cement embolus after percutaneous vertebroplasty: A case report. *Spine,* Vol.28, No.20, pp. E424-5, 1528-1159; 0362-2436

Galibert, P., Deramond, H., Rosat, P. & Le Gars, D. (1987). Preliminary note on the treatment of vertebral angioma by percutaneous acrylic vertebroplasty. [Note preliminaire sur le traitement des angiomes vertebraux par vertebroplastie acrylique percutanee] *Neuro-Chirurgie,* Vol.33, No.2, pp. 166-168, 0028-3770

Gangi, A., Dietemann, J. L., Guth, S., Steib, J. P. & Roy, C. (1999). Computed tomography (CT) and fluoroscopy-guided vertebroplasty: Results and complications in 187 patients. *Seminars in Interventional Radiology,* Vol.16, No.2, pp. 137-142, 0739-9529

Garfin, S. R., Yuan, H. A. & Reiley, M. A. (2001). New technologies in spine: Kyphoplasty and vertebroplasty for the treatment of painful osteoporotic compression fractures. *Spine,* Vol.26, No.14, pp. 1511-1515, 0362-2436

Gary, A. D. (2004). Amniotic fluid embolism. In L. C. Steven, A. B. Michael, G. R. Saabe & et al. (Eds.), *Text book of critical care obstetrics* (pp. 463-471) Blackwell.

Gauss, H. (1924). The pathology of fat embolism. *Archives of Surgery,* Vol.9, pp. 593-603, 0004-0010

Gigante, N. & Pierangeli, E. (2008). Minimally invasive anterior approach for kyphoplasty of the first thoracic vertebra in a patient with multiple myeloma. *Minimally Invasive Neurosurgery : MIN,* Vol.51, No.1, pp. 26-29, 0946-7211

Gill, N. S., Hamidjaja, L., Kandaswamy, C., Venugopal, C., Lesperance, R., & Balasubramanian, V. (2010). Incidence of cement pulmonary embolism after percutaneous vertebroplasty procedure [Abstract]. *American Journal of Respiratory Critical Care Medicine, 181* A1901.

Givica-Perez, A., Santana-Montesdeoca, J. M., Diaz-Sanchez, M., Martinez-Lagares, F. J. & Castaneda, W. R. (2001). Deliberate, repeated self-administration of metallic mercury injection: Case report and review of the literature. *European Radiology,* Vol.11, No.8, pp. 1351-1354, 0938-7994

Godeau, B., Schaeffer, A., Bachir, D., Fleury-Feith, J., Galacteros, F., Verra, F., Lebargy, F. (1996). Bronchoalveolar lavage in adult sickle cell patients with acute chest syndrome: Value for diagnostic assessment of fat embolism. *American Journal of Respiratory and Critical Care Medicine,* Vol.153, No.5, pp. 1691-1696, 1073-449X

Goldhaber, S. Z. (2004). Pulmonary embolism. *Lancet,* Vol.363, No.9417, pp. 1295-1305, 1474-547X; 0140-6736

Golpe, R., Marin, B. & Alonso, M. (1999). Lemierre's syndrome (necrobacillosis). *Postgraduate Medical Journal,* Vol.75, No.881, pp. 141-144, 0032-5473

Gossling, H. R. & Pellegrini, V. D.,Jr. (1982). Fat embolism syndrome: A review of the pathophysiology and physiological basis of treatment. *Clinical Orthopaedics and Related Research,* Vol.(165), No.165, pp. 68-82, 0009-921X

Gravante, G., Araco, A., Sorge, R., Araco, F., Nicoli, F., Caruso, R., . . . Cervelli, V. (2008). Pulmonary embolism after combined abdominoplasty and flank liposuction: A correlation with the amount of fat removed. *Annals of Plastic Surgery,* Vol.60, No.6, pp. 604-608, 1536-3708; 0148-7043

Grimes, D. A. & Cates, W.,Jr. (1977). Fatal amniotic fluid embolism during induced abortion, 1972-1975. *Southern Medical Journal,* Vol.70, No.11, pp. 1325-1326, 0038-4348

Grimes, D. A. & Schulz, K. F. (1985). Morbidity and mortality from second-trimester abortions. *The Journal of Reproductive Medicine,* Vol.30, No.7, pp. 505-514, 0024-7758

Guardia, S. N., Bilbao, J. M., Murray, D., Warren, R. E. & Sweet, J. (1989). Fat embolism in acute pancreatitis. *Archives of Pathology & Laboratory Medicine,* Vol.113, No.5, pp. 503-506, 0003-9985

Guidotti, R. J., Grimes, D. A. & Cates, W.,Jr. (1981). Fatal amniotic fluid embolism during legally induced abortion, united states, 1972 to 1978. *American Journal of Obstetrics and Gynecology,* Vol.141, No.3, pp. 257-261, 0002-9378

Guillevin, R., Vallee, J. N., Demeret, S., Sonneville, R., Bolgert, F., Mont'alverne, F., . . . Chiras, J. (2005). Cerebral fat embolism: Usefulness of magnetic resonance spectroscopy. *Annals of Neurology,* Vol.57, No.3, pp. 434-439, 0364-5134

Gurd, A. R. & Wilson, R. I. (1974). The fat embolism syndrome. *The Journal of Bone and Joint Surgery.British Volume,* Vol.56B, No.3, pp. 408-416, 0301-620X

Haber, L. M., Hawkins, E. P., Seilheimer, D. K. & Saleem, A. (1988). Fat overload syndrome. an autopsy study with evaluation of the coagulopathy. *American Journal of Clinical Pathology,* Vol.90, No.2, pp. 223-227, 0002-9173

Haines, J. & Wilkes, R. G. (2003). Non-fatal amniotic fluid embolism after cervical suture removal. *British Journal of Anaesthesia,* Vol.90, No.2, pp. 244-247, 0007-0912

Hamrick-Turner, J., Abbitt, P. L., Harrison, R. B. & Cranston, P. E. (1994). Diffuse lung calcifications following fat emboli and adult respiratory distress syndromes: CT findings. *Journal of Thoracic Imaging,* Vol.9, No.1, pp. 47-50, 0883-5993

Han, D., Lee, K. S., Franquet, T., Muller, N. L., Kim, T. S., Kim, H., . . . Byun, H. S. (2003). Thrombotic and nonthrombotic pulmonary arterial embolism: Spectrum of imaging findings. *Radiographics : A Review Publication of the Radiological Society of North America, Inc,* Vol.23, No.6, pp. 1521-1539, 1527-1323; 0271-5333

Hasaart, T. H. & Essed, G. G. (1983). Amniotic fluid embolism after transabdominal amniocentesis. *European Journal of Obstetrics, Gynecology, and Reproductive Biology,* Vol.16, No.1, pp. 25-30, 0301-2115

Hasan, M. Y., Kissoon, N., Khan, T. M., Saldajeno, V., Goldstein, J. & Murphy, S. P. (2001). Intraosseous infusion and pulmonary fat embolism. *Pediatric Critical Care Medicine : A Journal of the Society of Critical Care Medicine and the World Federation of Pediatric Intensive and Critical Care Societies,* Vol.2, No.2, pp. 133-138, 1529-7535

Hauck, S., Beisse, R. & Bu hren, V. (2005). Vertebroplasty and kyphoplasty in spinal trauma. *European Journal of Trauma,* Vol.31, pp. 453-463, 1439-0590; 1615-3146

Haymaker, W. & Davison, C. (1950). Fatalities resulting from exposure to simulated high altitudes in decompression chambers; a clinicopathologic study of five cases. *Journal of Neuropathology and Experimental Neurology,* Vol.9, No.1, pp. 29-59, illust, 0022-3069

Herndon, J. H. (1975). The syndrome of fat embolism. *Southern Medical Journal,* Vol.68, No.12, pp. 1577-1584, 0038-4348

Hodler, J., Peck, D. & Gilula, L. A. (2003). Midterm outcome after vertebroplasty: Predictive value of technical and patient-related factors. *Radiology,* Vol.227, No.3, pp. 662-668, 0033-8419

Honig, J. F., Brink, U. & Korabiowska, M. (2003). Severe granulomatous allergic tissue reaction after hyaluronic acid injection in the treatment of facial lines and its surgical correction. *The Journal of Craniofacial Surgery,* Vol.14, No.2, pp. 197-200, 1049-2275

Huang, R. M., Naidich, D. P., Lubat, E., Schinella, R., Garay, S. M. & McCauley, D. I. (1989). Septic pulmonary emboli: CT-radiographic correlation. *AJR.American Journal of Roentgenology,* Vol.153, No.1, pp. 41-45, 0361-803X

Hulman, G. (1988a). Fat macroglobule formation from chylomicrons and non-traumatic fat embolism. *Clinica Chimica Acta; International Journal of Clinical Chemistry,* Vol.177, No.2, pp. 173-178, 0009-8981

Hulman, G. (1988b). Pathogenesis of non-traumatic fat embolism. *Lancet,* Vol.1, No.8599, pp. 1366-1367, 0140-6736

Hutchinson, R. M., Merrick, M. V. & White, J. M. (1973). Fat embolism in sickle cell disease. *Journal of Clinical Pathology,* Vol.26, No.8, pp. 620-622, 0021-9746

Jackson, C. T. & Greendyke, R. M. (1965). Pulmonary and cerebral fat embolism after closed-chest cardiac massage. *Surgery, Gynecology & Obstetrics,* Vol.120, pp. 25-27, 0039-6087

Jacobson, D. M., Terrence, C. F. & Reinmuth, O. M. (1986). The neurologic manifestations of fat embolism. *Neurology,* Vol.36, No.6, pp. 847-851, 0028-3878

James, C. F., Feinglass, N. G., Menke, D. M., Grinton, S. F. & Papadimos, T. J. (2004). Massive amniotic fluid embolism: Diagnosis aided by emergency transesophageal echocardiography. *International Journal of Obstetric Anesthesia,* Vol.13, No.4, pp. 279-283, 0959-289X

Jang, J. S., Lee, S. H. & Jung, S. K. (2002). Pulmonary embolism of polymethylmethacrylate after percutaneous vertebroplasty: A report of three cases. *Spine,* Vol.27, No.19, pp. E416-8, 1528-1159; 0362-2436

Jenkins, K., Chung, F., Wennberg, R., Etchells, E. E. & Davey, R. (2002). Fat embolism syndrome and elective knee arthroplasty. *Canadian Journal of Anaesthesia = Journal Canadien d'Anesthesie,* Vol.49, No.1, pp. 19-24, 0832-610X

Johnson, M. J. & Lucas, G. L. (1996). Fat embolism syndrome. *Orthopedics,* Vol.19, No.1, pp. 41-8; discussion 48-9, 0147-7447

Jones, J. P.,Jr, Engleman, E. P. & Najarian, J. S. (1965). Systemic fat embolism after renal homotransplantation and treatment with corticosteroids. *The New England Journal of Medicine,* Vol.273, No.27, pp. 1453-1458, 0028-4793

Jorens, P. G., Van Marck, E., Snoeckx, A. & Parizel, P. M. (2009). Nonthrombotic pulmonary embolism. *The European Respiratory Journal : Official Journal of the European Society for Clinical Respiratory Physiology,* Vol.34, No.2, pp. 452-474, 1399-3003; 0903-1936

Judich, A., Kuriansky, J., Engelberg, I., Haik, J., Shabtai, M. & Czerniak, A. (1998). Amniotic fluid embolism following blunt abdominal trauma in pregnancy. *Injury,* Vol.29, No.6, pp. 475-477, 0020-1383

Kallenbach, J., Lewis, M., Zaltzman, M., Feldman, C., Orford, A. & Zwi, S. (1987). 'Low-dose' corticosteroid prophylaxis against fat embolism. *The Journal of Trauma,* Vol.27, No.10, pp. 1173-1176, 0022-5282

Kanayama, N., Yamazaki, T., Naruse, H., Sumimoto, K., Horiuchi, K. & Terao, T. (1992). Determining zinc coproporphyrin in maternal plasma--a new method for diagnosing amniotic fluid embolism. *Clinical Chemistry,* Vol.38, No.4, pp. 526-529, 0009-9147

Kane, R. D., Hawkins, H. K., Miller, J. A. & Noce, P. S. (1975). Microscopic pulmonary tumor emboli associated with dyspnea. *Cancer,* Vol.36, No.4, pp. 1473-1482, 0008-543X

Kearns, T. P. (1956). Fat embolism of the retina demonstrated by a flat retinal preparation. *American Journal of Ophthalmology,* Vol.41, No.1, pp. 1-2, 0002-9394

Kelekis, A. D., Martin, J. B., Somon, T., Wetzel, S. G., Dietrich, P. Y. & Ruefenacht, D. A. (2003). Radicular pain after vertebroplasty: Compression or irritation of the nerve root? initial experience with the "cooling system". *Spine,* Vol.28, No.14, pp. E265-9, 1528-1159; 0362-2436

Kim, S. Y., Seo, J. B., Do, K. H., Lee, J. S., Song, K. S. & Lim, T. H. (2005). Cardiac perforation caused by acrylic cement: A rare complication of percutaneous vertebroplasty. *AJR.American Journal of Roentgenology,* Vol.185, No.5, pp. 1245-1247, 0361-803X

Kim, Y. H., Oh, S. W. & Kim, J. S. (2002). Prevalence of fat embolism following bilateral simultaneous and unilateral total hip arthroplasty performed with or without cement : A prospective, randomized clinical study. *The Journal of Bone and Joint Surgery.American Volume,* Vol.84-A, No.8, pp. 1372-1379, 0021-9355

Kim, Y. J., Lee, J. W., Park, K. W., Yeom, J. S., Jeong, H. S., Park, J. M. & Kang, H. S. (2009). Pulmonary cement embolism after percutaneous vertebroplasty in osteoporotic vertebral compression fractures: Incidence, characteristics, and risk factors. *Radiology*, Vol.251, No.1, pp. 250-259, 1527-1315; 0033-8419

King, E. G., Weily, H. S., Genton, E. & Ashbaugh, D. G. (1971). Consumption coagulopathy in the canine oleic acid model of fat embolism. *Surgery*, Vol.69, No.4, pp. 533-541, 0039-6060

King, M. B. & Harmon, K. R. (1994). Unusual forms of pulmonary embolism. *Clinics in Chest Medicine*, Vol.15, No.3, pp. 561-580, 0272-5231

Kitchell, C. C. & Balogh, K. (1986). Pulmonary lipid emboli in association with long-term hyperalimentation. *Human Pathology*, Vol.17, No.1, pp. 83-85, 0046-8177

Kiyokawa, H., Utsumi, K., Minemura, K., Kasuga, I., Torii, Y., Yonemaru, M., . . . Toyama, K. (1995). Fat embolism syndrome caused by vegetable oil injection. *Internal Medicine (Tokyo, Japan)*, Vol.34, No.5, pp. 380-383, 0918-2918

Kjellin, I. B., Boechat, M. I., Vinuela, F., Westra, S. J. & Duckwiler, G. R. (2000). Pulmonary emboli following therapeutic embolization of cerebral arteriovenous malformations in children. *Pediatric Radiology*, Vol.30, No.4, pp. 279-283, 0301-0449

Knight, M., Tuffnell, D., Brocklehurst, P., Spark, P., Kurinczuk, J. J. & UK Obstetric Surveillance System. (2010). Incidence and risk factors for amniotic-fluid embolism. *Obstetrics and Gynecology*, Vol.115, No.5, pp. 910-917, 1873-233X; 0029-7844

Kobayashi, H., Ohi, H. & Terao, T. (1993). A simple, noninvasive, sensitive method for diagnosis of amniotic fluid embolism by monoclonal antibody TKH-2 that recognizes NeuAc alpha 2-6GalNAc. *American Journal of Obstetrics and Gynecology*, Vol.168, No.3 Pt 1, pp. 848-853, 0002-9378

Koegler, A., Sauder, P., Marolf, A. & Jaeger, A. (1994). Amniotic fluid embolism: A case with non-cardiogenic pulmonary edema. *Intensive Care Medicine*, Vol.20, No.1, pp. 45-46, 0342-4642

Koessler, M. J., Fabiani, R., Hamer, H. & Pitto, R. P. (2001). The clinical relevance of embolic events detected by transesophageal echocardiography during cemented total hip arthroplasty: A randomized clinical trial. *Anesthesia and Analgesia*, Vol.92, No.1, pp. 49-55, 0003-2999

Kramer, M. S., Rouleau, J., Baskett, T. F., Joseph, K. S. & Maternal Health Study Group of the Canadian Perinatal Surveillance System. (2006). Amniotic-fluid embolism and medical induction of labour: A retrospective, population-based cohort study. *Lancet*, Vol.368, No.9545, pp. 1444-1448, 1474-547X; 0140-6736

Krebs, J., Ferguson, S. J., Nuss, K., Leskosek, B., Hoerstrup, S. P., Goss, B. G., . . . Aebli, N. (2007). Plasma levels of endothelin-1 after a pulmonary embolism of bone marrow fat. *Acta Anaesthesiologica Scandinavica*, Vol.51, No.8, pp. 1107-1114, 0001-5172

Kropfl, A., Davies, J., Berger, U., Hertz, H. & Schlag, G. (1999). Intramedullary pressure and bone marrow fat extravasation in reamed and unreamed femoral nailing. *Journal of Orthopaedic Research : Official Publication of the Orthopaedic Research Society*, Vol.17, No.2, pp. 261-268, 0736-0266

Kwon, W. J., Jeong, Y. J., Kim, K. I., Lee, I. S., Jeon, U. B., Lee, S. H. & Kim, Y. D. (2007). Computed tomographic features of pulmonary septic emboli: Comparison of causative microorganisms. *Journal of Computer Assisted Tomography*, Vol.31, No.3, pp. 390-394, 0363-8715

Laforga, J. B. (1997). Amniotic fluid embolism. report of two cases with coagulation disorder. *Acta Obstetricia Et Gynecologica Scandinavica,* Vol.76, No.8, pp. 805-806, 0001-6349

Lang, C. T. & King, J. C. (2008). Maternal mortality in the united states. *Best Practice & Research.Clinical Obstetrics & Gynaecology,* Vol.22, No.3, pp. 517-531, 1521-6934

Laredo, J. D. & Hamze, B. (2005). Complications of percutaneous vertebroplasty and their prevention. *Seminars in Ultrasound, CT, and MR,* Vol.26, No.2, pp. 65-80, 0887-2171

Laub, D. R.,Jr & Laub, D. R. (1990). Fat embolism syndrome after liposuction: A case report and review of the literature. *Annals of Plastic Surgery,* Vol.25, No.1, pp. 48-52, 0148-7043

Lawson, H. W., Atrash, H. K. & Franks, A. L. (1990). Fatal pulmonary embolism during legal induced abortion in the united states from 1972 to 1985. *American Journal of Obstetrics and Gynecology,* Vol.162, No.4, pp. 986-990, 0002-9378

Lehman, E. P. & Moore, R. M. (1927). Fat embolism, including experimental production without trauma. *Archives of Surgery,* Vol.14, pp. 621, 0004-0010

Levy, D. (1990). The fat embolism syndrome. A review. *Clinical Orthopaedics and Related Research,* Vol.(261), No.261, pp. 281-286, 0009-921X

Lewis, G. (Ed.). (2007). *The confidential enquiry into maternal and child health (CEMACH). saving mothers' lives: Reviewing maternal deaths to make motherhood safer - 2003-2005. the seventh resport on confidential enquiries into maternal deaths in the united kingdom* CEMACH, London

Lim, S. H., Kim, H., Kim, H. K. & Baek, M. J. (2008). Multiple cardiac perforations and pulmonary embolism caused by cement leakage after percutaneous vertebroplasty. *European Journal of Cardio-Thoracic Surgery : Official Journal of the European Association for Cardio-Thoracic Surgery,* Vol.33, No.3, pp. 510-512, 1010-7940

Lindeque, B. G., Schoeman, H. S., Dommisse, G. F., Boeyens, M. C. & Vlok, A. L. (1987). Fat embolism and the fat embolism syndrome. A double-blind therapeutic study. *The Journal of Bone and Joint Surgery.British Volume,* Vol.69, No.1, pp. 128-131, 0301-620X

Lipton, J. H., Russell, J. A., Burgess, K. R. & Hwang, W. S. (1987). Fat embolization and pulmonary infiltrates after bone marrow transplantation. *Medical and Pediatric Oncology,* Vol.15, No.1, pp. 24-27, 0098-1532

Low, S. E. & Nicol, A. (2006). Talc induced pulmonary granulomatosis. *Journal of Clinical Pathology,* Vol.59, No.2, pp. 223, 0021-9746

Lozman, J., Deno, D. C., Feustel, P. J., Newell, J. C., Stratton, H. H., Sedransk, N., . . . Shah, D. M. (1986). Pulmonary and cardiovascular consequences of immediate fixation or conservative management of long-bone fractures. *Archives of Surgery (Chicago, Ill.: 1960),* Vol.121, No.9, pp. 992-999, 0004-0010

Lustig, L. R., Cusick, B. C., Cheung, S. W. & Lee, K. C. (1995). Lemierre's syndrome: Two cases of postanginal sepsis. *Otolaryngology--Head and Neck Surgery : Official Journal of American Academy of Otolaryngology-Head and Neck Surgery,* Vol.112, No.6, pp. 767-772, 0194-5998

Lynch, M. J. (1954). Nephrosis and fat embolism in acute hemorrhagic pancreatitis. *A.M.A.Archives of Internal Medicine,* Vol.94, No.5, pp. 709-717, 0888-2479

Macmahon, H. E. & Weiss, S. (1929). Carbon tetrachloride poisoning with macroscopic fat in the pulmonary artery. *The American Journal of Pathology,* Vol.5, No.6, pp. 623-630.3, 0002-9440

MacMillan, J. C., Milstein, S. H. & Samson, P. C. (1978). Clinical spectrum of septic pulmonary embolism and infarction. *The Journal of Thoracic and Cardiovascular Surgery,* Vol.75, No.5, pp. 670-679, 0022-5223

Maher, J. E., Wenstrom, K. D., Hauth, J. C. & Meis, P. J. (1994). Amniotic fluid embolism after saline amnioinfusion: Two cases and review of the literature. *Obstetrics and Gynecology,* Vol.83, No.5 Pt 2, pp. 851-854, 0029-7844

Manchanda, R. & Sriemevan, A. (2005). Anaphylactoid syndrome caused by amniotic fluid embolism following manual removal of placenta. *Journal of Obstetrics and Gynaecology : The Journal of the Institute of Obstetrics and Gynaecology,* Vol.25, No.2, pp. 201-202, 0144-3615

Marcus, B. J., Collins, K. A. & Harley, R. A. (2005). Ancillary studies in amniotic fluid embolism: A case report and review of the literature. *The American Journal of Forensic Medicine and Pathology,* Vol.26, No.1, pp. 92-95, 0195-7910

Margan, I., Urbancic, S., Voncina, D., Janezic, P., Mocivnik, M., Srebotnjak-Lipovec, D. & Stricevic, Z. (1984). Amniotic fluid embolism in multiple pregnancy in the second trimester of gestation. [Embolija amnijskom tekucinom kod viseplodne trudnoce u drugom tromjesecju gestacije] *Jugoslavenska Ginekologija i Opstetricija,* Vol.24, No.1-2, pp. 29-32, 0017-002X

Masson, R. G. & Ruggieri, J. (1985). Pulmonary microvascular cytology. A new diagnostic application of the pulmonary artery catheter. *Chest,* Vol.88, No.6, pp. 908-914, 0012-3692

Mays, E. T. (1970). The effect of surgical stress on plasma free fatty acids. *The Journal of Surgical Research,* Vol.10, No.7, pp. 315-319, 0022-4804

McCarthy, B., Mammen, E., Leblanc, L. P. & Wilson, R. F. (1973). Subclinical fat embolism: A prospective study of 50 patients with extremity fractures. *The Journal of Trauma,* Vol.13, No.1, pp. 9-16, 0022-5282

McDonald, R. J., Trout, A. T., Gray, L. A., Dispenzieri, A., Thielen, K. R. & Kallmes, D. F. (2008). Vertebroplasty in multiple myeloma: Outcomes in a large patient series. *AJNR.American Journal of Neuroradiology,* Vol.29, No.4, pp. 642-648, 1936-959X; 0195-6108

Meeke, R. I., Fitzpatrick, G. J. & Phelan, D. M. (1987). Cerebral oedema and the fat embolism syndrome. *Intensive Care Medicine,* Vol.13, No.4, pp. 291-292, 0342-4642

Mellor, A. & Soni, N. (2001). Fat embolism. *Anaesthesia,* Vol.56, No.2, pp. 145-154, 0003-2409

Metting, Z., Rodiger, L. A., Regtien, J. G. & van der Naalt, J. (2009). Delayed coma in head injury: Consider cerebral fat embolism. *Clinical Neurology and Neurosurgery,* Vol.111, No.7, pp. 597-600, 1872-6968; 0303-8467

Meyer, J. R. (1926). Embolia pulmonar amnio caseosa. *Brasil-Medico,* Vol.2, pp. 301-303, 0006-9205

Mimoz, O., Edouard, A., Beydon, L., Quillard, J., Verra, F., Fleury, J., . . . Samii, K. (1995). Contribution of bronchoalveolar lavage to the diagnosis of posttraumatic pulmonary fat embolism. *Intensive Care Medicine,* Vol.21, No.12, pp. 973-980, 0342-4642

Monticelli, F., Meyer, H. J. & Tutsch-Bauer, E. (2005). Fatal pulmonary cement embolism following percutaneous vertebroplasty (PVP). *Forensic Science International,* Vol.149, No.1, pp. 35-38, 0379-0738

Moore, J. & Baldisseri, M. R. (2005). Amniotic fluid embolism. *Critical Care Medicine,* Vol.33, No.10 Suppl, pp. S279-85, 0090-3493

Moreau, J. P. (1974). Fat embolism: A review and report of 100 cases. *Canadian Journal of Surgery.Journal Canadien De Chirurgie,* Vol.17, No.4, pp. 196-199, 0008-428X

Morgan, M. (1979). Amniotic fluid embolism. *Anaesthesia,* Vol.34, No.1, pp. 20-32, 0003-2409

Moylan, J. A., Birnbaum, M., Katz, A. & Everson, M. A. (1976). Fat emboli syndrome. *The Journal of Trauma,* Vol.16, No.5, pp. 341-347, 0022-5282

Murphy, P., Edelist, G., Byrick, R. J., Kay, J. C. & Mullen, J. B. (1997). Relationship of fat embolism to haemodynamic and echocardiographic changes during cemented arthroplasty. *Canadian Journal of Anaesthesia = Journal Canadien d'Anesthesie,* Vol.44, No.12, pp. 1293-1300, 0832-610X

Muth, C. M. & Shank, E. S. (2000). Gas embolism. *The New England Journal of Medicine,* Vol.342, No.7, pp. 476-482, 0028-4793

Nishio, H., Matsui, K., Miyazaki, T., Tamura, A., Iwata, M. & Suzuki, K. (2002). A fatal case of amniotic fluid embolism with elevation of serum mast cell tryptase. *Forensic Science International,* Vol.126, No.1, pp. 53-56, 0379-0738

Ober, W. B., Bruno, M. S., Simon, R. M. & Weiner, L. (1959). Hemoglobin S-C disease with fat embolism: Report of a patient dying in crisis: Autopsy findings. *The American Journal of Medicine,* Vol.27, pp. 647-658, 0002-9343

Oi, H., Kobayashi, H., Hirashima, Y., Yamazaki, T., Kobayashi, T. & Terao, T. (1998). Serological and immunohistochemical diagnosis of amniotic fluid embolism. *Seminars in Thrombosis and Hemostasis,* Vol.24, No.5, pp. 479-484, 0094-6176

Olcott, C.,4th, Robinson, A. J., Maxwell, T. M. & Griffin, H. A. (1973). Amniotic fluid embolism and disseminated intravascular coagulation after blunt abdominal trauma. *The Journal of Trauma,* Vol.13, No.8, pp. 737-740, 0022-5282

Oner, F. C., Verlaan, J. J., Verbout, A. J. & Dhert, W. J. (2006). Cement augmentation techniques in traumatic thoracolumbar spine fractures. *Spine,* Vol.31, No.11 Suppl, pp. S89-95; discussion S104, 1528-1159; 0362-2436

Padovani, B., Kasriel, O., Brunner, P. & Peretti-Viton, P. (1999). Pulmonary embolism caused by acrylic cement: A rare complication of percutaneous vertebroplasty. *AJNR.American Journal of Neuroradiology,* Vol.20, No.3, pp. 375-377, 0195-6108

Palmovic, V. & McCarroll, J. R. (1965). Fat embolism in trauma. *Archives of Pathology,* Vol.80, No.6, pp. 630-635, 0363-0153

Parisi, D. M., Koval, K. & Egol, K. (2002). Fat embolism syndrome. *American Journal of Orthopedics (Belle Mead, N.J.),* Vol.31, No.9, pp. 507-512, 1078-4519

Parizel, P. M., Demey, H. E., Veeckmans, G., Verstreken, F., Cras, P., Jorens, P. G. & De Schepper, A. M. (2001). Early diagnosis of cerebral fat embolism syndrome by diffusion-weighted MRI (starfield pattern). *Stroke; a Journal of Cerebral Circulation,* Vol.32, No.12, pp. 2942-2944, 1524-4628; 0039-2499

Pare, J. P., Cote, G. & Fraser, R. S. (1989). Long-term follow-up of drug abusers with intravenous talcosis. *The American Review of Respiratory Disease,* Vol.139, No.1, pp. 233-241, 0003-0805

Park, H. J., Jung, K. H., Kim, S. Y., Lee, J. H., Jeong, J. Y. & Kim, J. H. (2010). Hyaluronic acid pulmonary embolism: A critical consequence of an illegal cosmetic vaginal procedure. *Thorax,* Vol.65, No.4, pp. 360-361, 1468-3296; 0040-6376

Park, H. M., Ducret, R. P. & Brindley, D. C. (1986). Pulmonary imaging in fat embolism syndrome. *Clinical Nuclear Medicine,* Vol.11, No.7, pp. 521-522, 0363-9762

Parker, F. B.,Jr, Wax, S. D., Kusajima, K. & Webb, W. R. (1974). Hemodynamic and pathological findings in experimental fat embolism. *Archives of Surgery (Chicago, Ill.: 1960),* Vol.108, No.1, pp. 70-74, 0004-0010

Paterson, W. G., Grant, K. A., Grant, J. M. & McLean, N. (1977). The pathogenesis of amniotic fluid embolism with particular reference to transabdominal amniocentesis. *European Journal of Obstetrics, Gynecology, and Reproductive Biology,* Vol.7, No.5, pp. 319-324, 0301-2115

Patil, N. & Wakankar, H. (2008). Morbidity and mortality of simultaneous bilateral total knee arthroplasty. *Orthopedics,* Vol.31, No.8, pp. 780-9; quiz 790-1, 0147-7447

Peltier, L. F. (1965). The diagnosis of fat embolism. *Surgery, Gynecology & Obstetrics,* Vol.121, pp. 371-379, 0039-6087

Peltier, L. F. (1969). Fat embolism. A current concept. *Clinical Orthopaedics and Related Research,* Vol.66, pp. 241-253, 0009-921X

Peltier, L. F. (1984). Fat embolism. an appraisal of the problem. *Clinical Orthopaedics and Related Research,* Vol.(187), No.187, pp. 3-17, 0009-921X

Peltier, L. F. (1988). Fat embolism. A perspective. *Clinical Orthopaedics and Related Research,* Vol.(232), No.232, pp. 263-270, 0009-921X

Peltier, L. F., Collins, J. A., Evarts, C. M. & Sevitt, S. (1974). A panel by correspondence. fat embolism. *Archives of Surgery (Chicago, Ill.: 1960),* Vol.109, No.1, pp. 12-16, 0004-0010

Pelz, D. M., Lownie, S. P., Fox, A. J. & Hutton, L. C. (1995). Symptomatic pulmonary complications from liquid acrylate embolization of brain arteriovenous malformations. *AJNR.American Journal of Neuroradiology,* Vol.16, No.1, pp. 19-26, 0195-6108

Perrin, C., Jullien, V., Padovani, B. & Blaive, B. (1999). Percutaneous vertebroplasty complicated by pulmonary embolus of acrylic cement. [Une vertebroplastie percutanee compliquee d'une embolie pulmonaire de ciment acrylique] *Revue Des Maladies Respiratoires,* Vol.16, No.2, pp. 215-217, 0761-8425

Pitto, R. P., Hamer, H., Fabiani, R., Radespiel-Troeger, M. & Koessler, M. (2002). Prophylaxis against fat and bone-marrow embolism during total hip arthroplasty reduces the incidence of postoperative deep-vein thrombosis: A controlled, randomized clinical trial. *The Journal of Bone and Joint Surgery.American Volume,* Vol.84-A, No.1, pp. 39-48, 0021-9355

Pitto, R. P., Koessler, M. & Kuehle, J. W. (1999). Comparison of fixation of the femoral component without cement and fixation with use of a bone-vacuum cementing technique for the prevention of fat embolism during total hip arthroplasty. A prospective, randomized clinical trial. *The Journal of Bone and Joint Surgery.American Volume,* Vol.81, No.6, pp. 831-843, 0021-9355

Pitto, R. P., Schramm, M., Hohmann, D. & Kossler, M. (1999). Relevance of the drainage along the linea aspera for the reduction of fat embolism during cemented total hip arthroplasty. A prospective, randomized clinical trial. *Archives of Orthopaedic and Trauma Surgery,* Vol.119, No.3-4, pp. 146-150, 0936-8051

Platt, M. S., Kohler, L. J., Ruiz, R., Cohle, S. D. & Ravichandran, P. (2002). Deaths associated with liposuction: Case reports and review of the literature. *Journal of Forensic Sciences,* Vol.47, No.1, pp. 205-207, 0022-1198

Pluymakers, C., De Weerdt, A., Jacquemyn, Y., Colpaert, C., Van de Poel, E. & Jorens, P. G. (2007). Amniotic fluid embolism after surgical trauma: Two case reports and review of the literature. *Resuscitation,* Vol.72, No.2, pp. 324-332, 0300-9572

Prasad, B. G. R. & Howell, C. (September 2001). Cardiac arrest and cardiopulmonary resuscitation in pregnancy. In *MOET provider manual* (pp. 14:2-6)

Propp, D. A., Cline, D. & Hennenfent, B. R. (1988). Catheter embolism. *The Journal of Emergency Medicine,* Vol.6, No.1, pp. 17-21, 0736-4679

Pruszczyk, P., Torbicki, A., Pacho, R., Chlebus, M., Kuch-Wocial, A., Pruszynski, B. & Gurba, H. (1997). Noninvasive diagnosis of suspected severe pulmonary embolism: Transesophageal echocardiography vs spiral CT. *Chest,* Vol.112, No.3, pp. 722-728, 0012-3692

Rabah, R., Evans, R. W. & Yunis, E. J. (1987). Mineral oil embolization and lipid pneumonia in an infant treated for hirschsprung's disease. *Pediatric Pathology / Affiliated with the International Paediatric Pathology Association,* Vol.7, No.4, pp. 447-455, 0277-0938

Ratliff, J., Nguyen, T. & Heiss, J. (2001). Root and spinal cord compression from methylmethacrylate vertebroplasty. *Spine,* Vol.26, No.13, pp. E300-2, 0362-2436

Raulin, C., Greve, B., Hartschuh, W. & Soegding, K. (2000). Exudative granulomatous reaction to hyaluronic acid (hylaform). *Contact Dermatitis,* Vol.43, No.3, pp. 178-179, 0105-1873

Rauschmann, M. A., von Stechow, D., Thomann, K. D. & Scale, D. (2004). Complications of vertebroplasty. [Komplikationen in der Vertebroplastie] *Der Orthopade,* Vol.33, No.1, pp. 40-47, 0085-4530

Rayburg, M., Kalinyak, K. A., Towbin, A. J., Baker, P. B. & Joiner, C. H. (2010). Fatal bone marrow embolism in a child with hemoglobin SE disease. *American Journal of Hematology,* Vol.85, No.3, pp. 182-184, 1096-8652; 0361-8609

Richards, R. R. (1997). Fat embolism syndrome. *Canadian Journal of Surgery.Journal Canadien De Chirurgie,* Vol.40, No.5, pp. 334-339, 0008-428X

Richardson, J. D., Grover, F. L. & Trinkle, J. K. (1974). Intravenous catheter emboli. experience with twenty cases and collective review. *American Journal of Surgery,* Vol.128, No.6, pp. 722-727, 0002-9610

Righini, M., Sekoranja, L., Le Gal, G., Favre, I., Bounameaux, H. & Janssens, J. P. (2006). Pulmonary cement embolism after vertebroplasty. *Thrombosis and Haemostasis,* Vol.95, No.2, pp. 388-389, 0340-6245

Riordan, T. & Wilson, M. (2004). Lemierre's syndrome: More than a historical curiosa. *Postgraduate Medical Journal,* Vol.80, No.944, pp. 328-334, 0032-5473

Riska, E. B. & Myllynen, P. (1982). Fat embolism in patients with multiple injuries. *The Journal of Trauma,* Vol.22, No.11, pp. 891-894, 0022-5282

Riska, E. B., von Bonsdorff, H., Hakkinen, S., Jaroma, H., Kiviluoto, O. & Paavilainen, T. (1976). Prevention of fat embolism by early internal fixation of fractures in patients with multiple injuries. *Injury,* Vol.8, No.2, pp. 110-116, 0020-1383

Ritter, M., Mamlin, L. A., Melfi, C. A., Katz, B. P., Freund, D. A. & Arthur, D. S. (1997). Outcome implications for the timing of bilateral total knee arthroplasties. *Clinical*

Orthopaedics and Related Research, Vol.(345), No.345, pp. 99-105, 0009-921X
Robert, J. H., Hoffmeyer, P., Broquet, P. E., Cerutti, P. & Vasey, H. (1993). Fat embolism syndrome. *Orthopaedic Review,* Vol.22, No.5, pp. 567-571, 0094-6591
Roberts, C. L., Algert, C. S., Knight, M. & Morris, J. M. (2010). Amniotic fluid embolism in an australian population-based cohort. *BJOG : An International Journal of Obstetrics and Gynaecology,* Vol.117, No.11, pp. 1417-1421, 1471-0528; 1470-0328
Roberts, K. E., Hamele-Bena, D., Saqi, A., Stein, C. A. & Cole, R. P. (2003). Pulmonary tumor embolism: A review of the literature. *The American Journal of Medicine,* Vol.115, No.3, pp. 228-232, 0002-9343
Ross, A. P. (1970). The fat embolism syndrome: With special reference to the importance of hypoxia in the syndrome. *Annals of the Royal College of Surgeons of England,* Vol.46, No.3, pp. 159-171, 0035-8843
Ross, R. M. & Johnson, G. W. (1988). Fat embolism after liposuction. *Chest,* Vol.93, No.6, pp. 1294-1295, 0012-3692; 0012-3692
Rossi, S. E., Goodman, P. C. & Franquet, T. (2000). Nonthrombotic pulmonary emboli. *AJR.American Journal of Roentgenology,* Vol.174, No.6, pp. 1499-1508, 0361-803X
Sakuma, M., Sugimura, K., Nakamura, M., Takahashi, T., Kitamukai, O., Yazu, T., . . . Shirato, K. (2007). Unusual pulmonary embolism: Septic pulmonary embolism and amniotic fluid embolism. *Circulation Journal : Official Journal of the Japanese Circulation Society,* Vol.71, No.5, pp. 772-775, 1346-9843
Saldeen, T. (1970). Fat embolism and signs of intravascular coagulation in a posttraumatic autopsy material. *The Journal of Trauma,* Vol.10, No.4, pp. 273-286, 0022-5282
Sasano, N., Ishida, S., Tetsu, S., Takasu, H., Ishikawa, K., Sasano, H. & Katsuya, H. (2004). Cerebral fat embolism diagnosed by magnetic resonance imaging at one, eight, and 50 days after hip arthroplasty: A case report. *Canadian Journal of Anaesthesia = Journal Canadien d'Anesthesie,* Vol.51, No.9, pp. 875-879, 0832-610X
Satoh, H., Kurisu, K., Ohtani, M., Arita, K., Okabayashi, S., Nakahara, T., . . . Ohbayashi, N. (1997). Cerebral fat embolism studied by magnetic resonance imaging, transcranial doppler sonography, and single photon emission computed tomography: Case report. *The Journal of Trauma,* Vol.43, No.2, pp. 345-348, 0022-5282
Schmid, A., Tzur, A., Leshko, L. & Krieger, B. P. (2005). Silicone embolism syndrome: A case report, review of the literature, and comparison with fat embolism syndrome. *Chest,* Vol.127, No.6, pp. 2276-2281, 0012-3692
Schmidt, M. B. (1903). *Die verbreitungswege der karzinome und die beziehung generalisierter sarcome zu den leukaemischen neubildungen* G. Fischer, Vienna
Schmidt, R., Cakir, B., Mattes, T., Wegener, M., Puhl, W. & Richter, M. (2005). Cement leakage during vertebroplasty: An underestimated problem? *European Spine Journal : Official Publication of the European Spine Society, the European Spinal Deformity Society, and the European Section of the Cervical Spine Research Society,* Vol.14, No.5, pp. 466-473, 0940-6719
Schnaid, E., Lamprey, J. M., Viljoen, M. J., Joffe, B. I. & Seftel, H. C. (1987). The early biochemical and hormonal profile of patients with long bone fractures at risk of fat embolism syndrome. *The Journal of Trauma,* Vol.27, No.3, pp. 309-311, 0022-5282

Schoenes, B., Bremerich, D. H., Risteski, P. S., Thalhammer, A. & Meininger, D. (2008). Cardiac perforation after vertebroplasty. [Palacos im Herzen] *Der Anaesthesist,* Vol.57, No.2, pp. 147-150, 0003-2417

Schonfeld, S. A., Ploysongsang, Y., DiLisio, R., Crissman, J. D., Miller, E., Hammerschmidt, D. E. & Jacob, H. S. (1983). Fat embolism prophylaxis with corticosteroids. A prospective study in high-risk patients. *Annals of Internal Medicine,* Vol.99, No.4, pp. 438-443, 0003-4819

Schulz, F., Trubner, K. & Hildebrand, E. (1996). Fatal fat embolism in acute hepatic necrosis with associated fatty liver. *The American Journal of Forensic Medicine and Pathology,* Vol.17, No.3, pp. 264-268, 0195-7910

Sevitt, S. (1962). Pathophysiology of systemic embolism-- the brain. In S. Sevitt (Ed.), *Fat embolism* (pp. 143). London, UK: Butterworth.

Shareeff, M., Bhat, Y. M., Adabala, R. & Raoof, S. (2000). Shortness of breath after suicide attempt. *Chest,* Vol.118, No.3, pp. 837-838, 0012-3692

Shields, D. J. & Edwards, W. D. (1992). Pulmonary hypertension attributable to neoplastic emboli: An autopsy study of 20 cases and a review of the literature. *Cardiovascular Pathology,* Vol.1, pp. 279-287, 1054-8807

Shier, M. R. & Wilson, R. F. (1980). Fat embolism syndrome: Traumatic coagulopathy with respiratory distress. *Surgery Annual,* Vol.12, pp. 139-168, 0081-9638

Shier, M. R., Wilson, R. F., James, R. E., Riddle, J., Mammen, E. F. & Pedersen, H. E. (1977). Fat embolism prophylaxis: A study of four treatment modalities. *The Journal of Trauma,* Vol.17, No.8, pp. 621-629, 0022-5282

Shojai, R., Chau, C., Boubli, L. & D'Ercole, C. (2003). Amniotic fluid embolism during late term termination of pregnancy. *Prenatal Diagnosis,* Vol.23, No.11, pp. 950-951, 0197-3851

Sinave, C. P., Hardy, G. J. & Fardy, P. W. (1989). The lemierre syndrome: Suppurative thrombophlebitis of the internal jugular vein secondary to oropharyngeal infection. *Medicine,* Vol.68, No.2, pp. 85-94, 0025-7974

Soares, F. A., Pinto, A. P., Landell, G. A. & de Oliveira, J. A. (1993). Pulmonary tumor embolism to arterial vessels and carcinomatous lymphangitis. A comparative clinicopathological study. *Archives of Pathology & Laboratory Medicine,* Vol.117, No.8, pp. 827-831, 0003-9985

Son, K. H., Chung, J. H., Sun, K. & Son, H. S. (2008). Cardiac perforation and tricuspid regurgitation as a complication of percutaneous vertebroplasty. *European Journal of Cardio-Thoracic Surgery : Official Journal of the European Association for Cardio-Thoracic Surgery,* Vol.33, No.3, pp. 508-509, 1010-7940

Souders, J. E. (2000). Pulmonary air embolism. *Journal of Clinical Monitoring and Computing,* Vol.16, No.5-6, pp. 375-383, 1387-1307

Stanten, R. D., Iverson, L. I., Daugharty, T. M., Lovett, S. M., Terry, C. & Blumenstock, E. (2003). Amniotic fluid embolism causing catastrophic pulmonary vasoconstriction: Diagnosis by transesophageal echocardiogram and treatment by cardiopulmonary bypass. *Obstetrics and Gynecology,* Vol.102, No.3, pp. 496-498, 0029-7844

Stein, P. D., Yaekoub, A. Y., Matta, F. & Kleerekoper, M. (2008). Fat embolism syndrome. *The American Journal of the Medical Sciences,* Vol.336, No.6, pp. 472-477, 0002-9629

Steiner, P. E. & Lushbaugh, C. C. (1941). Maternal pulmolnary embolism by amniotic fluid as a cause of obstetric shock and unexpected deaths in obstetrics. *Journal of the American Medical Association,* Vol.117, pp. 1245-1254, 1341-1345, 0002-9955

Stoeger, A., Daniaux, M., Felber, S., Stockhammer, G., Aichner, F. & zur Nedden, D. (1998). MRI findings in cerebral fat embolism. *European Radiology,* Vol.8, No.9, pp. 1590-1593, 0938-7994

Stoffel, M., Wolf, I., Ringel, F., Stuer, C., Urbach, H. & Meyer, B. (2007). Treatment of painful osteoporotic compression and burst fractures using kyphoplasty: A prospective observational design. *Journal of Neurosurgery.Spine,* Vol.6, No.4, pp. 313-319, 1547-5654; 1547-5646

Stoltenberg, J. J. & Gustilo, R. B. (1979). The use of methylprednisolone and hypertonic glucose in the prophylaxis of fat embolism syndrome. *Clinical Orthopaedics and Related Research,* Vol.(143), No.143, pp. 211-221, 0009-921X

Stricker, K., Orler, R., Yen, K., Takala, J. & Luginbuhl, M. (2004). Severe hypercapnia due to pulmonary embolism of polymethylmethacrylate during vertebroplasty. *Anesthesia and Analgesia,* Vol.98, No.4, pp. 1184-6, table of contents, 0003-2999

Svenningsen, S., Nesse, O., Finsen, V., Hole, A. & Benum, P. (1987). Prevention of fat embolism syndrome in patients with femoral fractures--immediate or delayed operative fixation? *Annales Chirurgiae Et Gynaecologiae,* Vol.76, No.3, pp. 163-166, 0355-9521

Sviri, S., Woods, W. P. & van Heerden, P. V. (2004). Air embolism--a case series and review. *Critical Care and Resuscitation : Journal of the Australasian Academy of Critical Care Medicine,* Vol.6, No.4, pp. 271-276, 1441-2772

Szabo, G., Magyar, Z. & Reffy, A. (1977). The role of free fatty acids in pulmonary fat embolism. *Injury,* Vol.8, No.4, pp. 278-283, 0020-1383

Tachakra, S. C., Potts, D. & Idowu, A. (1990). Early operative fracture management of patients with multiple injuries. *The British Journal of Surgery,* Vol.77, No.10, pp. 1194, 0007-1323

Talbot, M. & Schemitsch, E. H. (2006). Fat embolism syndrome: History, definition, epidemiology. *Injury,* Vol.37 Suppl 4, pp. S3-7, 0020-1383

Talucci, R. C., Manning, J., Lampard, S., Bach, A. & Carrico, C. J. (1983). Early intramedullary nailing of femoral shaft fractures: A cause of fat embolism syndrome. *American Journal of Surgery,* Vol.146, No.1, pp. 107-111, 0002-9610

Tapson, V. F. (2008). Acute pulmonary embolism. *The New England Journal of Medicine,* Vol.358, No.10, pp. 1037-1052, 1533-4406; 0028-4793

Taviloglu, K. & Yanar, H. (2007). Fat embolism syndrome. *Surgery Today,* Vol.37, No.1, pp. 5-8, 0941-1291

ten Duis, H. J. (1997). The fat embolism syndrome. *Injury,* Vol.28, No.2, pp. 77-85, 0020-1383

ten Duis, H. J., Nijsten, M. W., Klasen, H. J. & Binnendijk, B. (1988). Fat embolism in patients with an isolated fracture of the femoral shaft. *The Journal of Trauma,* Vol.28, No.3, pp. 383-390, 0022-5282

Thomas, J. E. & Ayyar, D. R. (1972). Systemic fat embolism. A diagnostic profile in 24 patients. *Archives of Neurology,* Vol.26, No.6, pp. 517-523, 0003-9942

Tolentino, L. F., Tsai, S. F., Witt, M. D. & French, S. W. (2004). Fatal fat embolism following amphotericin B lipid complex injection. *Experimental and Molecular Pathology,* Vol.77, No.3, pp. 246-248, 0014-4800

Tozzi, P., Abdelmoumene, Y., Corno, A. F., Gersbach, P. A., Hoogewoud, H. M. & von Segesser, L. K. (2002). Management of pulmonary embolism during acrylic vertebroplasty. *The Annals of Thoracic Surgery,* Vol.74, No.5, pp. 1706-1708, 0003-4975

Tuffnell, D. J. (2005). United kingdom amniotic fluid embolism register. *BJOG : An International Journal of Obstetrics and Gynaecology,* Vol.112, No.12, pp. 1625-1629, 1470-0328

van Haeften, T. W., Strack van Schijndel, R. J. & Thijs, L. G. (1989). Severe lung damage after amniotic fluid embolism; a case with haemodynamic measurements. *The Netherlands Journal of Medicine,* Vol.35, No.5-6, pp. 317-320, 0300-2977

Van Liew, H. D., Conkin, J. & Burkard, M. E. (1993). The oxygen window and decompression bubbles: Estimates and significance. *Aviation, Space, and Environmental Medicine,* Vol.64, No.9 Pt 1, pp. 859-865, 0095-6562

Vas, W., Tuttle, R. J. & Zylak, C. J. (1980). Intravenous self-administration of metallic mercury. *Radiology,* Vol.137, No.2, pp. 313-315, 0033-8419

Vasconcelos, C., Gailloud, P., Beauchamp, N. J., Heck, D. V. & Murphy, K. J. (2002). Is percutaneous vertebroplasty without pretreatment venography safe? evaluation of 205 consecutives procedures. *AJNR.American Journal of Neuroradiology,* Vol.23, No.6, pp. 913-917, 0195-6108

Veinot, J. P., Ford, S. E. & Price, R. G. (1992). Subacute cor pulmonale due to tumor embolization. *Archives of Pathology & Laboratory Medicine,* Vol.116, No.2, pp. 131-134, 0003-9985

Verroust, N., Zegdi, R., Ciobotaru, V., Tsatsaris, V., Goffinet, F., Fabiani, J. N. & Mignon, A. (2007). Ventricular fibrillation during termination of pregnancy. *Lancet,* Vol.369, No.9576, pp. 1900, 1474-547X; 0140-6736

Vichinsky, E. P., Neumayr, L. D., Earles, A. N., Williams, R., Lennette, E. T., Dean, D., . . . Manci, E. A. (2000). Causes and outcomes of the acute chest syndrome in sickle cell disease. national acute chest syndrome study group. *The New England Journal of Medicine,* Vol.342, No.25, pp. 1855-1865, 0028-4793

Villa, A. & Sparacio, F. (2000). Severe pulmonary complications after silicone fluid injection. *The American Journal of Emergency Medicine,* Vol.18, No.3, pp. 336-337, 0735-6757

Wagner, E. (1865). Die fettembolie der lungen capillaren. *Arch Heilkunde,* Vol.6, pp. 146-147, 369-381, 481-491,

Weinhouse, G. L. (January 2011). Fat embolism syndrome. *UpToDate,*

Weisz, G. M. (1974). Fat embolism. *Current Problems in Surgery,* pp. 1-54, 0011-3840

Winterbauer, R. H., Elfenbein, I. B. & Ball, W. C.,Jr. (1968). Incidence and clinical significance of tumor embolization to the lungs. *The American Journal of Medicine,* Vol.45, No.2, pp. 271-290, 0002-9343

Wu, A. S. & Fourney, D. R. (2005). Supportive care aspects of vertebroplasty in patients with cancer. *Supportive Cancer Therapy,* Vol.2, No.2, pp. 98-104, 1543-2912

Yeom, J. S., Kim, W. J., Choy, W. S., Lee, C. K., Chang, B. S. & Kang, J. W. (2003). Leakage of cement in percutaneous transpedicular vertebroplasty for painful osteoporotic compression fractures. *The Journal of Bone and Joint Surgery.British Volume,* Vol.85, No.1, pp. 83-89, 0301-620X

Yoo, K. Y., Jeong, S. W., Yoon, W. & Lee, J. (2004). Acute respiratory distress syndrome associated with pulmonary cement embolism following percutaneous vertebroplasty with polymethylmethacrylate. *Spine,* Vol.29, No.14, pp. E294-7, 1528-1159; 0362-2436

6

Pathophysiology, Diagnosis and Treatment of Pulmonary Embolism Focusing on Thrombolysis – New approaches

Diana Mühl, Gábor Woth, Tamás Kiss,
Subhamay Ghosh and Jose E. Tanus-Santos
[1]*Department of Anaesthesia and Intensive Care, University of Pécs, Pécs*
[2]*Department of Pharmacology, Faculty of Medicine of Ribeirao Preto*
University of Sao Paulo, Ribeirao Preto, SP
[1]*Hungary*
[2]*Brazil*

1. Introduction

1.1 Incidence and mortality of pulmonary embolism

Pulmonary embolism (PE) is not a disease by itself but may have a venous thrombotic source and is therefore more precise if classified as venous thromboembolism (VTE). According to the international registry, the frequency of VTE is 150-200 new cases diagnosed per 100,000 inhabitants per year. Out of this, one third is diagnosed as primary PE (Oger, 2000; Walther et al., 2009). Following the diagnosis the average mortality is 11% in the first two months (Goldhaber et al., 1999). In the ICOPER study, the total mortality of PE in the first 3 months was 17.5%. However, in the long run the recurrent embolic episodes and lack of revascularisation caused progressive pulmonary hypertension (Goldhaber et al., 1999). The mortality of untreated PE is 30% and with adequate treatment can be reduced to 2-8% (Goldhaber, 1998). The hospital mortality of haemodynamically stable PE patients is overall 10% in general, 4% in the first 24 hours (Kline et al., 2003). Mortality of PE with respiratory and cardiovascular failure on hospital admission can be up to 95%. Hospital mortality is 80% in patients requiring mechanical ventilation and 77% in those who need cardiopulmonary resuscitation in the first 24 hours (Janata et al., 2002). Only 29% of fatal PE cases (verified at hospital autopsies) were previously diagnosed clinically. Based on these facts, the primary goal in PE management is a rapid and clear diagnosis followed by the appropriate treatment (S. Büchner & Th. Hachenberg, 2005).

1.2 Etiology

The source of PE in majority of cases can be due to the postoperative state, trauma injury, long term immobilization causing deep vein thrombosis (DVT), or congenital/acquired coagulation defect (Goldhaber & Morrison, 2002; Schürmann et al., 1992; Spöhr et al., 2005; Tapson, 2008). There are congenitally predisposed and non-influenced factors in the aetiology of VTE. Most important ones are: old age, family predisposition, genetic defects –

activated protein C resistance (Dahlbäck, 1995), 20210A mutation of factor II (Poort et al., 1996), hyperhomocysteinaemia (den Heijer et al., 1996), antithrombin III, protein C and protein S deficiency (Demers et al., 1992).
Aetiology can be divided into two groups:
a/ Congenital risk factors: Lack of anti-thrombin III (0.2%), lack of protein C (0.8%), lack of protein S (1.3%), Leiden point-mutation of factor V (3.0%), mutation of prothrombin G20210 A (2.3%) (Ageno et al., 2006).
b/ Acquired risk factors: DVT, phlebitis, immobilization, bed rest, post-traumatic and operative state, sepsis, diabetes, smoking, hypovolaemia, diuretic treatment, elevated plasma/blood viscosity, coagulation disorders (disseminated intravascular coagulation, heparin induced thrombocytopenia (HIT), drug induced coagulopathy (anticoncipient, oestrogen), obesity, sedentary lifestyle, pregnancy, postnatal state, cardiac insufficiency, heart valve disorders, artificial valves, central venous catheter, pacemaker electrode, tumour, old age, nephrosis syndrome (Goldhaber et al., 1997).

1.3 Pathophysiology

Based on the occlusion of the pulmonary vasculature we can differentiate between mild: <25%, intermediate: 25-50% and severe: >50% PE types. The pathophysiology of PE runs on two parallel pathways:

- *haemodynamic alterations*: The oxygen demand and workload on the right atrium increases with the afterload, while cardiac index decreases (even with normal arterial blood pressure and tachycardia) leading to systemic hypotension. The right intraatrial pressure increases and the pressure gradient between the right atrium and the aorta drops, pushing the intraventricular septa into the cavity of the left ventricle (LV) (D-sign). A severe shock with global cardiac ischemia can develop.
- *hypoxaemia*: Ventilation/perfusion (V/Q) disequilibrium rises. Areas with hypoperfusion have an increased V/Q, while it decreases on hypoventilated (atelectasis) or normally perfused regions. Low LV cardiac output results from shunt-perfusion and hypoxaemia (Nowak et al., 2007). Platelet released vasoactive substances cause vaso- and bronchospasm in the affected regions (Stratmann & Gregory, 2003; Wood, 2002; Konstantinides, 2005). Surfactant production impairs in the early phase of pulmonary hypertension. Due to shunt-perfusion, global arterial hypoxaemia develops with a decrease of arterial oxygen saturation (Konstantinides & Hasenfuss, 2004).

1.3.1 Risk stratification

Based on the haemodynamic symptoms,PE can be either *massive*, characterised by systolic blood pressure lower than 90 mmHg or a systolic blood pressure decrease > 40 mmHg, or *non-massive* which includes *submassive* severity characterised by increased right ventricular pressure (Torbicki et al., 2000).
The most recent PE guideline changed the definitions of various risk groups, according: high risk and non-high risk categories.
High risk definition: Shock and/or hypotension (systolic blood pressure <90 mmHg or a drop in blood pressure greater than 40 mmHg within 15 min. excluding other causes of shock (e.g. arrhythmia, hypovolaemia, sepsis etc.).
All others can be listed under *non-high risk* PE. Based on right ventricular (RV) pressure overload and myocardial injury, we can differentiate a subgroup, the *intermediate risk* PE patients without shock.

<table>
<tr><th colspan="2">Mortality risk</th><th colspan="4">Risk markers</th></tr>
<tr><th colspan="2"></th><th>shock/hypo tension</th><th>RV dysfunction</th><th>Myocardial injury</th><th>Potential treatment</th></tr>
<tr><td colspan="2">High>15%</td><td>+</td><td>(+)</td><td>(+)</td><td>Thrombolysis or embolectomy</td></tr>
<tr><td rowspan="4">Non high</td><td rowspan="3">Inter medi-ate 3-15%</td><td rowspan="3">-</td><td>+</td><td>+</td><td rowspan="3">Hospital admission</td></tr>
<tr><td>+</td><td>-</td></tr>
<tr><td>-</td><td>-</td></tr>
<tr><td>Low <1%</td><td>-</td><td>-</td><td>-</td><td>Early discharge or home treatment</td></tr>
</table>

(+) Presence of shock/hypotension it is not necessery confirm RV dysfunction

Table 1. Risk stratification according to the ESC 2008 guidelines.

The prognosis of the increased RV pressure (intermediate risk) group is worse than the normal RV pressure group (Torbicki et al., 2008).

The clinical probability of pulmonary embolism in outpatients (Wells et al., 2001)	**Score**
Clinical signs	
Deep vein thrombosis (DVT)	+3.0
Pulmonary embolism (PE) suspected from other signs or symptoms	+3.0
Hearth rate >100 / min	+1.5
Operation, immobilization, bed rest in the last 4 weeks	+1.5
Former DVT or PE	+1.5
Hemoptysis	+1.0
Malignancy (active or confirmed in the last 6 months)	+1.0
Probability of PE	
Small	< 2.0
Medium	2.0-6.0
High	> 6.0

Table 2. Clinical probability score

1.4 Pulmonary embolism diagnostic strategy

Acute PE, in the presence of shock/hypotension, RV dysfunction and myocardial injury causes high mortality risk. Rapid and clear diagnosis and appropriate therapy may help to improve survival of this critical condition.

1.4.1 Physical signs of PE

In the presence of typical physical signs (dyspnoea, chest pain, syncope, tachypnea, tachycardia, cough, hemoptysis, signs of DVT, cyanosis, etc.) the diagnosis of PE is 90% reliable, although the severity of symptoms do not correlate with the actual illness. About 10% of high-risk cases are recognised by radiology imaging and considered to be non-high risk according to physical symptoms.
Physical signs and symptoms: severe stabbing chest pain (52%), tachycardia (26%), cough (20%), cyanosis (15%) or paleness, increased perspiration, fever (38.5%), dyspnoea (with acute onset 80%), tachpnea (70%), hemoptysis (11%), mortal fear, syncope (19%), low blood pressure, haemodynamic failure with large vessel obstruction, arrhythmia (atrial or ventricular extrasystole, acute atrial fibrillation, flutter, etc.) (Miniati, Prediletto, Formichi, Marini, Di Ricco, Tonelli, Allescia & Pistolesi, 1999a; Stein & Henry, 1997).

1.4.2 Chest X-ray

According to the PISAPED study, occlusion of the hilar artery, oligaemia, wedge shaped infiltration against the pleural wall is detectable in 15-45% of all cases (Miniati, Prediletto, Formichi, Marini, Di Ricco, Tonelli, Allescia & Pistolesi, 1999b). In acute PE the typical X-ray signs can be weak or absent, but a single-sided elevation of the diaphragm, stripe-like atelectasis and the oedema of the affected pulmonary tissue (Westermark-sign) may develop with the prominence of the pulmonary artery. Occasionally unilateral pleural effusion is present. Chest X-ray is useful to exclude certain diagnoses.

1.4.3 Electrocardiography (ECG)

The most common alterations are: sinus tachycardia, $S_1Q_3T_3$ waveform (McGinn-White syndrome), acute P-pulmonale, negative T waves in V_{1-3} leads, incomplete or complete right bundle branch block, signs of RV strain, acute atrial fibrillation, atrio-ventricular conduction failures. Enlarged $S_IS_{II}S_{III}$ waveform develops after the dilatation of the right cavities causing the rotation of the cardiac axis. ECG signs are positive only in 50% of all patients (Torbicki et al., 2000; Torbicki et al., 2008; Geibel et al., 2005; Rodger, Makropoulos, et al., 2000).

1.4.4 Perfusion scintigraphy

Multiple studies have confirmed the benefit of perfusion scintigraphy as a non-invasive diagnostic procedure. It is necessary to combine perfusion scintigraphy with additional radiology imaging, like ventilation scintigraphy or chest X-ray. Various studies have confirmed that ventilation-perfusion scintigraphy has a positive predictive value of 88% (The PIOPED Investigators, 1990; Lee et al., 2005). The PISAPED study divided the probability of PE into 3 groups based on chest X-ray and perfusion scintigraphy results (Miniati et al., 1996). The sensitivity of perfusion scintigraphy is 92% with a positive predictive value of 92%. It has a negative predictive value of 88% with the specificity of 87%. Chronic pulmonary diseases caused perfusion defects may produce PE characteristic false results. To sum up, scintigraphy can help to exclude PE (error rate: 0.9%, confidence interval: 2.3%) (Kruip et al., 2003).

1.4.5 Angiography

According to the most recent PE guideline, the use of angiography is questionable as an invasive and hazardous intervention with mortality rate of 0.2%. The use of angiography is recommended in case of uncertain radiological imaging results. Non-invasive CT angiography offers comparable or better sensitivity (Wan et al., 2004; Agnelli et al., 2002).

1.4.6 Computed tomography, Multidetector Computed Tomography (MDCT)

The MDCT is a non-invasive approach, replacing angiography without the need of central venous access. It has a sensitivity of 83% and specificity of 96%. The negative predictive value of MDCT for PE is 89% in the intermediate and 96% in the low clinical risk groups. The cost-benefit and cost-life ratio increases significantly with the combination of MDCT and D-dimer assessment (Perrier et al., 2004; van Belle et al., 2006). With MDCT imaging one can visualise pulmonary vasculature up to the segmental level. An MDCT result showing a PE up to the segmental level could be taken as firm evidence (Eyer et al., 2005; Brunot et al., 2005; Righini et al., 2008; Ghaye et al., 2001; Perrier et al., 2004).

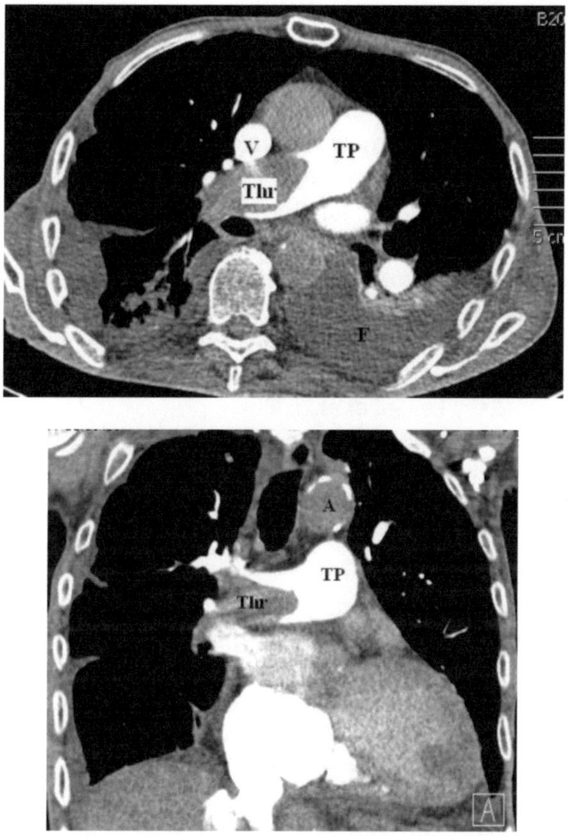

Fig. 1. Computed tomography image of acute pulmonary embolism.
(From authors own collection. A: aorta, TP: pulmonary trunk, F: thoracic effusion, Thr: clot)

1.4.7 Echocardiography

Transthoracic echocardiography

Echocardiography is a useful bedside non-invasive procedure in the differential diagnosis of various conditions (acute myocardial infarction, aortic dissection, pericardial tamponade, chest pain, valve dysfunction, hypovolaemia). The sensitivity of echocardiography is about 60-70% in PE. Negative results do not exclude PE. Acute massive PE has characteristic echocardiography signs: RV hypokinesis and/or dilatation, the end diastolic diameter of the RV in the parasternal short axis > 30 mm, or RV/LV end diastolic diameter ratio > 0.9, in the apical or subcostal axis, D-sign, increased pulmonary arterial pressure, dilatation of the inferior caval vein. A heart cavity thrombus, patent foramen ovale (with the risk of paradox thrombi), tricuspidal valve thrombosis or vegetation and floating clot in the right ventricle can also be visualised.

The positive echocardiographic result has a predictive value in haemodynamically stable patient, as the intermediate risk group has worse outcome (Konstantinides, 2008; Torbicki et al., 2003; Ferrari et al., 2005; Hsiao et al., 2006; Casazza et al., 2005; Bova et al., 2003; Miniati et al., 2001; Roy et al., 2005; Konstantinides et al., 1998).

Transoesophageal echocardiography

The transoesophageal echocardiography is a semi-invasive diagnostic procedure, which can be useful in mechanically ventilated patients. Benefits of the transoesophageal approach are: visualisation of thrombi in the pulmonary trunk and/or main pulmonary arteries and also in the caval vein. Possible tumours originating from the heart or floating into the cavities of the heart can also be visualised (Sanchez et al., 2008).

1.4.8 The diagnosis of DVT

With duplex ultrasound the clot is visible as a hyperechogenic signal. The procedure has 95-98% specificity. The sensitivity for PE is rather low, only 30-50% of PE cases present DVT with ultrasonography (Lee et al., 2005). The only validated verification method is the incomplete compressibility of the vein indicating the presence of the clot (Goldhaber & Morrison, 2002; Lee et al., 2005; Le Gal et al., 2006).

Although extremity CT can also aid the diagnosis of DVT, the increased irradiation, need of contrast agent and elevated costs contraindicate the use of CT scan in all cases (Brenner & Hall, 2007).

1.4.9 Laboratory diagnostics

Arterial blood gas analysis: Hypocapnia with hypoxaemia is characteristic for PE. About 20% of patients have a normal arterial oxygen tension and normal alveolar-arterial oxygen gradient (Rodger, Carrier, et al., 2000; Stein et al., 1996).

D-dimer is a fibrin degradation product. Quantitative ELISA or ELISA-like methods are 99% sensitive, if D-dimer concentration is above 500 μg/l. According to Dunn et al. the sensitivity for PE is 96.4%, with a negative predictive value of 99.6%, specificity 52.0% and positive predictive value 9.5%. Although the measurement is specific for fibrin, but the specificity of fibrin for VTE is considerably lower, the summarized specificity is only 40-65%. The D-dimer test can be positive in the following diseases: infections, tumours, necrosis, pregnancy, postnatal, postoperative state, sepsis, etc., therefore, it cannot be used generally. In emergency situations, the D-dimer test is useful to exclude PE from differential diagnosis. Segal recommended the inclusion of D-dimer into the Geneva and Wells score systems (Dunn et al., 2002; Segal, Eng, et al., 2007; Spannagl et al., 2005; Reber et al., 2004; van Belle et al., 2006).

Cardiac troponin T and B-type natriuretic peptide (BNP): Increased cardiac troponin and BNP levels are good indicators of impaired RV function. About 11-50% of PE patients show increased marker levels. Echocardiography results correlate showing a decreased RV function. Negative troponin results are good predictors of favourable outcome. Both markers are useful and independent predictors of the 30 days mortality. Impaired RV function with increased troponin and BNP are relative indications of thrombolysis (TL) therapy in the intermediate risk group (Giannitsis et al., 2000; Kostrubiec et al., 2005; Krüger et al., 2004; ten Wolde et al., 2004; Worth, 2009). The recommended therapeutic approach according to Kucher and Goldhaber based on these data (Kucher & Goldhaber, 2003):

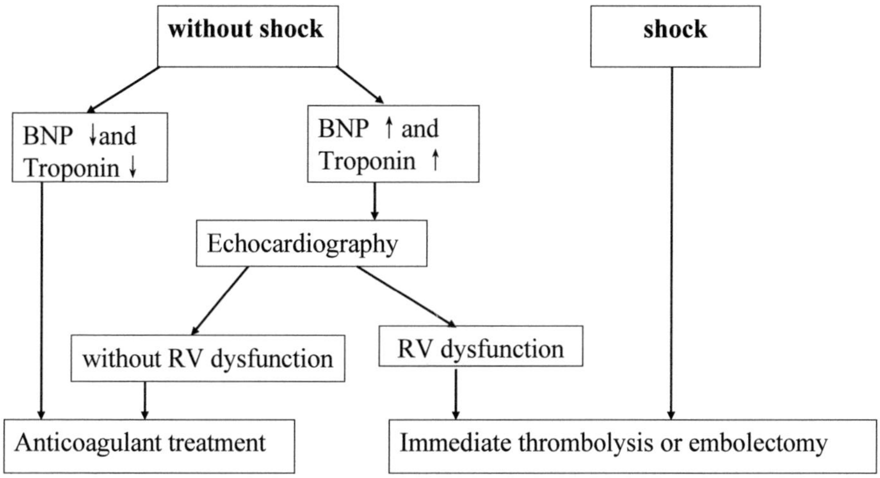

Fig. 2. Kucher and Goldhaber recommendation for the treatment of pulmonary embolism based on biomarkers and echocardiography.

Cases with severe haemodynamic shock present elevated lactate and metabolic acidosis due to global microcirculatory impairment and tissue hypoxaemia. These markers can predict poor outcome.

According to the recent guidelines, the diagnosis of PE is mainly based on the results of echocardiography, MDCT and biomarkers (Torbicki et al., 2008).

1.5 Therapy

1.5.1 Acute therapy

For main therapeutic recommendations, we follow the ESC 2008 guidelines (Torbicki et al., 2008). Anticoagulation therapy should be initiated upon suspicion of PE. 5000 IU Na-heparin is recommended as intravenous bolus if the patient had not already received Low Molecular Weight Heparin (LMWH) previously. Besides providing secure venous access, patients should receive immediate oxygen therapy through a 50% or 100% face mask. The indication of oxygen therapy is absolute, but mechanical ventilation should be used with caution. Mechanical ventilation may decrease the venous reflow and increases RV insufficiency, therefore, low tidal volume (7 ml/kg) ventilation and intravenous fluid therapy is recommended. The alveolar-arterial gas exchange can also be impaired as shunt-flow and cardiac output decrease (Singer, M; Webb, 2004; Sevransky et al., 2004). Capnometry is highly recommended during mechanical ventilation, as it may change due to thrombolysis

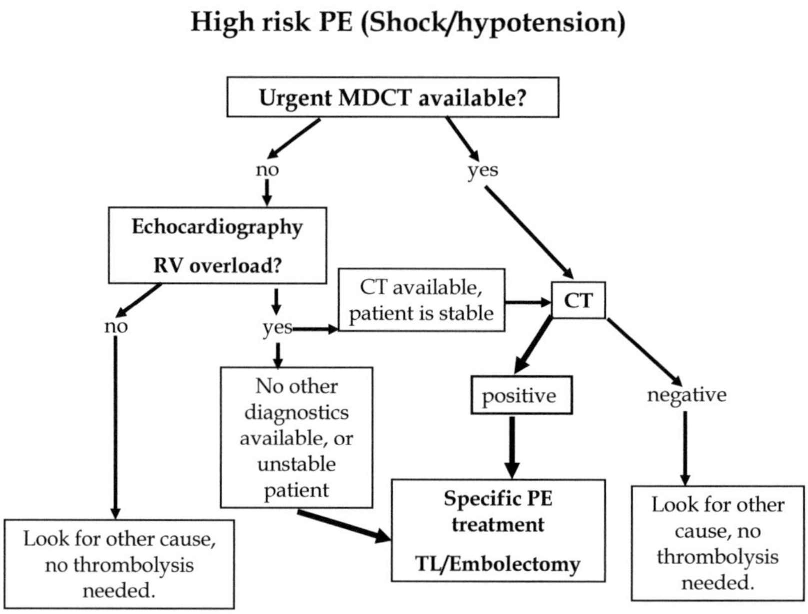

Fig. 3. The ESC 2008 guideline recommended diagnostic steps for high risk PE patients

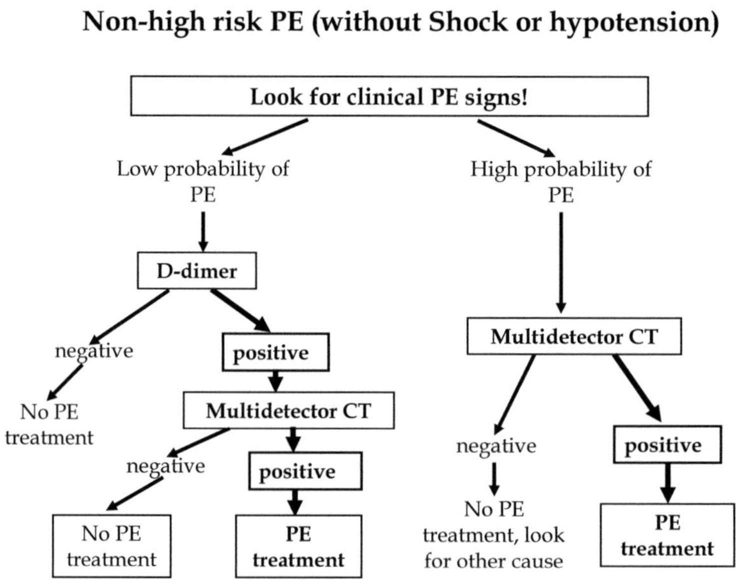

Fig. 4. The ESC 2008 guideline recommended diagnostic steps for non-high risk PE patients

or re-embolism. Morphine (or other opiate analgesic) can be administered as repeated intravenous bolus of 2 mg for analgesia. To achieve optimal haemorheological parameters and a desirable volume state, aggressive fluid resuscitation must be carried out intravenously in the acute phase (crystalloid 1.5-2 ml/kg/h). Early fluid resuscitation is recommended based on hypotension from the loss of LV end diastolic volume. Ozier et al.

measured the effect of 600 ml crystalloid infusion and found an increase of cardiac index from 1.7 to 2.0 l/min/m^2. Also, Mercat et al. found the same increase of cardiac index after the infusion of 500 ml dextrane. Modest fluid challenge is recommended, as fluid overload may depress contractility and decrease cardiac output (Kasper et al., 1997; Mercat et al., 1999; Ozier et al., 1984). If bronchospasm develops 200 mg intravenous theophyllin may be administered. If required, norepinephrine and/or dobutamine are the choice of positive inotropic drugs. Norepinephrine improve RV function with direct effect on contractility (Prewitt, 1990). Büchner primary recommends norepinephrine and dobutamine combination for haemodynamic shock (S. Büchner & Th. Hachenberg, 2005).

Elevated lactate levels indicate capillary perfusion impairment. The normalisation of lactate shows the resolution of the haemodynamic failure. Also, a radial arterial line is useful for continuous blood pressure monitoring and to draw frequent blood samples upon the verification of high-risk or non high-risk PE. Pulse contour cardiac output systems, like the "PiCCO"-system (Pulsion Medical Inc., Germany) is capable of continuous haemodynamic monitoring including cardiac output. Phosphodiesterase-III inhibitors (i.e. enoximon) and Ca-channel sensitizers (i.e. levosimendan) may have a beneficial effect, but insufficient clinical evidence is available yet (Nowak et al., 2007; Kerbaul et al., 2007). Also, the inhalation of nitrous oxide may improve the gas exchange of patients with PE (Torbicki et al., 2008).

If deep vein Doppler ultrasound suspects a floating, weak structure clot, thus re-embolisation may occur, a temporary placement of caval vein filter should be considered before TL.

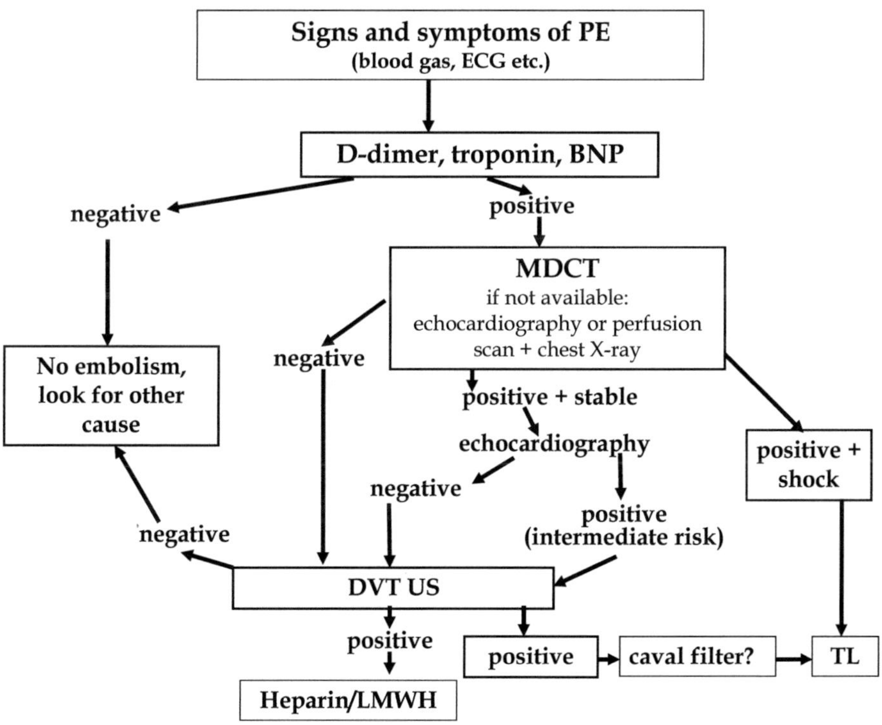

Fig. 5. The authors' own diagnostic and therapeutic approach (US: ultrasound)

1.5.2 Thrombolysis

Based on this complex classification a planned approach is essential. The aim of the management of acute severe PE is the resolution of the pulmonary artery obstruction. The most common procedure is TL, but invasive radiology procedures (clot fragmentation and vacuum evacuation, or selective TL through catheter arteriography, Class IIb C) or acute surgical embolectomy (Class I C) can also remove PE.

In critical patients with severe shock and confirmed PE the indication of urgent systemic TL is absolute (Class I A). The recommended medications and appropriate dosage is available in the current PE guideline (Table 3). The authors support the accelerated TL (rt-PA or SK) protocol in haemodynamically instable patients. According to our experience the ultra-high dose streptokinase is an economically reasonable and effective alternative to rt-PA (Sárosi et al., 1997; Sárosi et al., 1995).

Medication	Continuous TL	Accelerated TL
streptokinase (SK)	250,000 IU/30 min, following 100,000 IU/h for 12-24 hours	1.5 IU/2 hours
urokinase (UK)	4,400 IU/kg/10 min, following 4,400 IU/kg/h for 12-24 hours	3 IU/2 hours
rt-PA	100 mg/2 hours	0.6 mg/kg/15 min (max: 50 mg)

Table 3. Recommended thrombolytic regimens (Torbicki et al., 2008)

In the intermediate-risk group, with main arterial embolism and increased RV load, positive D-sign, elevated troponin and BNP levels but without haemodynamical impairment, TL is recommended only after considering relative contraindications and acquisition of written informed consent (Class IIb B).

Certain patient history *absolutely contraindicates TL*: haemorrhagic stroke, or stroke of unconfirmed origin, ischemic stroke in the last 6 months, central nervous system tumour, neuro, trauma, or general surgery intervention in the last 3 weeks, gastrointestinal bleeding in the last 30 days, known bleeding, or bleeding disorder.

The *relative contraindications* are: transient ischemic attack in the last 6 months, oral anticoagulation (vitamin K antagonists), pregnancy and the 1st week following labour, organ biopsy and non-compressible puncture, traumatic resuscitation, critical hypertension (RR_s > 180 mmHg), advanced liver disease, infective endocarditis, active peptic ulcer (Torbicki et al., 2008). In life-threatening situations, every contraindication can be considered to be relative.

The effectiveness of TL should be controlled between 12 and 24 hours by a second look MDCT or other available diagnostic procedure (perfusion lung scan or echocardiography). If the decrease of unperfused area does not improve by 30% following the first treatment cycle, TL should be repeated after 24 hours.

During *resuscitation*, chest compressions assist the mechanical fragmentation of clot and improve the infiltration of drugs into the clot. Urokinase 2-3 MIU, rt-PA 2 × 50 mg or streptokinase 1.5 MIU (may repeat once after 15 minutes) can be used for TL. Compressions should continue for at least 90 minutes during TL. As TL is beneficial in PE and also in acute myocardial infarction, no firm diagnostic evidence is needed for the treatment (Böttiger & Spöhr, 2003). One main advantage of TL is the possibility of prompt use and that it may improve overall microcirculation (Böttiger & Martin, 2001).

Based on our previous clinical investigations, in case of bleeding complications the repetitive measurement of clot formation factors (namely fibrinogen and plasminogen) may indicate the need of specific factor replacement or fresh frozen plasma infusion during or following TL. Major bleeding complications can be reduced below 5%, if factor replacement takes place in patients with fibrinogen levels below 1.5 g/l accompanied by minor bleeding disorder or fibrinogen levels < 0.6 g/l (Mühl et al., 2007).

Patients may not benefit from the TL of a more than 5-7 days old clot. Also, a second unsuccessful TL may indicate the presence of an older, connective tissue rich clot. Invasive radiology clot fragmentation and removal with or without selective TL should be used in these scenarios.

Anticoagulation therapy during TL: In the rt-PA group unfractionated heparin is recommended during TL (500-1000 IU/h, based on actual partial thromboplastin time (aPTT) levels on admission) (Segal, Streiff, et al., 2007).

Anticoagulation therapy after TL: Anticoagulant therapy starts after strepto- or urokinase TL with intravenous unfractionated heparin to maintain aPTT (check every 4 hours!) between 50-70 seconds for the first 48 hours and continues with a therapeutic dose of LMWH, if no further TL cycle is necessary. Using the "Heparin adjustment nomogram", the dose of Na-heparin is adjusted to reach a target aPTT (Torbicki et al., 2008).

Anticoagulant therapy should be provided with intravenous unfractionated heparin to maintain the aPTT between 60-70 seconds for 48 hours. If TL was effective it should be continued with a therapeutic dose of LMWH. Following TL, long term anticoagulation (acenocoumarol or warfarin) can start on day 3 or 4 (Torbicki et al., 2008; Kearon et al., 2008).

In case of unfractioned heparin use, the incidence of HIT is 1-3% (about 1% with LMWH), therefore regular platelet count check is recommended (Greinacher, 2009; Morris et al., 2007). In case of confirmed HIT, one should switch from heparin/LMWH therapy to: hirudin, lepirudin, danaparoid or fondaparinux.

One of the most common complication of TL is minor bleeding (arterial/venous port bleeding, haematuria, suffusions, e.t.c.), major bleeding occurs in 13% of cases. The incidence of intracranial haemorrhage is 1.8% (Spöhr et al., 2005), (Konstantinides et al., 2002; Goldhaber et al., 1993).

1.5.3 Catheter extraction and surgical embolectomy

Indications of percutaneous catheter embolectomy and fragmentation are unsuccessful systemic TL, contraindicatons of systemic lysis, PE with haemodynamic shock (resuscitation, mechanical ventilation), clot in the right heart, and also an alternative for the surgical embolectomy if no experienced team is available (Kucher et al., 2005; Uflacker, 2001).

Surgical embolectomy has a high mortality rate in the high-risk PE group. Indications are narrow, only patients with absolute systemic TL contraindications and in the absence of consent for TL may benefit from surgical intervention (Meneveau et al., 2006). Previous unsuccessful TL is not a contraindication for surgical embolectomy (Aklog et al., 2002).

1.5.4 Intravenous (caval) filter

Statistically there is no firm evidence of improved 12 days mortality of the caval filter use. Transient caval filters may be used up to 14 days. Late complications include migration and device thrombosis. Indications are not general; the main indication is suspected reoccurrence of PE and contraindication of long-term anticoagulation (Hann & Streiff, 2005). Also, venous filters for PE prophylaxis may be beneficial in trauma patients, but further studies are required to draw firm clinical evidence (Rajasekhar et al., 2011).

1.5.5 Follow-up after PE therapy

Following PE therapy, a switch from heparin/LMWH to oral anticoagulation is recommended. Oral anticoagulation should be continued for 6 months. Following, an extended diagnostic procedure should take place to elucidate possible genetic factors or acquired thrombophylia behind the development of PE. In case of irreversible complications or positive thrombotic predisposition, continuous oral anticoagulation is needed (Kearon et al., 2008).

2. A new approach to PE

2.1 The role of matrix metalloproteinases

Experimental evidence indicated that the pathophysiology of PE implies the activation of matrix metalloproteinases (MMPs) (Uzuelli et al., 2008; Dias-Junior et al., 2009; Souza-Costa et al., 2005; Souza-Costa et al., 2007; Palei et al., 2005; Fortuna et al., 2007). Indeed, hemodynamic derangements associated with this condition improved with the inhibition of MMPs. Neutrophil activation (Eagleton et al., 2002) and rapid release of granules containing large amounts of MMP-9 in inflammation (Van den Steen et al., 2002) and during PE explains how MMPs, especially MMP-9, are involved in pathophysiology of PE. The increased activity and levels of MMP-9 found in ischemic stroke, or the upregulation of the enzyme after cerebral ischemia are interestingly similar to PE (Asahi et al., 2000). The degradation of type IV collagen, laminin, and fibronectin by MMP-9, may contribute to hemorrhagic transformation after cardioembolic stroke as these components are the main structure of the vascular matrix (Rosell et al., 2008; Montaner et al., 2001). Also, tissue plasminogen activator (or alteplase) can amplify MMP-9 levels by upregulation, thus increasing ischemic brain damage (Wang et al., 2004; Burggraf et al., 2007; Ning et al., 2006; Tsuji et al., 2005). There is evidence, that increased plasmin concentration may activate MMPs. Previous experimental work by our group aimed to assess the levels of MMPs following fibrinolysis for acute PE. Circulating levels of MMPs were measured serially (MMP-9 and MMP-2). Their endogenous inhibitors, tissue inhibitor of metalloproteinase (TIMP)-1 and TIMP-2 were also measured in alteplase and in ultra-high dose streptokinase-treated patients with acute PE (Mühl et al., 2010).

2.2 Measurements and discussion of TIMP/MMP changes in PE

In our study MMP levels were assessed by sodium-dodecil-sulphate polyacrylamide gel electrophoresis, TIMP levels were measured with a commercially available ELISA kit (Mühl et al., 2010). Significant increases in pro-MMP-9 concentrations were found after TL therapy in both groups, but these were not associated with significant alterations in TIMP-1 levels. Pro-MMP-9/TIMP-1 ratio increased significantly. Interestingly, earlier increases in pro-MMP-9 levels and in pro-MMP-9/TIMP-1 ratio were found in subjects treated with streptokinase. From the 3rd day pro-MMP-9 levels and pro-MMP-9/TIMP-1 ratio returned to normal. No significant changes in pro-MMP-2 concentrations were measured after TL. Moreover, we found no significant changes in TIMP-2 concentrations or in pro-MMP-2/TIMP-2 ratio.

Although there is a lack of firm evidence, the possible explanation for increased MMP-9 levels during treatment with alteplase is the promotion of MMP-9 release by neutrophils (Cuadrado et al., 2008). According to our knowledge, no previous study has reported that streptokinase induces the release of MMP-9.

A slower increase of pro-MMP-9 was found in alteplase treated patients, but the precise explanation for this difference between fibrinolytic agents is not yet elucidated. There is significant interindividual variability in neutrophil degranulation (Cuadrado et al., 2008), therefore a multi-central study may draw firm evidence on this question.

No definitive conclusion can be drawn yet, but it is widely acknowledged that intracerebral hemorrhage is the most feared bleeding complication of TL (Arcasoy & Kreit, 1999). The use of alteplase enhanced MMP-9 levels, which has already been widely associated with hemorrhagic transformation after cardioembolic stroke (Rosell et al., 2008; Montaner et al., 2001). This observation offers an explanation for the hemorrhagic transformation during stroke.

It is possible that the MMP inhibitors may decrease the risk of intracerebral hemorrhage or other bleeding complication of TL for acute PE (Murata et al., 2008; Sumii & Lo, 2002; Machado et al., 2009) and may have beneficial hemodynamic effects (Fortuna et al., 2007; Palei et al., 2005).

3. Summary

Following risk stratification, prompt and specific diagnostics are life-saving in acute PE. Recommended diagnostic tools are biomarkers, MDCT and electrocardiography. Systemic TL is the first choice for high-risk PE patients, in case of contraindications surgical embolectomy or catheter clot fragmentation/removal should be considered. The fast resolution of haemodynamic shock indicates accelerated protocol systemic TL (rt-PA, SK or UK), as continuous TL dissolve clot slower and have a higher risk of bleeding disorder. The regular control of fibrinogen and plasminogen during and after TL, and clot formation factor supplement can reduce bleeding complications.

There is emerging evidence of the hypothesized role of the TIMP/MMP system in the development of bleeding complication. In future, pharmacological approach to MMP inhibition in human medicine may decrease the incidence of bleeding complications of TL.

4. References

Ageno, W., Squizzato, A., Garcia, D. & Imberti, D. (2006). Epidemiology and risk factors of venous thromboembolism. *Seminars in thrombosis and hemostasis*, Vol.32, No.7, (April 2007), pp. 651-8, ISSN 0094-6176

Agnelli, G., Becattini, C. & Kirschstein, T. (2002). Thrombolysis vs heparin in the treatment of pulmonary embolism: a clinical outcome-based meta-analysis. *Archives of internal medicine*, Vol.162, No.22, (December 2002), pp. 2537-41, ISSN 0003-9926

Aklog, L., Williams, C.S., Byrne, J.G. & Goldhaber, S.Z. (2002). Acute pulmonary embolectomy: a contemporary approach. *Circulation*, Vol.105, No.12, (March 2002), pp. 1416-9, ISSN 1524-4539

Arcasoy, S.M. & Kreit, J.W. (1999). Thrombolytic therapy of pulmonary embolism: a comprehensive review of current evidence. *Chest*, Vol.115, No.6, (June 1999), pp. 1695-707, ISSN 0012-3692

Asahi, M., Asahi, K., Jung, J.C., del Zoppo, G.J., Fini, M.E. & Lo, E.H. (2000). Role for matrix metalloproteinase 9 after focal cerebral ischemia: effects of gene knockout and enzyme inhibition with BB-94. *Journal of cerebral blood flow and metabolism: official journal of the International Society of Cerebral Blood Flow and Metabolism*, Vol.20, No.12, (December 2000), pp. 1681-9, ISSN 0271-678X

Bova, C., Greco, F., Misuraca, G., Serafini, O., Crocco, F., Greco, A. & Noto, A. (2003). Diagnostic utility of echocardiography in patients with suspected pulmonary embolism. *The American journal of emergency medicine*, Vol.21, No.3, (May 2003), pp. 180-3, ISSN 0735-6757

Brenner, D.J. & Hall, E.J. (2007). Computed tomography--an increasing source of radiation exposure. *The New England journal of medicine*, Vol.357, No.22, (November 2007), pp. 2277-84, ISSN 1533-4406

Brunot, S., Corneloup, O., Latrabe, V., Montaudon, M. & Laurent, F. (2005). Reproducibility of multi-detector spiral computed tomography in detection of sub-segmental acute pulmonary embolism. *European radiology*, Vol.15, No.10, (October 2005), pp. 2057-63, ISSN 0938-7994

Burggraf, D., Martens, H.K., Dichgans, M. & Hamann, G.F. (2007). Matrix metalloproteinase (MMP) induction and inhibition at different doses of recombinant tissue plasminogen activator following experimental stroke. *Thrombosis and haemostasis*, Vol.98, No.5, (November 2007), pp. 963-9, ISSN 0340-6245

Böttiger, B.W. & Martin, E. (2001). Thrombolytic therapy during cardiopulmonary resuscitation and the role of coagulation activation after cardiac arrest. *Current opinion in critical care*, Vol.7, No.3, (June 2001), pp. 176-83, ISSN 1070-5295

Böttiger, B.W. & Spöhr, F. (2003). The risk of thrombolysis in association with cardiopulmonary resuscitation: no reason to withhold this causal and effective therapy. *Journal of internal medicine*, Vol.253, No.2, (February 2003), pp. 99-101, ISSN 0954-6820

Büchner S., Pfeiffer B., Hachenberg T. (2005). Lungenembolie (CME 1/2/2005). *Anesth. Intensivmed.*, No.46, (2005), pp. 9-22.

Casazza, F., Bongarzoni, A., Capozi, A. & Agostoni, O. (2005). Regional right ventricular dysfunction in acute pulmonary embolism and right ventricular infarction. *European journal of echocardiography: the journal of the Working Group on Echocardiography of the European Society of Cardiology*, Vol.6, No.1, (January 2005), pp. 11-4, ISSN 1525-2167

Cuadrado, E., Ortega, L., Hernández-Guillamon, M., Penalba, A., Fernández-Cadenas, I., Rosell, A. & Montaner, J. (2008). Tissue plasminogen activator (t-PA) promotes neutrophil degranulation and MMP-9 release. *Journal of leukocyte biology*, Vol.84, No.1, (July 2008), pp. 207-14, ISSN 0741-5400

Dahlbäck, B. (1995). Inherited thrombophilia: resistance to activated protein C as a pathogenic factor of venous thromboembolism. *Blood*, Vol.85, No.3, (February 1995), pp. 607-14, ISSN 0006-4971

Demers, C., Ginsberg, J.S., Hirsh, J., Henderson, P. & Blajchman, M.A. (1992). Thrombosis in antithrombin-III-deficient persons. Report of a large kindred and literature review. *Annals of internal medicine*, Vol.116, No.9, (May 1992), pp. 754-61, ISSN 0003-4819

den Heijer, M., Koster, T., Blom, H.J., Bos, G.M., Briet, E., Reitsma, P.H., Vandenbroucke, J.P. & Rosendaal, F.R. (1996). Hyperhomocysteinemia as a risk factor for deep-vein thrombosis. *The New England journal of medicine,* Vol.334, No.12, (March 1996), pp. 759-62, ISSN 0028-4793

Dias-Junior, C.A., Cau, S.B.A., Oliveira, A.M., Castro, M.M., Montenegro, M.F., Gerlach, R.F. & Tanus-Santos, J.E. (2009). Nitrite or sildenafil, but not BAY 41-2272, blunt acute pulmonary embolism-induced increases in circulating matrix metalloproteinase-9 and oxidative stress. *Thrombosis research,* Vol.124, No.3, (January 2009), pp. 349-55, ISSN 1879-2472

Dunn, K.L., Wolf, J.P., Dorfman, D.M., Fitzpatrick, P., Baker, J.L. & Goldhaber, S.Z. (2002). Normal D-dimer levels in emergency department patients suspected of acute pulmonary embolism. *Journal of the American College of Cardiology,* Vol.40, No.8, (October 2002), pp. 1475-8, ISSN 0735-1097

Eagleton, M.J., Henke, P.K., Luke, C.E., Hawley, A.E., Bedi, A., Knipp, B.S., Wakefield, T.W. & Greenfield, L.J. (2002). Southern Association for Vascular Surgery William J. von Leibig Award. Inflammation and intimal hyperplasia associated with experimental pulmonary embolism. *Journal of vascular surgery: official publication, the Society for Vascular Surgery [and] International Society for Cardiovascular Surgery, North American Chapter,* Vol.36, No.3, (September 2002), pp. 581-8, ISSN 0741-5214

Eyer, B.A., Goodman, L.R. & Washington, L. (2005). Clinicians' response to radiologists' reports of isolated subsegmental pulmonary embolism or inconclusive interpretation of pulmonary embolism using MDCT. *AJR. American journal of roentgenology,* Vol.184, No.2, (February 2005), pp. 623-8, ISSN 0361-803X

Ferrari, E., Benhamou, M., Berthier, F. & Baudouy, M. (2005). Mobile thrombi of the right heart in pulmonary embolism: delayed disappearance after thrombolytic treatment. *Chest,* Vol.127, No.3, (March 2005), pp. 1051-3, ISSN 0012-3692

Fortuna, G.M., Figueiredo-Lopes, L., Dias-Junior, C.A.C., Gerlach, R.F. & Tanus-Santos, J.E. (2007). A role for matrix metalloproteinase-9 in the hemodynamic changes following acute pulmonary embolism. *International journal of cardiology,* Vol.114, No.1, (January 2007), pp. 22-7, ISSN 1874-1754

Geibel, A., Zehender, M., Kasper, W., Olschewski, M., Klima, C. & Konstantinides, S.V. (2005). Prognostic value of the ECG on admission in patients with acute major pulmonary embolism. *The European respiratory journal: official journal of the European Society for Clinical Respiratory Physiology,* Vol.25, No.5, (May 2005), pp. 843-8, ISSN 0903-1936

Ghaye, B., Szapiro, D., Mastora, I., Delannoy, V., Duhamel, A., Remy, J. & Remy-Jardin, M. (2001). Peripheral pulmonary arteries: how far in the lung does multi-detector row spiral CT allow analysis? *Radiology,* Vol.219, No.3, (June 2001), pp. 629-36, ISSN 0033-8419

Giannitsis, E., Müller-Bardorff, M., Kurowski, V., Weidtmann, B., Wiegand, U., Kampmann, M. & Katus, H.A. (2000). Independent prognostic value of cardiac troponin T in patients with confirmed pulmonary embolism. *Circulation,* Vol.102, No.2, (July 2000), pp. 211-7, ISSN 0009-7322

Goldhaber, S.Z. (1998). Pulmonary embolism. *The New England journal of medicine,* Vol.339, No.2, (July 1998), pp. 93-104, ISSN 0028-4793

Goldhaber, S.Z. & Morrison, R.B. (2002). Cardiology patient pages. Pulmonary embolism and deep vein thrombosis. *Circulation,* Vol.106, No.12, (September 2002), pp. 1436-8, ISSN 0009-7322

Goldhaber, S.Z., Grodstein, F., Stampfer, M.J., Manson, J.E., Colditz, G.A., Speizer, F.E., Willett, W.C. & Hennekens, C.H. (1997). A prospective study of risk factors for pulmonary embolism in women. *JAMA: the journal of the American Medical Association*, Vol.277, No.8, (February 1997), pp. 642-5, ISSN 1538-3598

Goldhaber, S.Z., Haire, W.D., Feldstein, M.L., Miller, M., Toltzis, R., Smith, J.L., Taveira da Silva, A.M., Come, P.C., Lee, R.T. & Parker, J.A. (1993). Alteplase versus heparin in acute pulmonary embolism: randomised trial assessing right-ventricular function and pulmonary perfusion. *Lancet*, Vol.341, No.8844, (February 1993), pp. 507-11, ISSN 0140-6736

Goldhaber, S.Z., Visani, L. & De Rosa, M. (1999). Acute pulmonary embolism: clinical outcomes in the International Cooperative Pulmonary Embolism Registry (ICOPER). *The Lancet*, Vol.353, No.9162, (April 1999), pp. 1386-1389, ISSN 0140-6736

Greinacher, A. (2009). Heparin-induced thrombocytopenia. *Journal of thrombosis and haemostasis: JTH*, Vol.7 Suppl 1, (July 2009), pp. 9-12, ISSN 1538-7836

Hann, C.L. & Streiff, M.B. (2005). The role of vena caval filters in the management of venous thromboembolism. *Blood reviews*, Vol.19, No.4, (July 2005), pp. 179-202, ISSN 0268-960X

Hsiao, S.-H., Chang, S.-M., Lee, C.-Y., Yang, S.-H., Lin, S.-K. & Chiou, K.-R. (2006). Usefulness of tissue Doppler parameters for identifying pulmonary embolism in patients with signs of pulmonary hypertension. *The American journal of cardiology*, Vol.98, No.5, (September 2006), pp. 685-90, ISSN 0002-9149

Janata, K., Holzer, M., Domanovits, H., Müllner, M., Bankier, A., Kurtaran, A., Bankl, H.C. & Laggner, A.N. (2002). Mortality of patients with pulmonary embolism. *Wiener klinische Wochenschrift*, Vol.114, No.17-18, (September 2002), pp. 766-72, 0043-5325

Kasper, W., Konstantinides, S., Geibel, A., Olschewski, M., Heinrich, F., Grosser, K.D., Rauber, K., Iversen, S., Redecker, M. & Kienast, J. (1997). Management strategies and determinants of outcome in acute major pulmonary embolism: results of a multicenter registry. *Journal of the American College of Cardiology*, Vol.30, No.5, (November 1997), pp. 1165-71, ISSN 0735-1097

Kearon, C., Kahn, S.R., Agnelli, G., Goldhaber, S., Raskob, G.E. & Comerota, A.J. (2008). Antithrombotic therapy for venous thromboembolic disease: American College of Chest Physicians Evidence-Based Clinical Practice Guidelines (8th Edition). *Chest*, Vol.133, No.6 Suppl, (June 2008), p. 454S-545S, ISSN 0012-3692

Kerbaul, F., Gariboldi, V., Giorgi, R., Mekkaoui, C., Guieu, R., Fesler, P., Gouin, F., Brimioulle, S. & Collart, F. (2007). Effects of levosimendan on acute pulmonary embolism-induced right ventricular failure. *Critical care medicine*, Vol.35, No.8, (August 2007), pp. 1948-54, ISSN 0090-3493

Kline, J.A., Hernandez-Nino, J., Newgard, C.D., Cowles, D.N., Jackson, R.E. & Courtney, D.M. (2003). Use of pulse oximetry to predict in-hospital complications in normotensive patients with pulmonary embolism. *The American journal of medicine*, Vol.115, No.3, (August 2003), pp. 203-8, ISSN 0002-9343

Konstantinides, S. (2008). Clinical practice. Acute pulmonary embolism. *The New England journal of medicine*, Vol.359, No.26, (December 2008), pp. 2804-13, ISSN 0028-4793

Konstantinides, S. (2005). Pulmonary embolism: impact of right ventricular dysfunction. *Current opinion in cardiology*, Vol.20, No.6, (November 2005), pp. 496-501, ISSN 0268-4705

Konstantinides, S. & Hasenfuss, G. (2004). [Acute cor pulmonale in pulmonary embolism. An important prognostic factor and a critical parameter for the choice of a therapeutic strategy]. *Der Internist*, Vol.45, No.10, (October 2004), pp. 1155-62, ISSN 0020-9554

Konstantinides, S., Geibel, A., Heusel, G., Heinrich, F. & Kasper, W. (2002). Heparin plus alteplase compared with heparin alone in patients with submassive pulmonary embolism. *The New England journal of medicine*, Vol.347, No.15, (October 2002), pp. 1143-50, ISSN 0028-4793

Konstantinides, S., Geibel, A., Kasper, W., Olschewski, M., Blümel, L. & Just, H. (1998). Patent foramen ovale is an important predictor of adverse outcome in patients with major pulmonary embolism. *Circulation*, Vol.97, No.19, (May 1998), pp. 1946-51, ISSN 0009-7322

Kostrubiec, M., Pruszczyk, P., Bochowicz, A., Pacho, R., Szulc, M., Kaczynska, A., Styczynski, G., Kuch-Wocial, A., Abramczyk, P., Bartoszewicz, Z., Berent, H. & Kuczynska, K. (2005). Biomarker-based risk assessment model in acute pulmonary embolism. *European heart journal*, Vol.26, No.20, (October 2005), pp. 2166-72, ISSN 0195-668X

Kruip, M.J.H.A., Leclercq, M.G.L., van der Heul, C., Prins, M.H. & Büller, H.R. (2003). Diagnostic strategies for excluding pulmonary embolism in clinical outcome studies. A systematic review. *Annals of internal medicine*, Vol.138, No.12, (June 2003), pp. 941-51, ISSN 0003-4819

Krüger, S., Graf, J., Merx, M.W., Koch, K.C., Kunz, D., Hanrath, P. & Janssens, U. (2004). Brain natriuretic peptide predicts right heart failure in patients with acute pulmonary embolism. *American heart journal*, Vol.147, No.1, (January 2004), pp. 60-5, ISSN 0002-8703

Kucher, N. & Goldhaber, S.Z. (2003). Cardiac biomarkers for risk stratification of patients with acute pulmonary embolism. *Circulation*, Vol.108, No.18, (November 2003), pp. 2191-4 ISSN 0009-7322

Kucher, N., Windecker, S., Banz, Y., Schmitz-Rode, T., Mettler, D., Meier, B. & Hess, O.M. (2005). Percutaneous catheter thrombectomy device for acute pulmonary embolism: in vitro and in vivo testing. *Radiology*, Vol.236, No.3, (September 2005), pp. 852-8, ISSN 0033-8419

Lee, C.H., Hankey, G.J., Ho, W.K. & Eikelboom, J.W. (2005). Venous thromboembolism: diagnosis and management of pulmonary embolism. *The Medical journal of Australia*, Vol.182, No.11, (June 2005), pp. 569-74, ISSN 0025-729X

Le Gal, G., Righini, M., Sanchez, O., Roy, P.-M., Baba-Ahmed, M., Perrier, A. & Bounameaux, H. (2006). A positive compression ultrasonography of the lower limb veins is highly predictive of pulmonary embolism on computed tomography in suspected patients. *Thrombosis and haemostasis*, Vol.95, No.6, (June 2006), pp. 963-6, ISSN 0340-6245

Machado, L.S., Sazonova, I.Y., Kozak, A., Wiley, D.C., El-Remessy, A.B., Ergul, A., Hess, D.C., Waller, J.L. & Fagan, S.C. (2009). Minocycline and tissue-type plasminogen activator for stroke: assessment of interaction potential. *Stroke; a journal of cerebral circulation*, Vol.40, No.9, (September 2009), pp. 3028-33, ISSN 0039-2499

Meneveau, N., Séronde, M.-F., Blonde, M.-C., Legalery, P., Didier-Petit, K., Briand, F., Caulfield, F., Schiele, F., Bernard, Y. & Bassand, J.-P. (2006). Management of unsuccessful thrombolysis in acute massive pulmonary embolism. *Chest*, Vol.129, No.4, (April 2006), pp. 1043-50, ISSN 0012-3692

Mercat, A., Diehl, J.L., Meyer, G., Teboul, J.L. & Sors, H. (1999). Hemodynamic effects of fluid loading in acute massive pulmonary embolism. *Critical care medicine*, Vol.27, No.3, (March 1999), pp. 540-4, ISSN 0090-3493

Miniati, M., Monti, S., Pratali, L., Di Ricco, G., Marini, C., Formichi, B., Prediletto, R., Michelassi, C., Di Lorenzo, M., Tonelli, L. & Pistolesi, M. (2001). Value of transthoracic echocardiography in the diagnosis of pulmonary embolism: results of a prospective study in unselected patients. *The American journal of medicine*, Vol.110, No.7, (May 2001), pp. 528-35, ISSN 0002-9343

Miniati, M., Pistolesi, M., Marini, C., Di Ricco, G., Formichi, B., Prediletto, R., Allescia, G., Tonelli, L., Sostman, H.D. & Giuntini, C. (1996). Value of perfusion lung scan in the diagnosis of pulmonary embolism: results of the Prospective Investigative Study of Acute Pulmonary Embolism Diagnosis (PISA-PED). *American journal of respiratory and critical care medicine*, Vol.154, No.5, (November 1996), pp. 1387-93, ISSN 1073-449X

Miniati, M., Prediletto, R., Formichi, B., Marini, C., Di Ricco, G., Tonelli, L., Allescia, G. & Pistolesi, M. (1999). Accuracy of clinical assessment in the diagnosis of pulmonary embolism. *American journal of respiratory and critical care medicine*, Vol.159, No.3, (March 1999), pp. 864-71, ISSN 1073-449X

Montaner, J., Alvarez-Sabín, J., Molina, C.A., Anglés, A., Abilleira, S., Arenillas, J. & Monasterio, J. (2001). Matrix metalloproteinase expression is related to hemorrhagic transformation after cardioembolic stroke. *Stroke; a journal of cerebral circulation*, Vol.32, No.12, (December 2001), pp. 2762-7, ISSN 0039-2499

Morris, T.A., Castrejon, S., Devendra, G. & Gamst, A.C. (2007). No difference in risk for thrombocytopenia during treatment of pulmonary embolism and deep venous thrombosis with either low-molecular-weight heparin or unfractionated heparin: a metaanalysis. *Chest*, Vol.132, No.4, (October 2007), pp. 1131-9, ISSN 0012-3692

Murata, Y., Rosell, A., Scannevin, R.H., Rhodes, K.J., Wang, X. & Lo, E.H. (2008). Extension of the thrombolytic time window with minocycline in experimental stroke. *Stroke; a journal of cerebral circulation*, Vol.39, No.12, (December 2008), pp. 3372-7, ISSN 0039-2499

Mühl, D., Füredi, R., Gecse, K., Ghosh, S., Falusi, B., Bogár, L., Roth, E. & Lantos, J. (2007). Time course of platelet aggregation during thrombolytic treatment of massive pulmonary embolism. *Blood coagulation & fibrinolysis: an international journal in haemostasis and thrombosis*, Vol.18, No.7, (October 2007), pp. 661-7, ISSN 0957-5235

Mühl, D., Ghosh, S., Uzuelli, J.A., Lantos, J. & Tanus-Santos, J.E. (2010). Increases in circulating matrix metalloproteinase-9 levels following fibrinolysis for acute pulmonary embolism. *Thrombosis research*, Vol.125, No.6, (June 2010), pp. 549-53, ISSN 0049-3848

Ning, M., Furie, K.L., Koroshetz, W.J., Lee, H., Barron, M., Lederer, M., Wang, X., Zhu, M., Sorensen, A.G., Lo, E.H. & Kelly, P.J. (2006). Association between tPA therapy and raised early matrix metalloproteinase-9 in acute stroke. *Neurology*, Vol.66, No.10, (May 2006), pp. 1550-5, ISSN 0028-3878

Nowak, F.G., Halbfass, P. & Hoffmann, E. (2007). [Pulmonary embolism: clinical relevance, requirements for diagnostic and therapeutic strategies]. *Der Radiologe*, Vol.47, No.8, (August 2007), pp. 663-72, ISSN 0033-832X

Oger, E. (2000). Incidence of venous thromboembolism: a community-based study in Western France. EPI-GETBP Study Group. Groupe d'Etude de la Thrombose de Bretagne Occidentale. *Thrombosis and haemostasis*, Vol.83, No.5, (May 2000), pp. 657-60, ISSN 0340-6245

Ozier, Y., Dubourg, O., Farcot, J.C., Bazin, M., Jardin, F. & Margairaz, A. (1984). Circulatory failure in acute pulmonary embolism. *Intensive care medicine*, Vol.10, No.2, (1984), pp. 91-7, ISSN 0342-4642

Palei, A.C.T., Zaneti, R.A.G., Fortuna, G.M., Gerlach, R.F. & Tanus-Santos, J.E. (2005). Hemodynamic benefits of matrix metalloproteinase-9 inhibition by doxycycline during experimental acute pulmonary embolism. *Angiology*, Vol.56, No.5, (September-October 2005), pp. 611-7, ISSN 0003-3197

Perrier, A., Roy, P.-M., Aujesky, D., Chagnon, I., Howarth, N., Gourdier, A.-L., Leftheriotis, G., Barghouth, G., Cornuz, J., Hayoz, D. & Bounameaux, H. (2004). Diagnosing pulmonary embolism in outpatients with clinical assessment, D-dimer measurement, venous ultrasound, and helical computed tomography: a multicenter management study. *The American journal of medicine*, Vol.116, No.5, (March 2004), pp. 291-9, ISSN 0002-9343

Poort, S.R., Rosendaal, F.R., Reitsma, P.H. & Bertina, R.M. (1996). A common genetic variation in the 3'-untranslated region of the prothrombin gene is associated with elevated plasma prothrombin levels and an increase in venous thrombosis. *Blood*, Vol.88, No.10, (November 1996), pp. 3698-703, ISSN 0006-4971

Prewitt, R.M. (1990). Hemodynamic management in pulmonary embolism and acute hypoxemic respiratory failure. *Critical care medicine*, Vol.18, No.1 Pt 2, (January 1990), pp. S61-9, ISSN 0090-3493

Rajasekhar, A., Lottenberg, R., Lottenberg, L., Liu, H. & Ang, D. (2011). Pulmonary embolism prophylaxis with inferior vena cava filters in trauma patients: a systematic review using the meta-analysis of observational studies in epidemiology (MOOSE) guidelines. *Journal of thrombosis and thrombolysis*, Vol.32, No.1, (July 2011), pp. 40-6, ISSN 0929-5305

Reber, G., Bounameaux, H., Perrier, A. & De Moerloose, P. (2004). A new rapid point-of-care D-dimer enzyme-linked immunosorbent assay (Stratus CS D-dimer) for the exclusion of venous thromboembolism. *Blood coagulation & fibrinolysis: an international journal in haemostasis and thrombosis*, Vol.15, No.5, (July 2004), pp. 435-8, ISSN 0957-5235

Righini, M., Le Gal, G., Aujesky, D., Roy, P.-M., Sanchez, O., Verschuren, F., Rutschmann, O., Nonent, M., Cornuz, J., Thys, F., Le Manach, C.P., Revel, M.-P., Poletti, P.-A., Meyer, G., Mottier, D., Perneger, T., Bounameaux, H. & Perrier, A. (2008). Diagnosis of pulmonary embolism by multidetector CT alone or combined with venous ultrasonography of the leg: a randomised non-inferiority trial. *Lancet*, Vol.371, No.9621, (April 2008), pp. 1343-52, ISSN 0140-6736

Rodger, M., Makropoulos, D., Turek, M., Quevillon, J., Raymond, F., Rasuli, P. & Wells, P.S. (2000). Diagnostic value of the electrocardiogram in suspected pulmonary embolism. *The American journal of cardiology*, Vol.86, No.7, (October 2000), pp. 807-9, A10, ISSN 0002-9149

Rodger, M.A., Carrier, M., Jones, G.N., Rasuli, P., Raymond, F., Djunaedi, H. & Wells, P.S. (2000). Diagnostic value of arterial blood gas measurement in suspected pulmonary embolism. *American journal of respiratory and critical care medicine*, Vol.162, No.6, (December 2000), pp. 2105-8, ISSN 1073-449X

Rosell, A., Cuadrado, E., Ortega-Aznar, A., Hernández-Guillamon, M., Lo, E.H. & Montaner, J. (2008). MMP-9-positive neutrophil infiltration is associated to blood-brain barrier breakdown and basal lamina type IV collagen degradation during hemorrhagic transformation after human ischemic stroke. *Stroke; a journal of cerebral circulation*, Vol.39, No.4, (April 2008), pp. 1121-6, ISSN 0039-2499

Roy, P.-M., Colombet, I., Durieux, P., Chatellier, G., Sors, H. & Meyer, G. (2005). Systematic review and meta-analysis of strategies for the diagnosis of suspected pulmonary embolism. *British medical journal*, Vol.331, No.7511, (July 2005), p. 259, ISSN 0959-8138

Sanchez, O., Trinquart, L., Colombet, I., Durieux, P., Huisman, M.V., Chatellier, G. & Meyer, G. (2008). Prognostic value of right ventricular dysfunction in patients with haemodynamically stable pulmonary embolism: a systematic review. *European heart journal*, Vol.29, No.12, (June 2008), pp. 1569-77, ISSN 0195-668X

Schürmann, M., Stiegler, H., Riel, K.A. & Schildberg, F.W. (1992). [Lung embolisms in a surgical patient sample. A retrospective study over 9 years]. *Der Chirurg; Zeitschrift für alle Gebiete der operativen Medizen*, Vol.63, No.10, (October 1992), pp. 811-6, ISSN 0009-4722

Segal, J.B., Eng, J., Tamariz, L.J. & Bass, E.B. (2007). Review of the evidence on diagnosis of deep venous thrombosis and pulmonary embolism. *Annals of family medicine*, Vol.5, No.1, (February 2007), pp. 63-73, ISSN 1544-1709

Segal, J.B., Streiff, M.B., Hofmann, L.V., Hoffman, L.V., Thornton, K. & Bass, E.B. (2007). Management of venous thromboembolism: a systematic review for a practice guideline. *Annals of internal medicine*, Vol.146, No.3, (February 2007), pp. 211-22, ISSN 0003-4819

Sevransky, J.E., Levy, M.M. & Marini, J.J. (2004). Mechanical ventilation in sepsis-induced acute lung injury/acute respiratory distress syndrome: an evidence-based review. *Critical care medicine*, Vol.32, No.11 Suppl, (November 2004), pp. S548-53, ISSN 0090-3493

Singer, M; Webb, A. (2004). Pulmonary embolism. In *Oxford handbook of critical care*. p. 296-, ISBN 0192-6319-0X

Souza-Costa, D.C., Figueiredo-Lopes, L., Alves-Filho, J.C., Semprini, M.C., Gerlach, R.F., Cunha, F.Q. & Tanus-Santos, J.E. (2007). Protective effects of atorvastatin in rat models of acute pulmonary embolism: involvement of matrix metalloproteinase-9. *Critical care medicine*, Vol.35, No.1, (January 2007), pp. 239-45, ISSN 0090-3493

Souza-Costa, D.C., Zerbini, T., Palei, A.C., Gerlach, R.F. & Tanus-Santos, J.E. (2005). L-arginine attenuates acute pulmonary embolism-induced increases in lung matrix metalloproteinase-2 and matrix metalloproteinase-9. *Chest*, Vol.128, No.5, (November 2005), pp. 3705-10, ISSN 0012-3692

Spannagl, M., Haverkate, F., Reinauer, H. & Meijer, P. (2005). The performance of quantitative D-dimer assays in laboratory routine. *Blood coagulation & fibrinolysis: an international journal in haemostasis and thrombosis*, Vol.16, No.6, (September 2005), pp. 439-43, ISSN 0957-5235

Spöhr, F., Böttiger, B.W. & Walther, A. (2005). [Errors and risks in perioperative thrombolysis therapy]. *Der Anaesthesist*, Vol.54, No.5, (May 2005), pp. 485-94, ISSN 0003-2417

Stein, P.D. & Henry, J.W. (1997). Clinical characteristics of patients with acute pulmonary embolism stratified according to their presenting syndromes. *Chest*, Vol.112, No.4, (October 1997), pp. 974-9, ISSN 0012-3692

Stein, P.D., Goldhaber, S.Z., Henry, J.W. & Miller, A.C. (1996). Arterial blood gas analysis in the assessment of suspected acute pulmonary embolism. *Chest*, Vol.109, No.1, (January 1996), pp. 78-81, ISSN 0012-3692

Stratmann, G. & Gregory, G.A. (2003). Neurogenic and humoral vasoconstriction in acute pulmonary thromboembolism. *Anesthesia and analgesia*, Vol.97, No.2, (August 2003), pp. 341-54, ISSN 0003-2999

Sumii, T. & Lo, E.H. (2002). Involvement of matrix metalloproteinase in thrombolysis-associated hemorrhagic transformation after embolic focal ischemia in rats. *Stroke; a journal of cerebral circulation*, Vol.33, No.3, (March 2002), pp. 831-6, ISSN 0039-2499

Sárosi, I., Mühl, D., Bogár, L., Battyányi, I., Horváth, L. & Nemessányi, Z. (1995). [Treatment possibilities for extensive pulmonary embolism as an alternative to the Trendelenburg operation]. *Orvosi hetilap*, Vol.136, No.47, (November 1995), pp. 2553-9, ISSN 0030-6002

Sárosi, I., Mühl, D., Tekeres, M., Debreceni, G., Kónyi, A., Szabó, A., Farkasfalvi, K., Battyányi, I. & Horváth, L. (1997). [Lifesaving thrombolysis--in the light of contraindications]. *Orvosi hetilap*, Vol.138, No.49, (December 1997), pp. 3105-9, ISSN 0030-6002

Tapson, V.F. (2008). Acute pulmonary embolism. *The New England journal of medicine*, Vol.358, No.10, (March 2008), pp. 1037-52, ISSN 0028-4793

ten Wolde, M., Söhne, M., Quak, E., Mac Gillavry, M.R. & Büller, H.R. (2004). Prognostic value of echocardiographically assessed right ventricular dysfunction in patients with pulmonary embolism. *Archives of internal medicine*, Vol.164, No.15, (August 2004), pp. 1685-9, ISSN 0003-9926

The PIOPED Investigators. (1990). Value of the ventilation/perfusion scan in acute pulmonary embolism. Results of the prospective investigation of pulmonary embolism diagnosis (PIOPED). *JAMA: the journal of the American Medical Association*, Vol.263, No.20, (May 1990), pp. 2753-9, ISSN 0098-7484

Torbicki, A., van Beek, E.J.R., Charbonnier, B., Meyer, G., Morpurgo, M., Palla, A. & Perrier, A. (2000). Guidelines on diagnosis and management of acute pulmonary embolism. Task Force on Pulmonary Embolism, European Society of Cardiology. *European heart journal*, Vol.21, No.16, (August 2000), pp. 1301-36, ISSN 0195-668X

Torbicki, A., Galié, N., Covezzoli, A., Rossi, E., De Rosa, M. & Goldhaber, S.Z. (2003). Right heart thrombi in pulmonary embolism: results from the International Cooperative Pulmonary Embolism Registry. *Journal of the American College of Cardiology*, Vol.41, No.12, (June 2003), pp. 2245-51, ISSN 0735-1097

Torbicki, A., Perrier, A., Konstantinides, S., Agnelli, G., Galiè, N., Pruszczyk, P., Bengel, F., Brady, A.J.B., Ferreira, D., Janssens, U., Klepetko, W., Mayer, E., Remy-Jardin, M. & Bassand, J.-P. (2008). Guidelines on the diagnosis and management of acute pulmonary embolism: the Task Force for the Diagnosis and Management of Acute Pulmonary Embolism of the European Society of Cardiology (ESC). *European heart journal*, Vol.29, No.18, (September 2008), pp. 2276-315, ISSN 0735-1097

Tsuji, K., Aoki, T., Tejima, E., Arai, K., Lee, S.-R., Atochin, D.N., Huang, P.L., Wang, X., Montaner, J. & Lo, E.H. (2005). Tissue plasminogen activator promotes matrix metalloproteinase-9 upregulation after focal cerebral ischemia. *Stroke; a journal of cerebral circulation*, Vol.36, No.9, (September 2005), pp. 1954-9, ISSN 0039-2499

Uflacker, R. (2001). Interventional therapy for pulmonary embolism. *Journal of vascular and interventional radiology: JVIR*, Vol.12, No.2, (February 2001), pp. 147-64, ISSN 1051-0443

Uzuelli, J.A., Dias-Junior, C.A.C. & Tanus-Santos, J.E. (2008). Severity dependent increases in circulating cardiac troponin I and MMP-9 concentrations after experimental acute pulmonary thromboembolism. *Clinica chimica acta; international journal of clinical chemistry*, Vol.388, No.1-2, (February 2008), pp. 184-8, ISSN 0009-8981

van Belle, A., Büller, H.R., Huisman, M.V., Huisman, P.M., Kaasjager, K., Kamphuisen, P.W., Kramer, M.H.H., Kruip, M.J.H.A., Kwakkel-van Erp, J.M., Leebeek, F.W.G., Nijkeuter, M., Prins, M.H., Sohne, M. & Tick, L.W. (2006). Effectiveness of managing suspected pulmonary embolism using an algorithm combining clinical probability, D-dimer testing, and computed tomography. *JAMA: the journal of the American Medical Association*, Vol.295, No.2, (January 2006), pp. 172-9, ISSN 1538-3598

Van den Steen, P.E., Dubois, B., Nelissen, I., Rudd, P.M., Dwek, R.A. & Opdenakker, G. (2002). Biochemistry and molecular biology of gelatinase B or matrix metalloproteinase-9 (MMP-9). *Critical reviews in biochemistry and molecular biology*, Vol.37, No.6, (December 2002), pp. 375-536, ISSN 1040-9238

Walther, A., Schellhaass, A., Böttiger, B.W. & Konstantinides, S. (2009). [Diagnosis, therapy and secondary prophylaxis of acute pulmonary embolism. Presentation of and commentary on the new ESC 2008 guidelines]. *Der Anaesthesist*, Vol.58, No.10, (October 2009), pp. 1048-54, ISSN 0003-2417

Wan, S., Quinlan, D.J., Agnelli, G. & Eikelboom, J.W. (2004). Thrombolysis compared with heparin for the initial treatment of pulmonary embolism: a meta-analysis of the randomized controlled trials. *Circulation*, Vol.110, No.6, (August 2004), pp. 744-9, ISSN 0009-7322

Wang, X., Tsuji, K., Lee, S.-R., Ning, M., Furie, K.L., Buchan, A.M. & Lo, E.H. (2004). Mechanisms of hemorrhagic transformation after tissue plasminogen activator reperfusion therapy for ischemic stroke. *Stroke; a journal of cerebral circulation*, Vol.35, No.11 Suppl 1, (November 2004), pp. 2726-30, ISSN 0039-2499

Wells, P.S., Anderson, D.R., Rodger, M., Stiell, I., Dreyer, J.F., Barnes, D., Forgie, M., Kovacs, G., Ward, J. & Kovacs, M.J. (2001). Excluding pulmonary embolism at the bedside without diagnostic imaging: management of patients with suspected pulmonary embolism presenting to the emergency department by using a simple clinical model and d-dimer. *Annals of internal medicine*, Vol.135, No.2, (July 2001), pp. 98-107, ISSN 0003-4819

Wood, K.E. (2002). Major pulmonary embolism: review of a pathophysiologic approach to the golden hour of hemodynamically significant pulmonary embolism. *Chest*, Vol.121, No.3, (March 2002), pp. 877-905, ISSN 0012-3692

Worth, H. (2009). Aktuelles Management der akuten Lungenembolie. *Der Pneumologe*, Vol.6, No.6, (November 2009), pp. 378-389, ISSN 1613-5636

7

Ventilation Perfusion Single Photon Emission Tomography (V/Q SPECT) in the Diagnosis of Pulmonary Embolism

Michel Leblanc
Nuclear Medicine Department
Centre Hospitalier Régional de Trois-Rivières
University of Montreal
University of Sherbrooke
Canada

1. Introduction

Pulmonary embolism (PE) is a frequent and potentially lethal disease caused by the migration of a thrombus to the pulmonary circulation, typically from the venous system of the lower limbs. Unfortunately, there are no specific sets of symptoms which accurately predict or exclude the diagnosis. Therefore, in clinical practice, the diagnosis always strongly relies on imaging. On the other hand, clinical evaluation can predict the probability of embolism in a specific patient. This information can be used to select which patient can benefit most from imaging studies.

Historically, pulmonary angiography and planar ventilation perfusion (V/Q) scintigraphy were the main techniques available for identification of PE. Although traditionally viewed as the gold standard, pulmonary angiography is an invasive technique that suffers from significant limitations. It is not considered anymore as a suitable gold standard(Baile, King et al. 2000). V/Q scintigraphy was used extensively as a non-invasive alternative. It has a high sensitivity and a high negative predictive value. Unfortunately, the technique suffers from a large number of indeterminate studies in which the diagnosis of PE cannot be reliably confirmed or excluded. Indeed, in the PIOPED study, as much as 72% of cases were in that category. Although later studies substantially improved those numbers, the level of indeterminate findings remains high.

It is in that context that computed tomography pulmonary angiography (CTPA) emerged as an alternative non-invasive technique. CTPA carries the advantages of a much lower rate of indeterminate study and the ability to diagnose alternate conditions for the patient's symptoms. Also, the binary interpretation ("positive" vs "negative") was much more acceptable to physicians than the rather complex probabilistic system of V/Q scintigraphy. As such, it has become the principal imaging technique worldwide for the diagnosis of PE. In most centers, conventional planar V/Q scintigraphy is now a secondary technique used mainly when there are contraindications to CTPA or when CTPA is non-diagnostic or not available.

Nonetheless, CTPA also suffers from significant limitations. There are contraindications such as impaired renal function and allergies. The radiation dose is very high, especially to the female breast. Also, the performance of CTPA in terms of sensitivity and specificity is far from optimal, especially when judged according to the results of the PIOPED II study, which showed significant inaccuracies when the CTPA result was not in line with the clinical probability.

Therefore, there is still a need for other techniques. In that context, Ventilation Perfusion Single Photon Emission Computed Tomography (V/Q SPECT) is rapidly emerging as an interesting alternative. V/Q SPECT is a natural 3D tomographic extension of the conventional V/Q planar technique. It is used in many centers in Europe, Australia and Canada as well as in Asia. Its use in the United States has unfortunately been limited by the absence of FDA approval of Technegas, a superior ventilation imaging agent which is essential for the implementation of V/Q SPECT.

2. Basis of emboli detection by nuclear techniques

The major physiological consequence of PE is occlusion of a part of the pulmonary circulation. Usually, ventilation is preserved, resulting in increased dead space. Therefore, altered perfusion with normal ventilation is the usual consequence of PE. There are situations in which ventilation can be altered such as secondary lung infarct or atelectasis. In those cases, the chest x-ray is usually abnormal.

Nuclear techniques for the evaluation of regional ventilation and perfusion have existed for several decades. Ventilation is usually studied by inhalation of a radioactive gas or radioactive nebulised particles. Perfusion is studied by intravenous injection of radioactive particles (typically macroaggregates of albumin) which are trapped in the pulmonary circulation. In both cases, the distribution of radioactivity on the images is absolutely proportional to ventilation and perfusion. By comparing regional perfusion and ventilation, PE can be diagnosed as areas of absent perfusion with normal ventilation.

3. Technical aspects of V/Q SPECT

SPECT technique requires a ventilation agent which will distribute proportionately to true ventilation in the lungs. Also, once distributed, the agent has to remain fixed for the full period of the acquisition. Therefore, SPECT technique with a gas (xenon-133 or Krypton-81m) is not feasible with current technology, except if a steady state method is used which is complex and not practical in disease situations since it requires a high degree of patient collaboration with ventilation during the whole acquisition period. Therefore, evaluation of ventilation with gaseous agents is always done with a very limited number of planar views (often 1 or 2) and modern tomographic techniques (SPECT) are not clinically available.

SPECT is possible with radio-aerosols, such as DTPA-Tc99m, since these particles become impacted in the lung and their position remains relatively stable during the acquisition time. However, these aerosols, created by nebulisation, produce particles that are rather large (0,5 to 2,0 μm), that tend to deposit in the central airways to a certain degree, especially in chronic obstructive pulmonary disease (COPD). This leads to artefacts in the SPECT reconstruction and poor peripheral lung penetration. Images of suboptimal quality are produced, particularly in diseased lungs, in which mismatches can be missed or underestimated using these conventional aerosols.

Therefore, the use of newer generation ventilation agents such as Technegas is highly preferable. Technegas is an aerosol with very small technetium labelled solid graphite particles that are generated at high temperature using a specialized oven. The particle sizes are typically 0,005 to 0,2 μm and have a high alveolar penetration index. Ventilation distribution is highly related to those obtained with Krypton 81m (Peltier, De Faucal et al. 1990; Cook and Clarke 1992). The term pseudogas has been used to describe the agent, a reflection of the fact that its behaviour during inspiration is close to that of a true gas. The superiority of Technegas to conventional DTPA aerosols has been demonstrated in COPD (Yogi et al. 2010). There is limited central deposition except in severe COPD. Underestimation of true ventilation is not a problem. The particles are cleared from the lungs with a biological half-life of about 5 1/2 days. The agent is thus ideal for SPECT evaluation of true ventilation.

The perfusion technique has not changed significantly in last decades. It is accomplished by micro-embolization with radio-labelled particles injected into a peripheral vein. The particles are labelled with technetium-99m. Particle size is about 15 to 100μm. For a typical exam, about 400,000 labelled particles are injected. However, since there are about 300 million pre-capillary arterioles and 280 billion pulmonary capillaries, a very small percentage of the pulmonary circulation will be occluded. SPECT technique for perfusion is readily accomplished without artefacts.

In a clinical setting, ventilation is usually performed first with a smaller dose of radioactivity. Typically, the patient is asked to inhale Technegas through a tube set until the desired quantity of radioactivity is present in the lungs, typically 20-50 mega Becquerels (MBq). Usually, 2 to 5 breaths are required. The activity can be standardized in each department either through counting directly under the scintillation camera or with a portable Geiger counter. Patients are then positioned under the camera for image acquisition.

The perfusion study is then performed with a higher dose of radioactivity. In most centers, a ratio of perfusion to ventilation activity of 4 to 1 is considered adequate. The injected dose should be tailored to insure such a ratio. Administered intravenous dose of labelled particles will typically be in the range of 100 to 250 MBq for most patients. Both ventilation and perfusion should be performed in the supine position to minimize regional gradients.

4. SPECT acquisition protocol

The protocol can be tailored to a certain point to the preference of the different centers. The number of tomographic steps should be at least 64 while 128 are considered optimal. Higher radiation doses will permit either higher-quality images or faster acquisition times. If a lower dose range is preferred, a general-purpose collimator which has a higher sensitivity (but a lower resolution) can be used. With such a collimator, using a 64 X 64 matrix, acquisition time can be as low as 5 second per step with perfusion and 10 seconds per step in ventilation in a 128 step protocol with 20-25 MBq in ventilation and 100-120 MBq in perfusion (Palmer, Bitzen et al. 2001). Using a high-resolution collimator and a matrix of 128 X 128 will produce higher-quality images at the expense of a higher radiation dose and longer acquisition times. Depending on the number of steps, the activity will be more in the range of 35-40 MBq in ventilation and 180-200 MBq in perfusion and the time per step will be 15-20 seconds in ventilation and 7-10 seconds in perfusion. Reconstruction of the data should be iterative using OSEM (ordered subset expectation maximization). Eight subsets and two iterations are recommended. Using a higher number of subsets and iterations may produce sharper images but noise will also be increased. However, every center can optimize their protocol.

Image display should strive to match precisely each ventilation slice with the corresponding perfusion slice in all three planes (transverse, coronal, sagittal). This can be easily done either by not moving the patient or bed position between ventilation and perfusion or, alternatively, by using commercially available software which will co-register each set of images.

5. Image interpretation

In a normal patient, perfusion and ventilation are both homogeneous (figure1). There is usually a ventilation and perfusion gradient which increases from the anterosuperior to the posteroinferior region of the lungs. There is often a thin band of hyperventilation located in the lower two thirds of the posterior aspect of both lungs. The normal indentations of the mediastinum should be recognized.

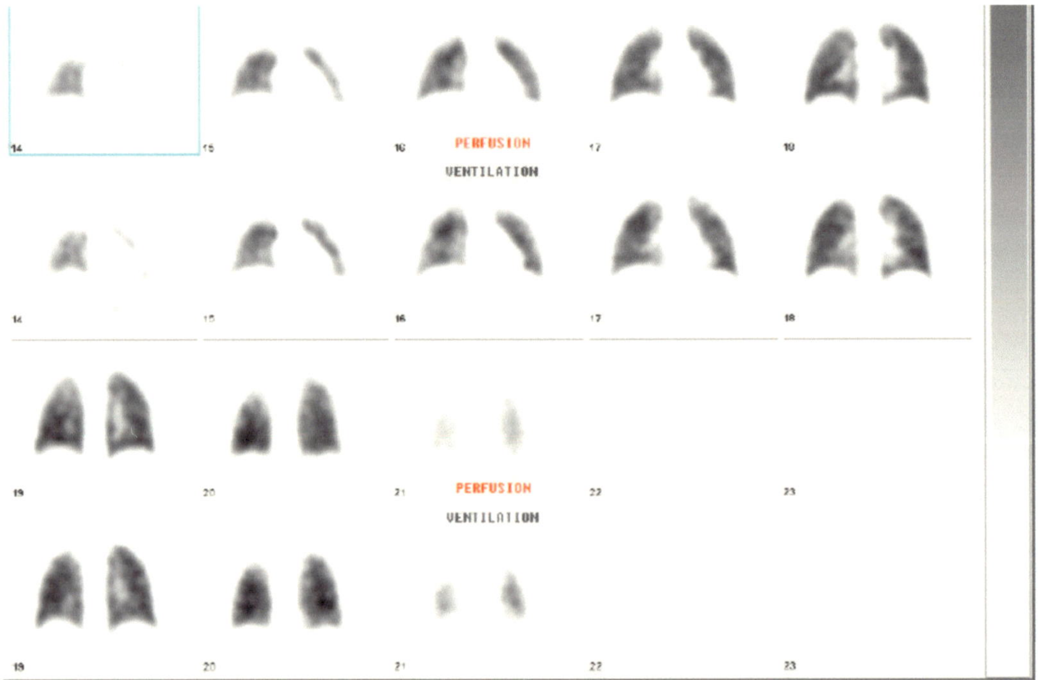

Fig. 1. Normal perfusion and ventilation coronal SPECT slices.

Non-segmental partial mismatches (preserved ventilation with abnormal perfusion) can occur in normal subjects. Physiologically, they are explained by the fact that ventilation with Technegas is usually evaluated with deep breathing. Such deep breathing can temporarily overcome partially compressed lung and result in hyperventilation. Those lung sections are usually poorly ventilated with tidal breathing. Since perfusion will be physiologically matched to tidal breathing, this explains the potential for partial mismatches. Perfusion is usually maintained to some degree (figure 2). The most common areas are the medial postero-inferior regions of both lungs because of compression by the mediastinum in the supine position. Both the inferior and posterior costal phrenic angles are also often subject to this phenomenon (figure 3). Also, the superior portion of the large fissure may be the site of a small mismatch. None of these anomalies follow the topography of normal lung vessels.

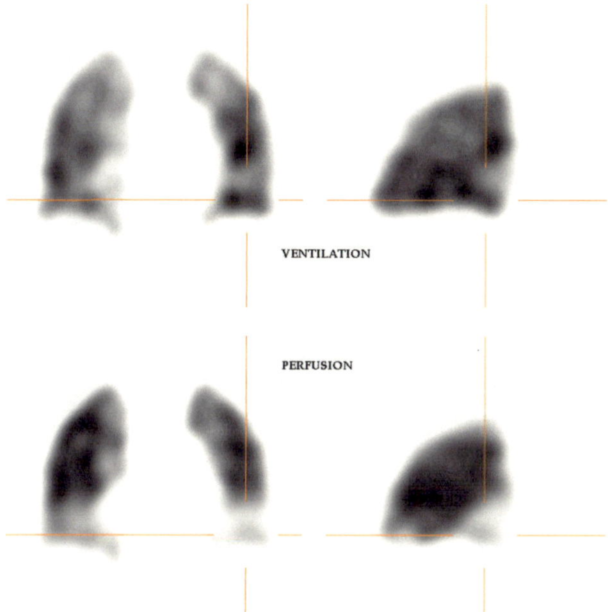

Fig. 2. Passive atelectasis (coronal and sagittal slice triangulation). Note non-segmental partial mismatch.

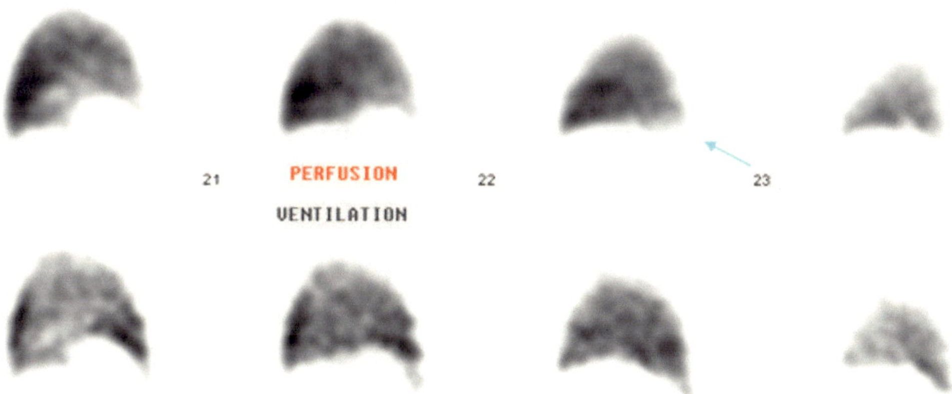

Fig. 3. Sagittal SPECT slices showing non-embolic mismatch at posterior costophrenic angle caused by lung compression.

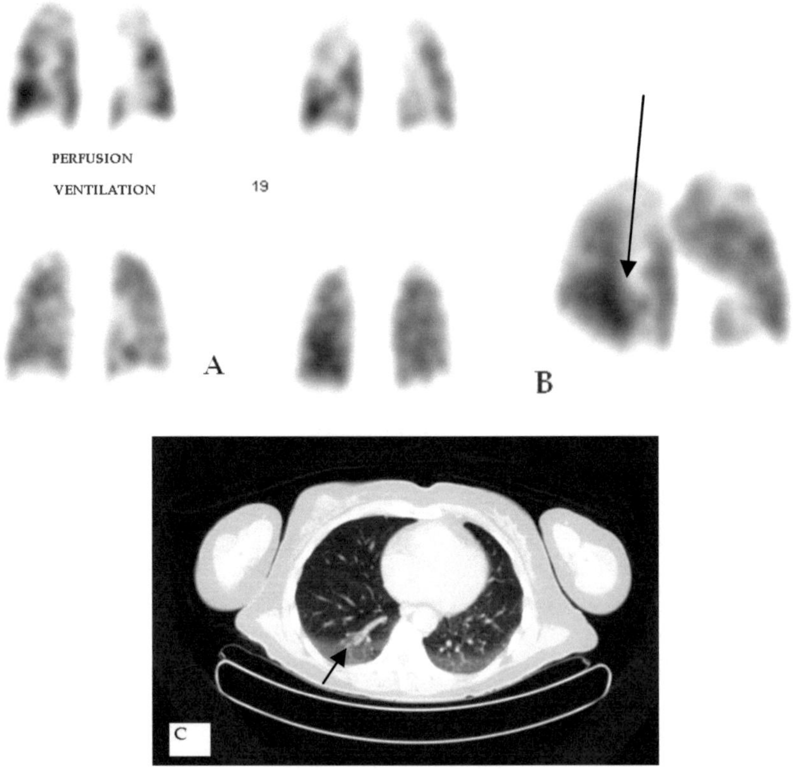

Fig. 4. Gravity dependant atelectasis. (A) Coronal slices centered on posterior surface of the lungs show diffuse shallow non segmental partial mismatches. (B) Excerpt from a 3D reconstruction of perfusion in oblique view showing a topography totally incompatible with a vascular origin. (C) CT of another patient showing the typical pattern of gravity dependent atelectasis on posterior surfaces.

In some patients, gravity dependent atelectasis can result in widespread partial mismatches on the posterior surface of both lungs. This pattern is usually easily recognized by the occurrence of multiple shallow perfusion defects which are often in a linear pattern (figure 4). A 3D display will often best demonstrate the topography.

PE is diagnosed when there is a severe and well demarcated perfusion defect which is pleural-based and clearly larger at the periphery (typically wedge-shaped, triangular or half-oval). Small size partial defects that are not well defined are much less specific and should be ignored in most acute settings, even if they are partially mismatched. The defect should clearly follow an orientation compatible with known pulmonary vascular anatomy. Ventilation should be normal or at least much better preserved than perfusion. One such large sub-segmental defect is sufficient for the diagnosis (figure 5 & 6). There are however multiple mismatched regions in most cases (figures 7, 8 & 12). For smaller sub-segmental defects, at least two are required for a confident diagnosis (figure 9 & 11). Distal PE is usually totally occlusive. However, more proximal PE (i.e.: lobar) can be partially occlusive and the perfusion defect may at times be moderate. It should be remembered that an isolated whole lung mismatch is usually not caused by PE but rather by compression of the main pulmonary artery by a mediastinal or hilar lesion.

The preceding discussion applies only to acute pulmonary embolism. In the sub-acute or chronic phases, when partial reperfusion has occurred, the aspect can vary considerably and interpretation can be less straightforward because strange shaped partial mismatches can occasionally be seen in this setting.

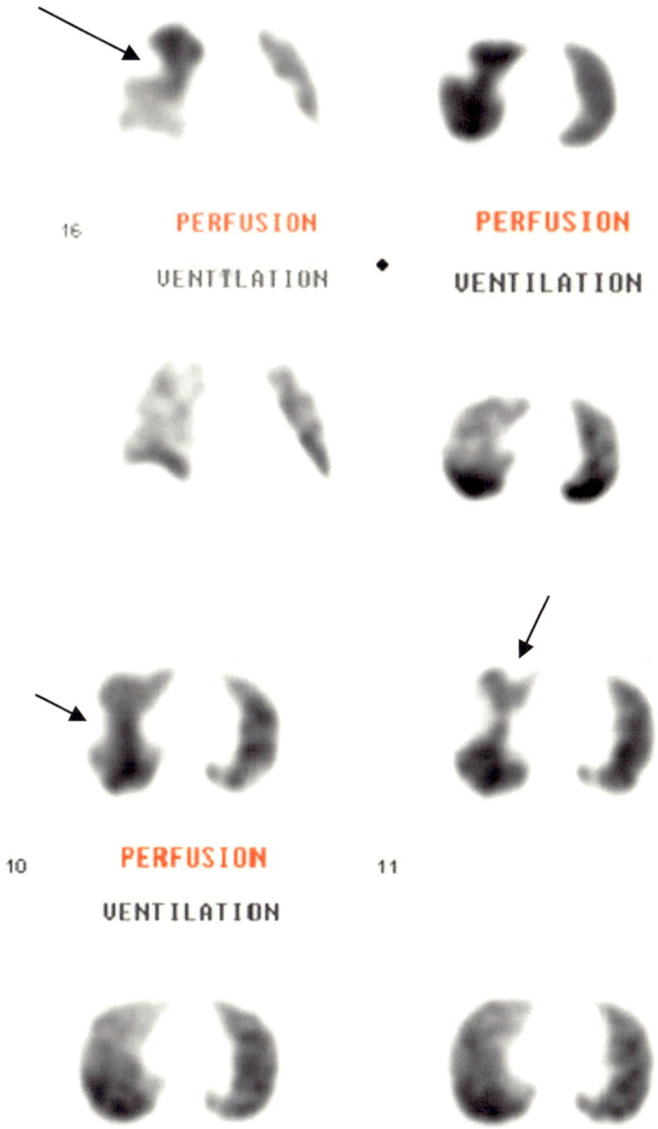

Fig. 5. Typical wedge-shaped emboli in two different patients (coronal and transverse slices)

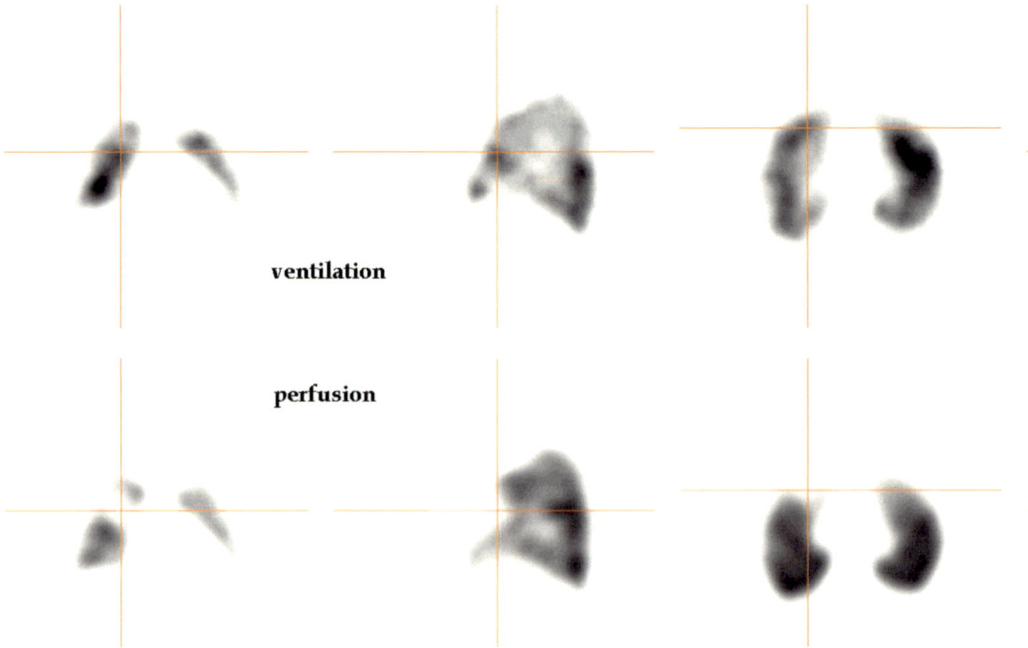

Fig. 6. Typical embolus, coronal, sagittal and transverse slice triangulation.

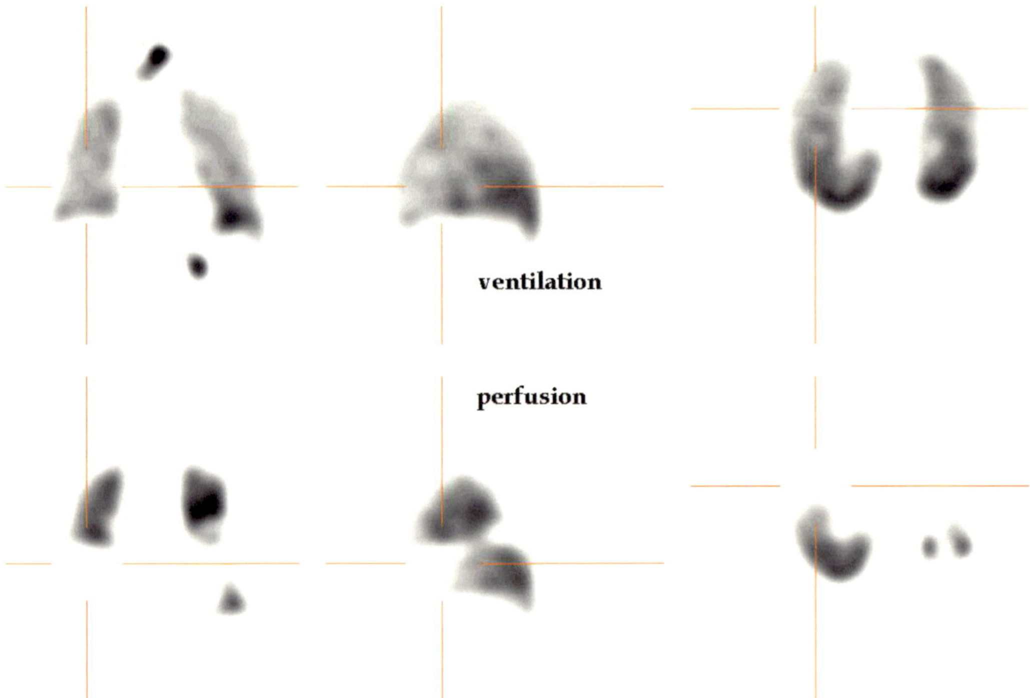

Fig. 7. Multiple emboli.

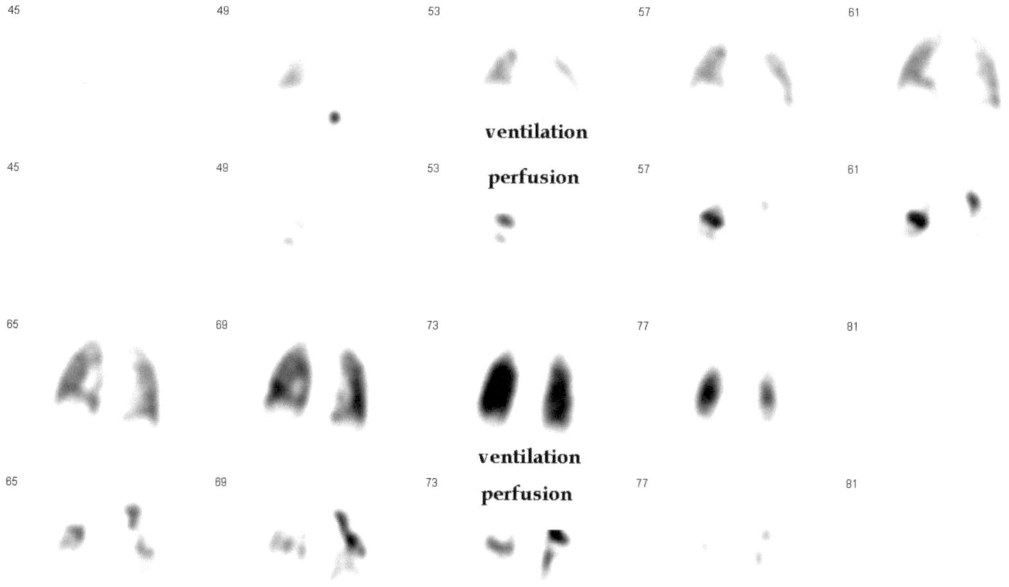

Fig. 8. Massive embolism (co-registered coronal slices). Ventilation slices are on 1st and 3rd row. Corresponding perfusion slices on 2nd and 4th row show massive areas of vascular amputation with preserved ventilation.

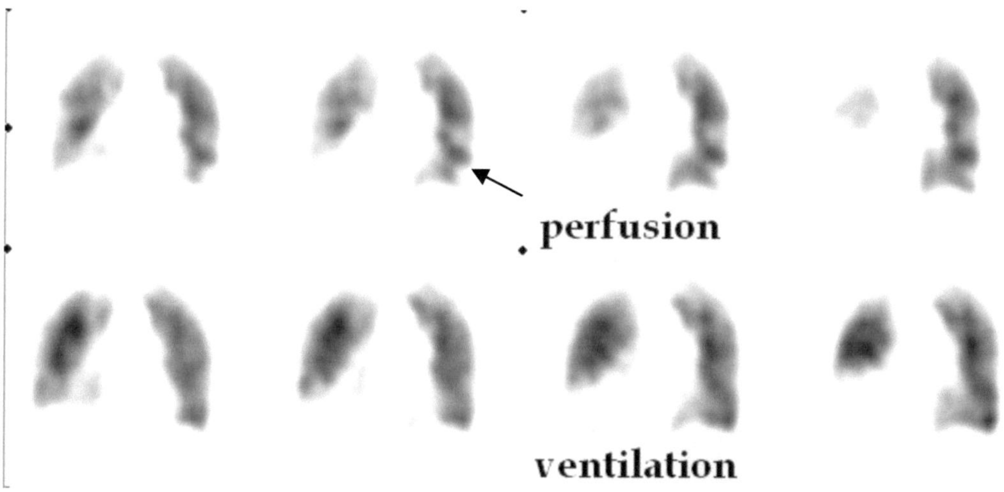

Fig. 9. Small left sub-segmental embolus. Pleural effusion is noted on the right side (co-registered coronal slices)

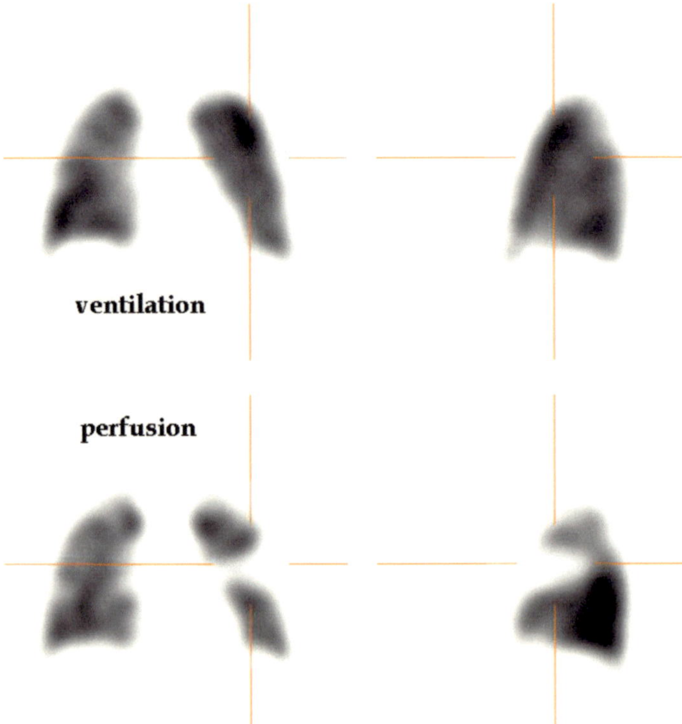

Fig. 10. Typical wedge-shaped embolus.

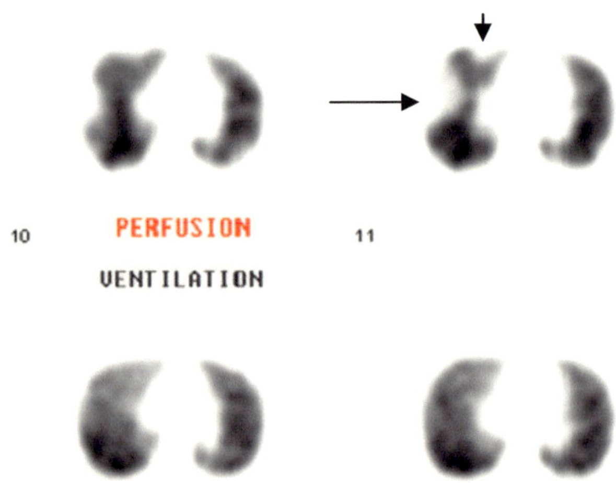

Fig. 11. Example of segmental (long arrow) and subsegmental (short arrow) emboli.

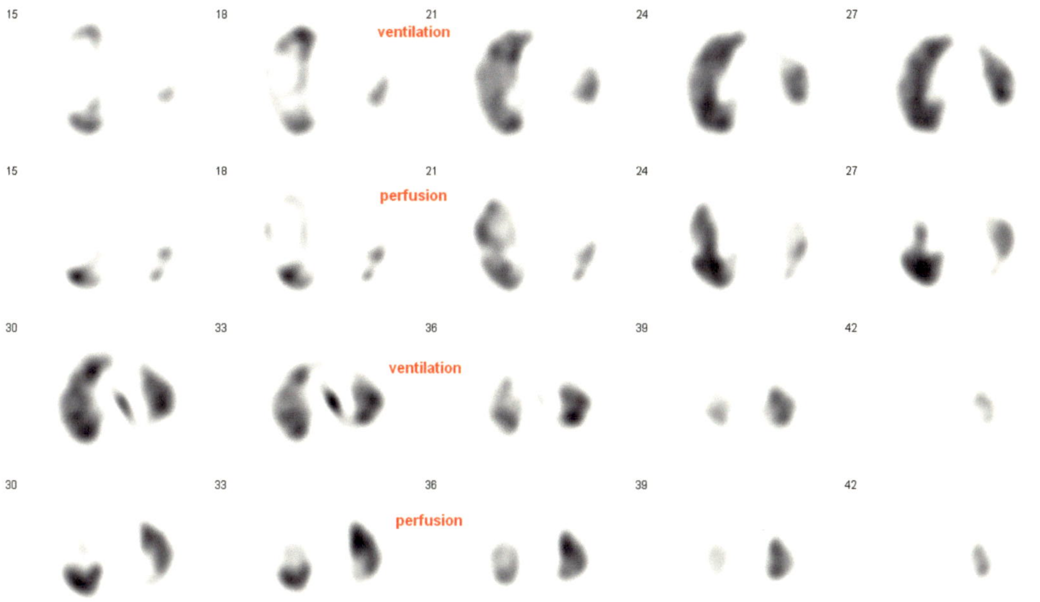

Fig. 12. Transverse slices showing multiple right sided emboli. Pleural effusion on left.

Probabilistic interpretation with classification of cases into "normal", "low", "indeterminate" or "high" probability which is still in use with planar scintigraphy is absolutely not warranted with V/Q SPECT. Indeed, there has been no study to specifically address the validity of probabilistic interpretation with V/Q SPECT. Therefore, using a probabilistic interpretation in that context has no scientific basis. All authors that have published on the subject have used a straightforward positive-negative approach and it is the only one that is acceptable. It makes no sense to use a mode of interpretation that has been motivated by the use of an inferior ventilation agent (xenon-133) in a single planar view, associated with planar perfusion imaging. As for any other type of imaging, a very narrow indeterminate category can be acceptable for highly atypical cases.

Causes of non-embolic pathological mismatches are well known and are essentially the same with V/Q SPECT as they are with the conventional planar V/Q scintigraphy. They may be the source of false-positive readings. Septic, fat or amniotic fluid embolization may occasionally occur in specific settings. The mismatches are usually small. Intravenous illicit drug use may occasionally result in small sized mismatches, although larger mismatches may occur. Vasculitis can be considered when clinically appropriate. A compression of a segmental or sub-segmental branch of the pulmonary artery by a lung nodule can be rarely seen. Much more frequent is a very large mismatch caused by a compression of hilar or mediastinal origin. Small partial mismatches can also occur in emphysematous bullae (Figure 13) because of occasional penetration of Technegas. However, the mismatch does not usually have a vascular pattern and is typically located at the apex. Lung scarring or fibrosis can also cause small or partial mismatches. Rarely, asthma can present with some strange looking small but multiple partial mismatches, presumably because there can be a lag time between restoration of regional ventilation and adjustment of the physiologically matched perfusion anomaly (figure 14). In such cases, V/Q SPECT will normalise after 24 hours of aerosol therapy.

It is therefore highly recommended that image interpretation is made with full knowledge of the clinical data and that correlation should be made with a recent chest x-ray. Correlation with existing anterior thoracic CT may be helpful in selected pathological cases. In this manner, high specificity can be achieved. Also, equivocal cases should be interpreted in light of the pre-test probability and knowledge of prior pulmonary pathology. Evidently, knowledge of prior PE or venous thrombotic disease is essential for the correct interpretation of positive cases. This type of interpretation ("holistic" or "Gestalt") is now considered as standard in most parts of the world and has been officially endorsed by the guidelines of the European Association of nuclear medicine (Bajc, Neilly et al. 2009).

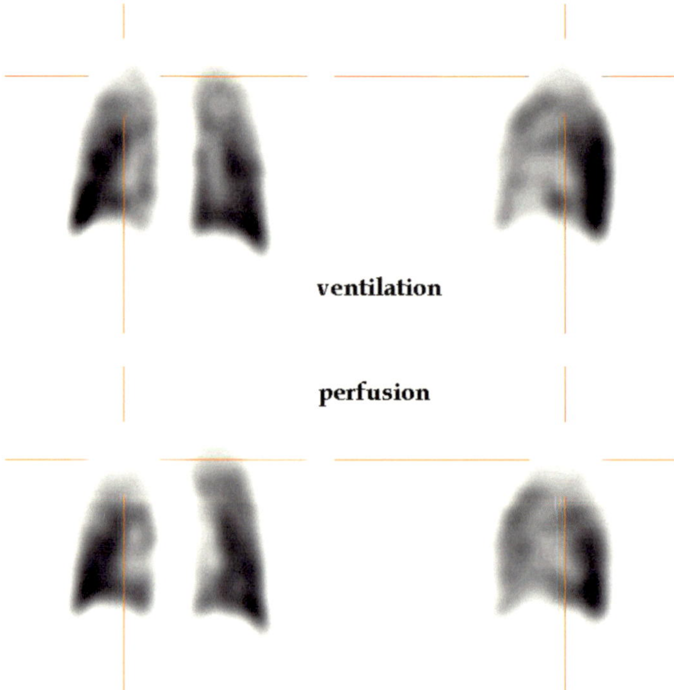

Fig. 13. Small apical mismatch caused by a bullae. This should be suspected in all non-segmental apical mismatch, although scarring may also cause a similar image.

6. Some non-embolic pathological patterns that can be recognized on V/Q SPECT

Although other pulmonary pathologies are not an indication for V/Q SPECT, diagnostic patterns have been described and validated for several situations and their recognition can provide useful information to the referring physician.

6.1 COPD

In COPD, ventilation is usually diffusely more affected than perfusion. The exact configuration depends on the severity of the process as well as the relative contribution of emphysema and bronchitis (figures 15 to 17). With a relatively pure bronchitis, the changes

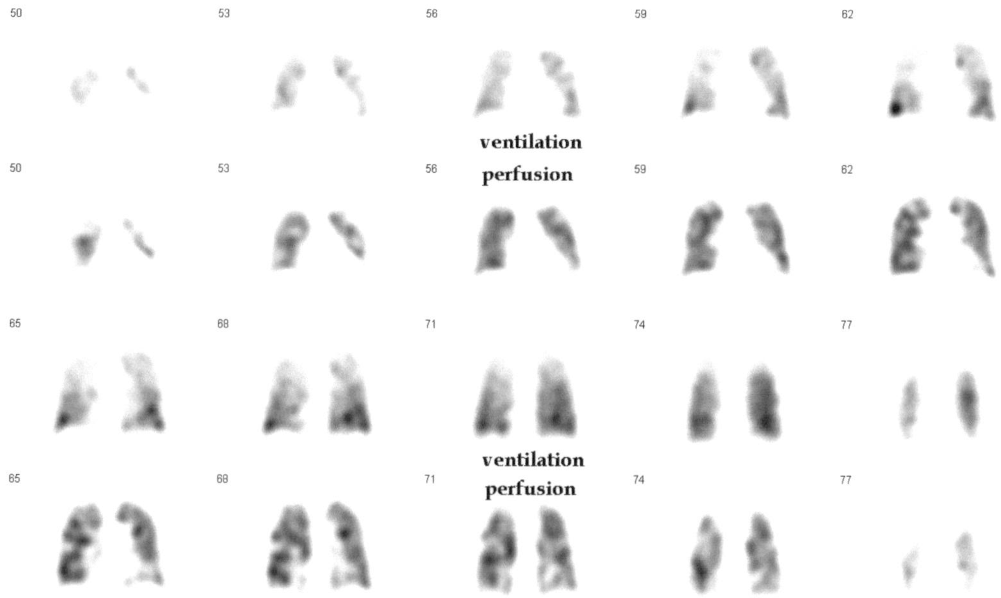

Fig. 14. Asthma, acute attack (retrospective diagnosis). Aerosol therapy was begun before V/Q SPECT. Notice multiple non-vascular looking partial mismatches.

are mainly seen on the ventilation part of this study. Distribution is heterogeneous and, in the more severe cases, there may be focal deposition of Technegas in Airways. With advanced disease, there may be widespread focal deposition. On the other hand, perfusion is usually better preserved. With a pattern of relatively pure and advanced emphysema, perfusion and ventilation are more matched, reflecting mainly focal architectural pulmonary changes. It has been demonstrated that the degree of heterogeneity on the ventilation study, as well as the degree of heterogeneity of perfusion and ventilation matching, are both proportional to the severity of COPD. In fact, these measures appear to be more sensitive to the presence of COPD than high-resolution CT which, despite its higher resolution, has a limited capacity for the detection of airway closure. However, heterogeneous distribution of ventilation and perfusion can also be found in pulmonary oedema, lung fibrosis and infectious or non-infectious diffuse lung inflammation.

6.2 Cardiac failure and volume overload

Although pulmonary oedema is usually well demonstrated on a chest x-ray, in the early stages of volume overload the only sign will be vascular redistribution to the upper lung zone. On a V/Q SPECT study, this is very easily appreciated. Typically, the examination being performed in a supine position, redistribution will be most marked anteriorly and superiorly and will usually be much more apparent on perfusion then on ventilation (figure 18). In the earliest stages, the ventilation gradient will be totally preserved which produces a rather large scale partial mismatch. It is important that this pattern be recognized and not confused with bilateral partially occluding inferior lobar PE. It should be noted that cardiac failure is not the only cause of vascular redistribution. Volume overload, whether iatrogenic or caused by hepatic of renal failure may produce the same images.

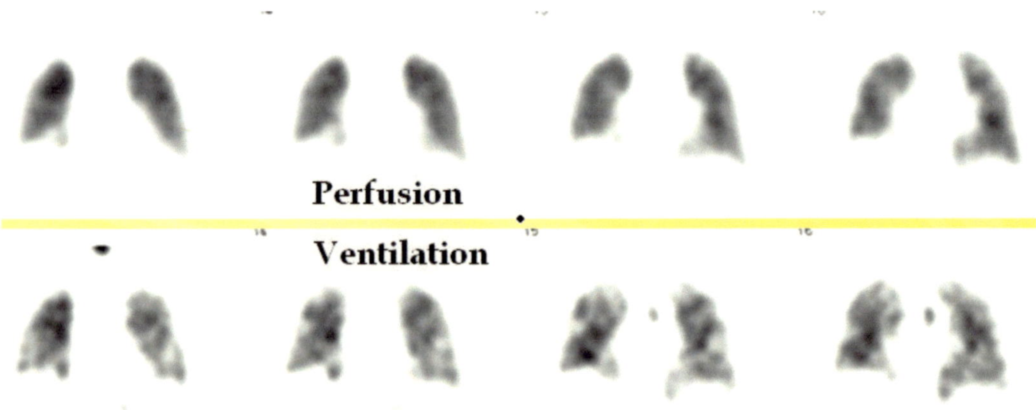

Fig. 15. Mild to moderate COPD (selected coronal slices). Diffusely mottled ventilation with better preservation of perfusion.

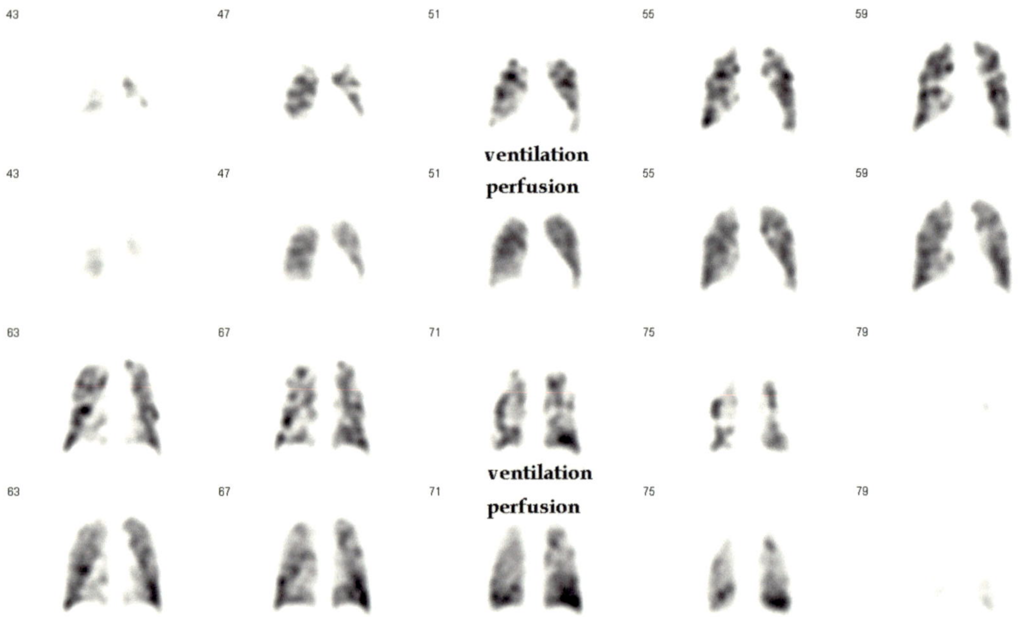

Fig. 16. Moderate COPD. Focal deposition of Technegas with heterogeneous ventilation. Perfusion is also mottled but to a lesser degree.

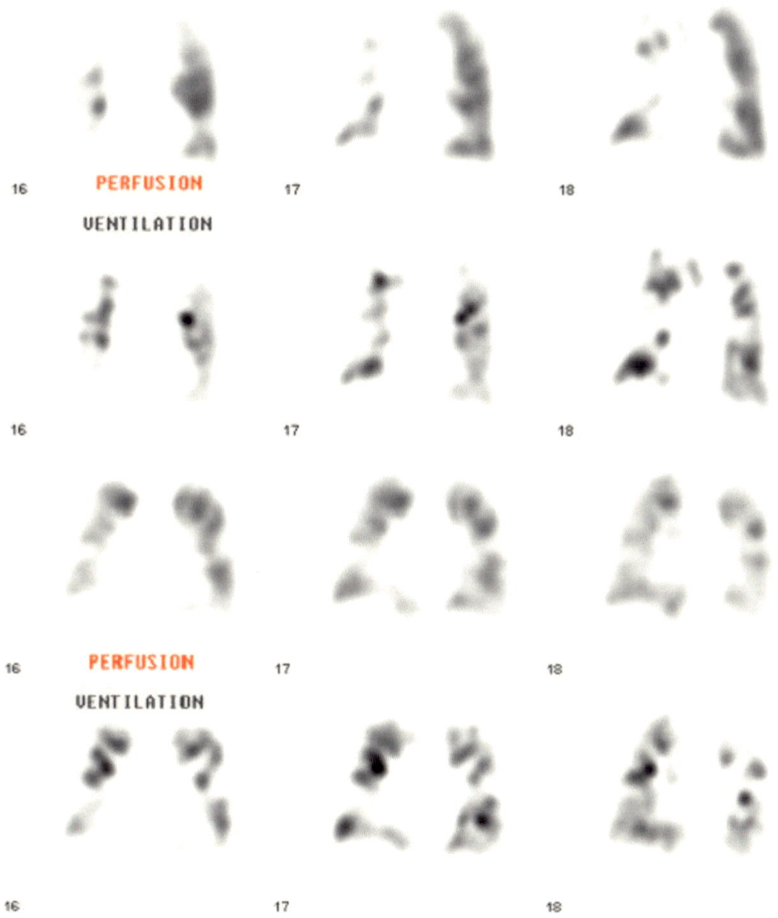

Fig. 17. Severe COPD. Multiple matched perfusion and ventilation defects associated with focal deposition on ventilation.

6.3 Pneumonia and atelectasis

In most cases, ventilation will be totally absent while perfusion will be partially preserved at least to some extent. Sometimes, a pattern of total reverse mismatch will be observed (absent ventilation with normal perfusion). It is unusual for PE to present with absent ventilation and some degree of residual perfusion. Also, in many cases of pneumonia, the distribution of the defect will not be compatible with a vascular anomaly (not pleural based, trans-segmental or orientation not compatible with vascular anatomy). Preservation of some perfusion in the presence of an x-ray anomaly favours a non-embolic cause (figure 19).

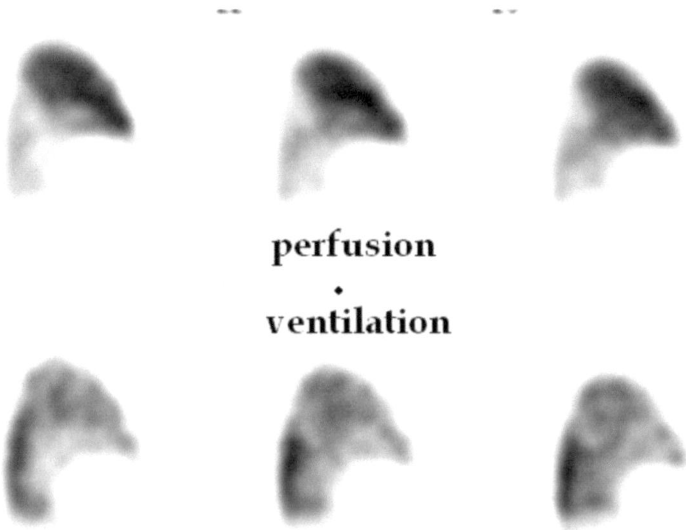

Fig. 18. Cardiac failure (volume overload). Note vascular redistribution to the super-anterior regions while normal gradient is preserved in ventilation.

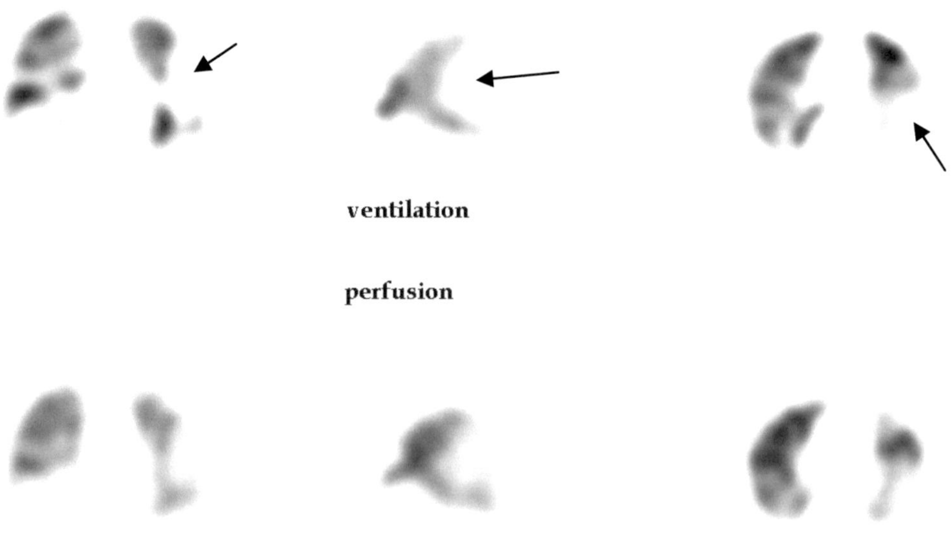

Fig. 19. Pneumonia (triangulation in coronal, sagittal and tranverse slices). Note the large trans-segmental defect. Absent ventilation with some partial residual perfusion.

6.4 Interstitial pneumonitis

Some recent work suggests that usual interstitial pneumonitis (UIP) can give rise to a rather specific pattern of sub pleural mismatch of crescent shape (Suga, Kawakami et al. 2009). The posterior surfaces of the lungs have to be excluded from the analysis however because in a supine position, this phenomenon is frequently observed because of gravity dependent atelectasis.

6.5 Pleural effusion

Pleural effusions of significant size are usually well recognized on V/Q SPECT. On transverse sections, the patient being in a supine position, the lung is displaced in the anterior direction as the effusion occupies the posterior region. On sagittal slices, there is loss of posterior angle. The perfusion and ventilation are typically matched although a thin band of hyperventilation is common at the lung-effusion interface because of compressed lung tissue. It is not uncommon however that the perfusion is better preserved. In that case, there is failure of the vasoconstriction reflex combined with lung compression which cannot be overcome by deep inspiration. For confident interpretation of a non-embolic effusion, there should not be any mismatches elsewhere and there should not be any hint of a wedge-shaped perfusion defect underlying the effusion (mismatched or not) (figures 20 and 21).

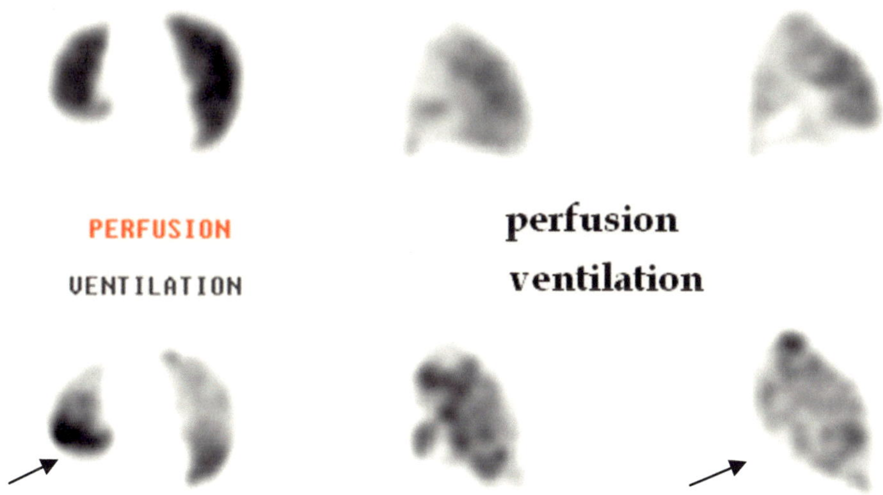

Fig. 20. Pleural effusion. Left: transverse slices show upward displacement of lung on both ventilation and perfusion, creating a non-segmental defect. Note band of hyperventilation indicating partially compressed lung. Right: sagittal slices in another patient show relatively preserved perfusion but absent ventilation. In this case, the effusion does not permit lung expansion.

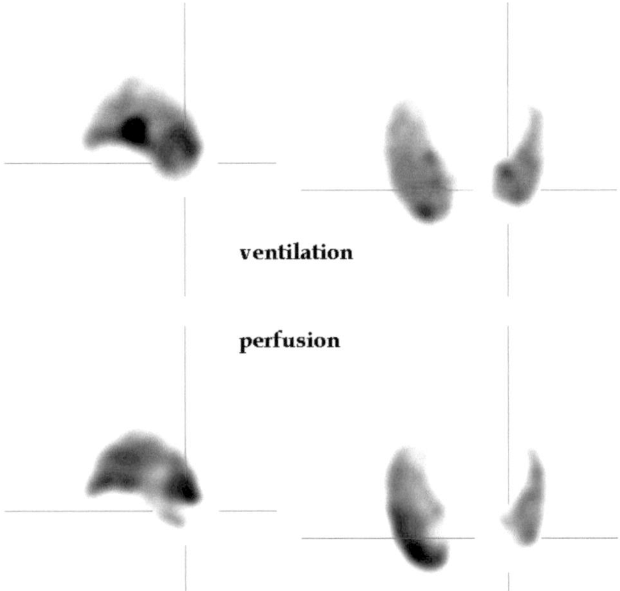

Fig. 21. Pleural effusion caused by embolism (sagittal and transverse slices). Note upward displacement of right lung by the effusion with an underlying. wedge shaped sub-segmental mismatched defect.

6.6 Reverse mismatches

In most physiological and pathological conditions, ventilation and perfusion are matched. This is accomplished by the pulmonary vasoconstriction reflex which diverts blood away from poorly ventilated areas to prevent a right to left shunt equivalent. Indeed, perfusion of non-ventilated areas causes non-oxygenated blood to return to the arterial circulation and this has a profound impact on the arterial oxygen pressure (figure 22). Failure of the vasoconstriction reflex is not an uncommon finding on V/Q SPECT imaging. It is often seen in the context of pneumonia (established or pre-radiological), atelectasis or bronchial mucous plug in COPD patients. It is important to report this finding as it represents an obvious cause to the patient's oxygen saturation problems. Reverse mismatch in the context of emboli is extremely uncommon as it requires causation of a ventilation anomaly which persists with reperfusion, without any other mismatches elsewhere. It is theoretically possible in the sub acute phase.

7. Validation of V/Q SPECT

7.1 Theoretical basis

SPECT has proven advantageous in just about every field in nuclear medicine. It is now standard procedure either as the sole examination (myocardial perfusion imaging and brain imaging) or a very useful adjunct to just about every other organ imaging (bone, gallium, white blood cell, liver, hemangioma, somatostatin). The theoretical advantages in lung imaging are the same as they are in every other organ: suppression of overlapping structures, better imaging contrast and 3-D representation of the data. Better depiction of sub-segmental and even some segmental defects is expected, resulting in better sensitivity.

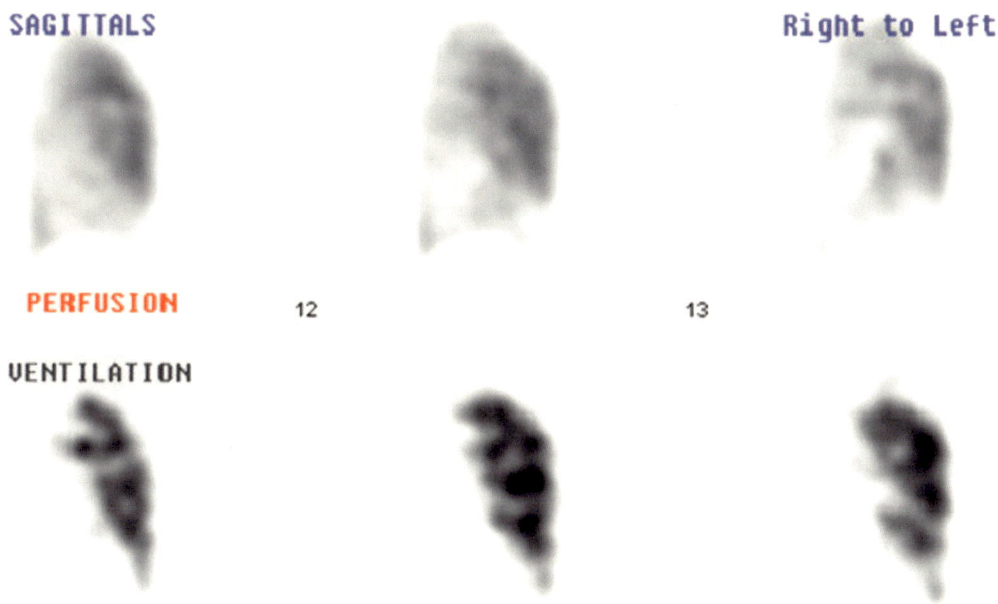

Fig. 22. Reverse mismatch. Sagittal slices show absent ventilation to inferior lobe with relative preservation of perfusion. In such a case, there is a huge amount of un-oxygenated blood returned to the arterial circulation, causing hypoxemia. In this case, a mucous plug in a COPD patient was the culprit.

Also, with 3-D data, the assignment of a defect to a vascular or non-vascular origin is much easier which will result in both better specificity and a much lower rate of indeterminate study.

7.2 Computer modeling

The superiority of V/Q SPECT (sensitivity 97%) to planar imaging (sensitivity 77%) was tested in a computer model which clearly predicted much better accuracy with V/Q SPECT (Magnussen, Chicco et al. 1999). It is very interesting to note that this model accurately predicted the results of clinical studies which would appear several years later.

7.3 Animal studies

The technique was also tested in a pig model with artificially produced small size emboli (Bajc, Bitzen et al. 2002). Again, the superiority of V/Q SPECT to planar imaging was clearly demonstrated, as sensitivity for V/Q SPECT was 91% while it was 64% for planar imaging for the same emboli. Specificity was also better for SPECT (87% vs 79%). It should be mentioned that a similar model had been employed earlier for validation of invasive pulmonary angiography and that the performance numbers in terms of sensitivity and specificity were no better than that obtained with V/Q SPECT (Baile, King et al. 2000).

7.4 Validation with alternative perfusion techniques

New generation techniques to measure regional perfusion independently (by opposition to simply visualizing the artery and the thrombus) by means of perfusion thoracic CT (Wildberger, Klotz et al. 2005) or nuclear magnetic resonance (NMR) (Kluge, Gerriets et al. 2006) have correlated very well with V/Q SPECT measures of regional perfusion. Indeed, work with those techniques suggests that embolism is almost always totally occlusive and that inclusion of perfusion data enhances sensitivity over an approach based purely on luminology.

7.5 Clinical studies

It is beyond the scope of this chapter to review individually all studies. However, even if proof of superiority of V/Q SPECT to planar imaging seems redundant, it has been proven clinically, with V/Q SPECT having an edge in sensitivity of more than 20% while still maintaining better specificity (Gutte, Mortensen et al. 2010; Bajc, Olsson et al. 2004). The negative predictive value of V/Q SPECT (the ability to reliably exclude PE) has been validated and is excellent, in the order of 98-99%, even in the presence of abnormal perfusion with a nonvascular pattern (Leblanc, Leveillee et al. 2007). Sensitivity is in the range of 96-99% and specificity hovers between 85% and 98%, depending on the study. The rate of non-diagnostic studies is 1-3%. Comparison to CTPA is unfortunately limited because of the lack of a large-scale prospective study comparing both techniques. A detailed discussion on each of the available studies can be found elsewhere (Leblanc and Paul 2010). However, all published studies have demonstrated that V/Q SPECT performs at least as well as CTPA for the diagnosis of pulmonary embolism (Reinartz, Wildberger et al. 2004; Suga, Yasuhiko et al. 2008; Gutte, Mortensen et al. 2009; Miles, Rogers et al. 2009).

8. V/Q SPECT and CTPA: Relative advantages and limitations

8.1 Diagnostic performance

Although a large randomized prospective study comparing the two techniques is not available, the pooled published results suggest at this point that V/Q SPECT may have an edge in sensitivity while CTPA may have an edge on specificity. Better sensitivity of V/Q SPECT can be attributed essentially to sub-segmental embolism. Indeed, to visualize directly a thrombus in a sub-segmental vessel is difficult even with the latest CTPA technology. Also, existing literature suggest that inter-observer agreement is very low for sub-segmental embolism with CTPA (Ghanima, Nielssen et al. 2007). Since V/Q SPECT visualizes the resulting perfusion defect, it has a clear advantage. Indeed, even for a small sub-segmental defect implicating 25% of a segment, the pleural base of the defect will have at least 3 cm, a dimension easily resolved by the SPECT technique. On the other hand, since CTPA directly visualizes a filling defect, it is less prone to false positive studies since most (but not all) filling defects will represent embolus. This may not be true of sub-segmental emboli because the poor inter-observer agreement in this setting suggests limited specificity. Causes of false-positive mismatches on V/Q SPECT have been discussed earlier. Causes of false-positive filling defect on CTPA do exist and have been discussed elsewhere (Kuriakose and Patel 2010). Indeterminate interpretation is usually low for CTPA and is generally related to technical factors. It is also very low for V/Q SPECT, occurring in less than 5% of cases in all published studies. Finally, different studies have proven that both techniques have a high negative predictive value (capacity to exclude) for PE (Leblanc, Leveillee et al. 2007).

8.2 Radiation dose

Estimated radiation dose is a complex subject and a detailed discussion is beyond the scope of this chapter and can be found elsewhere (Schembri, Miller et al. 2010). However, there is little doubt that when comparing state-of-the-art technology for both modalities, incurred radiation dose is much higher with CTPA and this is particularly true of the female breast. Depending on the exact protocol that is employed, total radiation dose for CTPA is in the range of 8-20 milliSievert (mSv) while it is 2,0 - 3,5 mSv for V/Q SPECT. The dose to the female breast varies between 10 and 70 mSv for CTPA (equivalent to 10-25 mammograms or 100-400 chest x-rays) while the corresponding breast dose for V/Q SPECT is less than 1,5 mSv.

8.3 Contraindications and technical success rate

There are no contraindications to V/Q SPECT imaging. Some degree of prudence is required in cases of severe pulmonary hypertension (the number of particle injected should be limited) and reasonable efforts should be made to limit the dose during pregnancy, but any patient may undergo V/Q SPECT as long as he can tolerate a supine position for 20 min. Allergies are virtually nonexistent. There are no known deleterious effects on any organ system.

On the other hand, CTPA has specific contraindications. Allergies are relatively frequent and, depending on the severity, constitute an absolute or relative contraindication. If the decision is made to proceed with the study, patients must be prepared appropriately. Also, because of the injection of contrast, renal failure is a possible complication especially in patients with established underlying renal disease. In some subgroups, the risk of renal failure requiring dialysis is extremely high.

Performance in pregnancy has also been reviewed (Ridge, McDermott et al. 2009). The radiation dose to the foetus is very low for both techniques (< 1mSv) although it is significantly lower for CTPA. However, at this level, there is no increased risk for either technique. On the other hand, it is clear that the technical performance of CTPA in pregnancy is poor, with as many as one third of the studies being technically inadequate. This is probably due to increased pressure in the inferior vena cava during pregnancy with aspiration of large amounts of non-opacified blood during inspiration that interferes with optimal mixing of contrast coming from the superior vena cava. There are no technical limits to V/Q SPECT during pregnancy. Therefore, V/Q SPECT should be the preferred modality in this situation, especially considering the very high breast radiation dose given with CTPA in young patients with actively proliferating breasts.

High-quality imaging with CTPA requires accurate timing for contrast injection. In most studies, the technical failure rate hovers between 5 and 10%. The technical success rate for

VQ SPECT is extremely high, with failure occurring in less then 1% of cases in all studies. Using Technegas as a ventilation agent, it is possible to ventilate patients on mechanical ventilation.

8.4 Performance in difficult patients: COPD and abnormal x-ray

The presence of COPD is generally thought to decrease the usefulness of V/Q scanning. However, this stems from the use of a planar technique using an inferior ventilation agent (xenon-133) interpreted in probabilistic terms according to the PIOPED scheme. This is much less true with V/Q SPECT in which a superior ventilation agent is used (technegas) and determination of the nature of a vascular defect is much easier. In COPD, ventilation is often much more affected than perfusion and is it is generally possible to distinguish vascular from nonvascular type defects following the definition outlined above for PE. Also, in COPD, emboli will always follow vascular flow which, by definition, always corresponds to residual ventilated areas, thus permitting the identification of a mismatch. However, in cases of very severe COPD where there are very few residual normally ventilated regions, interpretation may be more difficult and theoretically, sensitivity may be decreased. There are however no studies to prove this point.

There are no data suggesting that the performance of CTPA is altered by the presence of severe COPD. Therefore, in severe COPD, with a high pre-test likelihood of PE and with a V/Q SPECT difficult to interpret, CTPA may be warranted.

The presence of an abnormal lung x-ray causes special problems in nuclear imaging. Embolism detection is based on a mismatch between ventilation and perfusion. Ventilation is rarely possible in the presence of atelectasis, consolidations or marked infiltrate. Since embolism may create secondary atelectasis or lung infarcts, detection of PE on the basis of a mismatch may not be possible in that specific scenario. It must be stressed however that an x-ray anomaly does not preclude exclusion of PE by V/Q SPECT. Significant residual perfusion at the site of the chest x-ray anomaly or the presence of a nonvascular or non-pleural-based defect associated with the anomaly are reliable signs for the absence of PE. Also, PE is generally thought to be much more often multiple than single. Therefore, in most cases, you would expect identification of a mismatch away from the x-ray anomaly. Indeed, with the published data, using mismatching as the sole criteria for the presence of PE, the sensitivity of V/Q SPECT has been excellent. Nevertheless, there are no data on the incidence of solitary PE associated with a radiological anomaly. Therefore, if the anomaly has a vascular pattern on the perfusion study and the perfusion defect is complete, CTPA should be performed if the pre-test probability is significant. For lower pre-test probabilities, lower limb Doppler studies are probably sufficient. The presence of an x-ray anomaly is not thought to alter the capacity of CTPA to diagnose PE accurately. Altered sensitivity is unlikely since there are several studies confirming a high negative predictive value for CTPA. However, in the absence of a suitable gold standard, there is no data to evaluate the specificity of CTPA in that setting.

8.5 Chronic PE and follow-up studies

The sensitivity of CTPA for the detection of chronic pulmonary embolism has been proven to be poor, with a sensitivity of probably not much more than 50%. The sensitivity of V/Q SPECT for the detection of chronic PE is excellent, probably on the order of 95%(Tunariu, Gibbs et al. 2007). Specificity is in the same range. Therefore, chronic PE cannot be reliably excluded by CTPA and V/Q SPECT should always be performed if this diagnosis is suspected. It is to be noted that in chronic PE, mismatches may not have the typical vascular shape it usually has in acute PE because of partial reperfusion.

From the previous discussion, it is obvious that follow-up studies using CTPA may be of limited value. Conversely, the evolution of the perfusion defects on serial V/Q SPECT is very easy to follow and resolution or persistence of perfusion anomalies is easily identified. Follow-up studies are very important in PE, especially for the larger embolic processes which are at risk for later pulmonary hypertension. Also, since there is a risk of relapse, follow-up studies need to be done to have a baseline to evaluate this dynamic process. Therefore, even if the initial diagnosis has been made by CTPA, an initial V/Q SPECT study is very valuable. Also, it should be pointed out that it seems difficult to justify the higher radiation dose and contrast agent of CTPA solely for follow-up purposes. There are of course some signs that permit distinction by CTPA of acute and chronic embolism but differentiation between the two conditions is far from being always easy (Castaner, Gallardo et al. 2009).

8.6 Alternate diagnosis

The capacity to provide an alternate explanation for the patient's symptoms is certainly one of CTPA's strong points. This subject has been recently reviewed extensively (Hall, Truitt et al. 2009). An alternate diagnosis for the symptoms (not previously known) can be expected in approximately 1/3 of patients undergoing CTPA for the exclusion of PE. However, a substantial number of those anomalies are also visualized on a chest x-ray and there is some concern that those that are not visualized on a standard x-ray may be of limited clinical consequence. However, for some alternate diagnosis (aortic dissection) CTPA is essential. Also, some tumours will obviously be visualized only on chest CT. As mentioned above, some diagnostic patterns other than PE can be recognized on V/Q SPECT. Early cardiac failure, identification of a large area of reverse mismatch and underestimation of the severity of COPD constitute the most frequent alternative explanations for the symptoms that are not apparent on a standard chest x-ray. Such alternate findings are frequent, occurring in nearly 40% of patients in one study (Bajc, Olsson et al. 2004). However, COPD in often known beforehand and the scope of potential diagnosis is narrower than with CTPA. It is to be noted that approximately 1/4 of patients undergoing CTPA will have incidental findings not related to the acute symptomatic episode that will require follow-up. Most of these findings are pulmonary nodules or thoracic adenopathy. The vast majority will prove benign on follow-up and thus, there is a potential for the generation of multiple follow-up studies with extra costs, extra radiation dose and significant concern for patients. Such incidental findings are inexistent for V/Q SPECT.

9. Future directions

Technical enhancements which are under study at this point for V/Q SPECT include respiratory gating, SPECT-CT technique and quantitative evaluation of ventilation perfusion ratio.

Respiratory gating takes advantage of the fact that image acquisition can be timed electronically with a device that identifies the patient's respiratory movements. This has the potential to create images of better quality, especially for the lung regions closer to the diaphragm where movement during acquisition causes some blurring. Better images have been confirmed in at least one study. Since the majority of emboli are in the lower lung fields, this enhancement may be significant for some patients (Suga, Yasuhiko et al. 2008).

In recent years, hybrid machines, called SPECT-CT, that combine a nuclear camera with a standard CT have become available. Those machines permit acquisition of physiological nuclear medicine data and anatomical CT images that can be perfectly registered. Therefore, physiological anomalies (in the case of lung imaging, ventilation or perfusion anomalies) can be mapped directly on the anatomical images. The potential of this technique is mainly to enhance the specificity of V/Q SPECT, as potential causes of false-positive imaging can be readily identified with this technique (Roach, Gradinscak et al. 2010). There is however the drawback of the higher radiation dose although most protocols will use a low-dose CT.

Quantitative evaluation of the ventilation and perfusion ratios has been the subject of physiological evaluation in normal patients but also in different pathological settings including embolism (Palmer, Bitzen et al. 2001). This type of evaluation has the potential to enhance reading accuracy in embolism, accurately quantify the volume of lung affected by the embolic process and to pinpoint patterns which may be indicative of other types of lung pathology (Suga, Kawakami et al.) (figures 23 to 25). Basically, relative matching of perfusion is illustrated by a color display to show areas of normal matching, mismatches (altered perfusion with preserved ventilation) and reverse mismatches (altered ventilation with preserved perfusion).

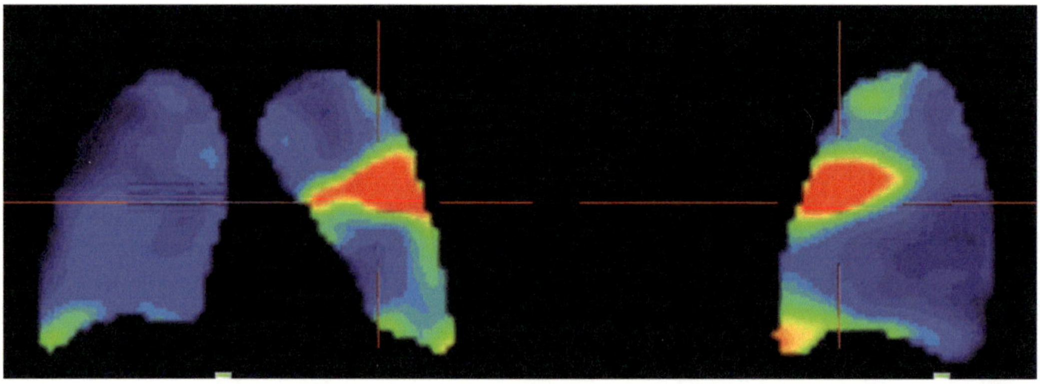

Fig. 23. V/Q quotient of embolism, coronal (left) and sagittal (right) slices. Red indicates the area of complete mismatch, while blue shows normally matched regions.

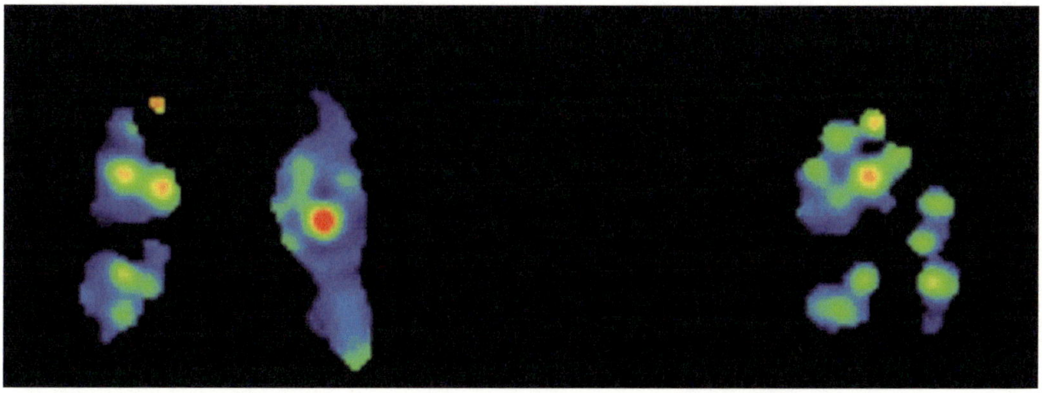

Fig. 24. V/Q quotient of severe COPD, coronal (left) and sagittal (right) slices. Black indicates reverse mismatched areas, green indicates partial mismatches while blue indicates normally matched areas. Widespread areas of non-matched perfusion and ventilation are typical of established COPD.

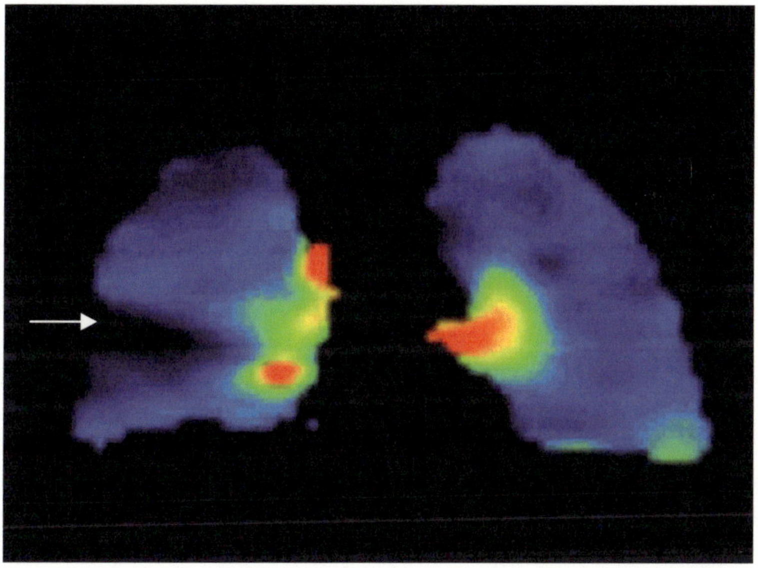

Fig. 25. V/Q quotient of pneumonia, coronal slice. Note wedge shaped area in black indicating reverse mismatch.

10. Role of V/Q SPECT in PE

Given the high sensitivity associated with a low indeterminate rate, absence of contraindications and low radiation dose, V/Q SPECT seems ideally suited to be the initial

screening test for PE in most clinical settings. It should be the test of choice in all cases with a clear chest x-ray (or minor alterations), and most probably in cases of X-rays with a single anomaly. It should be the test of choice in cases associated with pregnancy.
Consideration for CTPA as an initial test should be in cases of severe radiological anomalies or cases for which it is clear from the clinical presentation that a chest CT will be mandatory anyway (to exclude a non-embolic aetiology, when a chest X-ray is deemed insufficient). Cross over to the alternate technique (whether V/Q SPECT or CTPA was used first) should be considered for all equivocal cases and for cases with very strong disagreement between the imaging result and the clinical data. In those cases, lower limb Doppler studies may also be useful. For patients with moderate chest x-ray anomalies there is insufficient data for recommendations at this point but the performance of V/Q SPECT in that setting has been encouraging.

11. Conclusion

V/Q SPECT has proven its value in the setting of PE. It should totally replace planar V/Q scintigraphy in all settings, except in rare cases when a patient cannot tolerate supine imaging. It has significant advantages over CTPA in several common situations and its excellent sensitivity associated with a better safety profile and lower radiation dose makes it the ideal routine screening technique for PE.

12. References

Baile, E. M.,. King, G.G.et al. (2000). Spiral computed tomography is comparable to angiography for thediagnosis of pulmonary embolism. *American Journal of Respiratory and critical care medicine* 161(3 Pt 1): 1010-5

Bajc, M., Bitzen, U. et al. (2002). Lung ventilation/perfusion SPECT in the artificially embolized pig. *Journal of Nuclear Medicine* 43(5): 640-7.

Bajc, M., Neilly, J.B. et al. (2009). EANM guidelines for ventilation/perfusion scintigraphy : Part 1. Pulmonary imaging with ventilation/perfusion single photon emission tomography. *European Journal of Nuclear Medicine and Molecular Imaging* 36(8): 1356-70.

Bajc, M., Olsson, C.G. et al. (2004). Diagnostic evaluation of planar and tomographic ventilation/perfusion lung images in patients with suspected pulmonary emboli. *Clinical Physiology and functional Imaging* 24(5): 249-56.

Castaner, E., Gallardo, X. et al. (2009). CT diagnosis of chronic pulmonary thromboembolism. *Radiographics* 29(1): 31-50; discussion 50-3.

Cook, G. and Clarke S.E.(1992). An evaluation of Technegas as a ventilation agent compared with krypton-81 m in the scintigraphic diagnosis of pulmonary embolism. *European Journal of Nuclear Medicine* 19(9): 770-4.

Ghanima, W., Nielssen B.E., et al. (2007). Multidetector computed tomography (MDCT) in the diagnosis of pulmonary embolism: interobserver agreement among radiologists with varied levels of experience. *Acta Radiologica* 48(2): 165-70.

Gutte, H., Mortensen, J. et al. (2009). Detection of pulmonary embolism with combined ventilation-perfusion SPECT and low-dose CT: head-to-head comparison with multidetector CT angiography. *Journal of Nuclear Medicine* 50(12): 1987-92.

Gutte, H., Mortensen, J. et al. (2010). Comparison of V/Q SPECT and planar V/Q lung scintigraphy in diagnosing acute pulmonary embolism. *Nuclear Medicine Communications* 31(1): 82-6.

Hall, W. B., Truitt, S.G. et al. (2009). The prevalence of clinically relevant incidental findings on chest computed tomographic angiograms ordered to diagnose pulmonary embolism. *Archives of Internal Medicine* 169(21): 1961-5.

Kluge, A., Gerriets, T. et al. (2006). Pulmonary perfusion in acute pulmonary embolism: agreement of MRI and SPECT for lobar, segmental and subsegmental perfusion defects. *Acta Radiologica* 47(9): 933-40.

Kuriakose, J. and Patel, S. (2010). Acute pulmonary embolism. *Radiologic Clinics of North America* 48(1): 31-50.

Leblanc, M., Leveillee, F. et al. (2007). Prospective evaluation of the negative predictive value of V/Q SPECT using 99mTc-Technegas. *Nuclear Medicine Communications* 28(8): 667-72.

Leblanc, M. and Paul, N. (2010). V/Q SPECT and computed tomographic pulmonary angiography. *Seminar of Nuclear Medicine* 40(6): 426-41.

Magnussen, J. S., Chicco, P. et al. (1999). Single-photon emission tomography of a computerised model of pulmonary embolism. *European Journal of Nuclear Meicine* 26(11): 1430-8.

Miles, S., Rogers, K.M. et al. (2009). A comparison of single-photon emission CT lung scintigraphy and CT pulmonary angiography for the diagnosis of pulmonary embolism. *Chest* 136(6): 1546-53.

Palmer, J., Bitzen, U. et al. (2001). Comprehensive ventilation/perfusion SPECT. *Journal of Nuclear Medicine* 42(8): 1288-94.

Peltier, P., De Faucal, P. et al. (1990). Comparison of technetium-99m aerosol and krypton-81m in ventilation studies for the diagnosis of pulmonary embolism. *Nuclear Medicine Communications* 11(9): 631-8.

Reinartz, P., Wildberger, J.E. et al. (2004). Tomographic imaging in the diagnosis of pulmonary embolism: a comparison between V/Q lung scintigraphy in SPECT technique and multislice spiral CT. *Journal of Nuclear Medicine* 45(9): 1501-8.

Ridge, C. A., McDermott, S. et al. (2009). Pulmonary embolism in pregnancy: comparison of pulmonary CT angiography and lung scintigraphy. *American Journal of Roentgenology* 193(5): 1223-7.

Roach, P. J., Gradinscak, D.J. et al, (2010). SPECT/CT in V/Q scanning. *Seminar of Nuclear Medicine* 40(6): 455-66.

Schembri, G. P., Miller, A. E. et al, (2010). Radiation dosimetry and safety issues in the investigation of pulmonary embolism. *Seminar of Nuclear Medicine* 40(6): 442-54.

Suga, K., Kawakami, Y. et al, (2010). Lung ventilation-perfusion imbalance in pulmonary emphysema: assessment with automated V/Q quotient SPECT. *Annals of Nuclear Medicine* 24(4): 269-77.

Suga, K., Kawakami, Y. et al. (2009). Characteristic crescentic subpleural lung zones with high ventilation (V)/perfusion (Q) ratios in interstitial pneumonia on V/Q quotient SPECT. *Nuclear Medicine Communications* 30(11): 881-9.

Suga, K., Yasuhiko, K. et al. (2008). Relation between lung perfusion defects and intravascular clots in acute pulmonary thromboembolism: assessment with breath-hold SPECT-CT pulmonary angiography fusion images. *European Journal of Radiology* 67(3): 472-80.

Tunariu, N., Gibbs, S.J. et al. (2007). Ventilation-perfusion scintigraphy is more sensitive than multidetector CTPA in detecting chronic thromboembolic pulmonary disease as a treatable cause of pulmonary hypertension. *Journal of Nuclear Medicine* 48(5): 680-4.

Wildberger, J. E., Klotz, E. et al. (2005). Multislice computed tomography perfusion imaging for visualization of acute pulmonary embolism: animal experience. *European Radiology* 15(7): 1378-86.

Yogi, J., Jonson B., et al. (2010). Ventilation-perfusion SPECT with 99mTc-DTPA versus Technegas: a head-to- study in obstructive and nonobstructive disease. Journal of Nuclear Medicine 51(5): 735-741

8

Risk Stratification of Submassive Pulmonary Embolism: The Role of Chest Computed Tomography as an Alternative to Echocardiography

Won Young Kim, Shin Ahn and Choong Wook Lee
University of Ulsan College of Medicine; Asan Medical Center
Korea

1. Introduction

Acute pulmonary embolism (PE) is a common and potentially fatal disease (Goldhaber et al., 1999). The most frequent cause of death within 30 days is right ventricular (RV) failure (Goldhaber & Elliott, 2003). Rapid risk stratification is paramount for identifying high-risk patients and for helping to select the appropriate treatment strategy. According to European guidelines (Torbicki et al., 2008), high-risk PE (formerly 'massive' PE) implies the presence of shock or hemodynamic instability (mortality >15%) (Goldhaber et al., 1999). Non high-risk PE can be further stratified by the presence of markers of RV dysfunction and/or myocardial injury as intermediate- and low-risk PE. Intermediate-risk PE (formerly 'sub-massive' PE) is diagnosed by the presence of at least one marker of RV dysfunction or myocardial injury. Low-risk PE (formerly 'non-massive' PE) is diagnosed when RV dysfunction markers are negative (mortality <1%). Reperfusion therapy, including thrombolysis or surgical embolectomy, is indicated for patients with high-risk PE. However, the risks and benefits of reperfusion therapy for patients with intermediate risk PE are less clear. Based on pathophysiological knowledge of the impact of RV dysfunction on acute PE, risk stratification is based on imaging modalities for the visualization of RV dysfunction. Therefore, echocardiographic assessment of RV dysfunction in acute PE may predict early mortality, and may guide decisions regarding reperfusion therapy (Grifoni et al., 2000; Kucher et al., 2005). Echocardiography, however, is time-consuming, operator-dependent, and not always available in an emergency situation, and echocardiographic criteria for assessing RV have not yet been determined. The development of narrow collimation, multi–detector row computed tomography (CT) imaging, and modern workstations for image postprocessing and analysis have made CT pulmonary angiography the modality of choice for the assessment of patients with pulmonary emboli (Ghaye et al., 2006; Schoepf & Costello, 2004). At times, CT is more rapidly accessible in emergency settings, and is more widely available than echocardiography. CT enables the direct visualization of emboli and provides information about cardiac morphology. CT findings, including RV enlargement, the ratio of RV diameter to the diameter of the left ventricle (LV) (RV/LV ratio), interventricular septal bowing, and pulmonary vascular obstruction score, have been associated with early mortality and clinical outcomes (Araoz et al., 2003; Collomb et al., 2003; Coutance et al., 2011; Ghuysen et al., 2005;

Jimenez et al., 2010; Lu et al., 2009; Qanadli et al., 2001; Sanchez et al., 2008; Schoepf & Costello, 2004; van der Meer et al., 2005; Wu et al., 2004).

This chapter will focus on recent studies comparing CT and echocardiographic findings of RV dysfunction. The data obtained in these trials provide the background for emerging risk stratification algorithms, which we hope will lead to the use of chest CT as an alternative to echocardiography in the successful identification of RV dysfunction.

2. Echocardiographic assessment of right ventricular dysfunction

Transthoracic echocardiography is a noninvasive tool that can be easily utilized at the bedside, even in hemodynamically compromised patients. It can help diagnose conditions that mimic acute PE but are treated differently, such as acute myocardial infarction, aortic dissection, and pericardial tamponade. Although echocardiography is not recommended for the diagnosis of PE, it can detect or exclude RV dysfunction. Moreover, echocardiography is an important tool for risk stratification in patients with PE because RV dysfunction on an echocardiogram is a powerful and independent predictor of mortality (Ribeiro et al., 1997; Torbicki et al., 2003). Echocardiographic findings suggesting RV dysfunction have been reported to occur in at least 25% of patients with PE (Kreit, 2004). A meta-analysis found that patients with echocardiographic signs of RV dysfunction were at greater than two-fold higher risk of PE-related mortality than patients without signs of RV dysfunction (ten Wolde et al., 2004). Importantly, patients with normal echocardiographic findings had excellent outcomes, with in-hospital PE-related mortality rates <1% in most of the reported series. A recent systemic review (Fremont et al., 2008) identified five studies that evaluated the prognostic role of echocardiography in diagnosing RV dysfunction. The unadjusted relative risk of RV dysfunction for predicting death was 2.5 (95% CI 1.2-5.5).

Echocardiography, however, has limitations, including restricted availability and relatively high cost. Moreover, in some patients, including those with chronic obstructive pulmonary disease or morbid obesity, it is difficult to adequately image the RV free wall with a transthoracic approach. More importantly, the lack of a clear echocardiographic definition of RV dysfunction is problematic (ten Wolde et al., 2004). A meta-analysis of eight studies that compared the impact of RV dysfunction measured by echocardiography and CT found that the presence of echocardiographically determined RV dysfunction in patients with sub-massive PE was associated with increased short-term mortality (OR 2.36, 95% CI: 1.3-43), but that corresponding pooled negative and positive likelihood ratios independent of death rates were unsatisfactory for clinical usefulness in risk stratification (Coutance et al., 2011). Unfortunately, the echocardiographic criteria of RV dysfunction differ among published studies and have included RV dilatation, hypokinesis, increased RV/LV diameter ratio and increased velocity of the tricuspid regurgitation jet. Thus, since there is no universal echocardiographic definition of RV dysfunction, only a completely normal result should be considered as defining low-risk PE. This is particularly important because, in some of trials, echocardiographic signs of RV pressure overload alone (such as increased tricuspid insufficiency peak gradient and decreased acceleration time of RV ejection) were considered sufficient to classify a patient as having RV dysfunction.

2.1 Echocardiographic findings of right ventricular dysfunction

RV dysfunction is diagnosed by the presence of RV dilatation, defined as a RV/LV end-diastolic dimension ratio >0.6 on a parasternal long-axis view or >0.9 on a four-chamber

view (Fig. 1); as RV systolic free wall hypokinesis (McConnell sign); or as systolic pulmonary arterial hypertension, defined as a tricuspid regurgitant velocity >2.6 m/s (Goldhaber, 2002). Indirect signs of RV pressure overload include a flattened interventricular septum, paradoxical systolic motion of the interventricular septum toward the LV, and a dilated inferior vena cava with reduced respiratory variability (Table 1).
Signs of RV dysfunction have been found in 40-70% of patients with PE, and numerous studies have demonstrated that echocardiography is a useful tool for estimating the prognosis of normotensive patients with acute PE (Goldhaber et al., 1999; Ribeiro et al., 1997; Grifoni et al., 2001). A recent meta-analysis found that echocardiographic evidence of RV dysfunction was associated with a significantly elevated risk of death during the acute phase of PE (OR, 2.5; 95% CI, 1.2-5.5%) (Sanchez et al., 2008). However, since large populations of patients with signs of RV dysfunction have low mortality rates, echocardiographic detection of RV dysfunction alone does not justify more aggressive treatment strategies (Goldhaber et al., 1999; Konstantinides, 2008). More importantly, definitions of RV dysfunction differed greatly among these studies, and patients with chronic obstructive pulmonary disease were not excluded (Jimenez et al., 2007). In addition, it is difficult to differentiate chronic from acute RV overload based on standardized criteria (e.g. RV free wall thickness > 6 mm or tricuspid valve regurgitation jet velocity > 2.6 m/sec).

2.1.1 Echocardiographic RV/LV ratio

A retrospective study of 950 patients showed that the echocardiographic RV/LV ratio was prognostic in the evaluation of PE, with a critical cutoff for prediction of in-hospital mortality of 0.9 (Fremont et al., 2008). Echocardiograms were electrocardiogram (ECG)-gated to allow end-diastolic diameter measurement on the R wave. The minor axes of the RV and LV were measured in apical 4-chamber views from the septum to the lateral wall endothelium at their widest point just above the mitral valve and tricuspid valve annulus. The prognostic value of this easily measurable echocardiographic parameter was independent of patient history and clinical data. Multivariate analysis showed that the independent predictors of in-hospital mortality included systolic BP < 90 mm Hg (odds ratio [OR], 10.73; p < 0.0001), history of left heart failure (OR, 8.99; p < 0.0001), and RV/LV ratio > 0.9 (OR, 2.66; p < 0.01).

2.1.2 Echocardiographic RV hypokinesis

Moderate or severe RV free-wall hypokinesis may be accompanied by relatively normal contraction and "sparing" of the RV apex, a phenomenon called the McConnell sign (McConnell et al., 1996). In patients with PE, the McConnell sign had a sensitivity of 77%, a specificity of 94%, a positive predictive value of 71%, and a negative predictive value of 96%. This sign appeared useful in distinguishing between RV dysfunction due to PE and dysfunction due to other conditions, such as primary pulmonary hypertension. For patients with RV hypokinesis due to acute PE, the excursion diminished markedly when measured in the middle of the RV free wall. However, the excursion improved progressively when segments closer to the apex were measured. This pattern of regional RV dysfunction appeared highly specific for acute PE; in patients with RV dysfunction due to primary pulmonary hypertension, RV hypokinesis was not improved when apical segments were assessed.

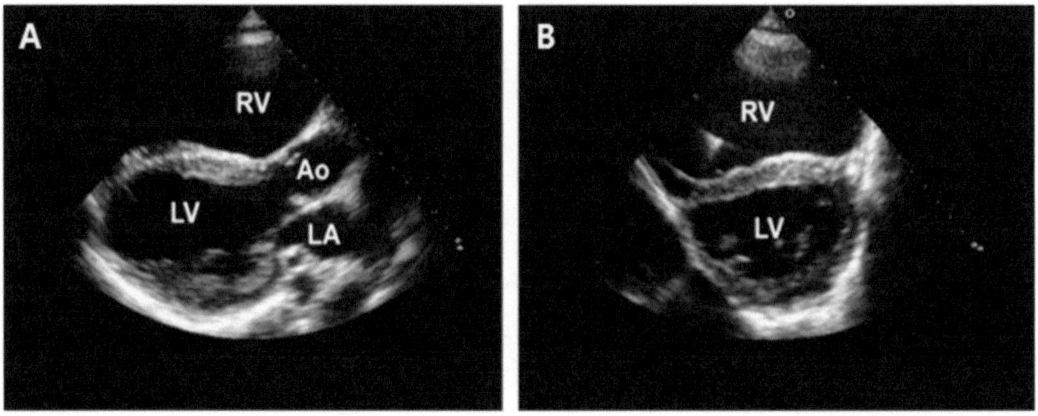

RV: right ventricle; LV: left ventricle; Ao: aorta; LA: left atrium

Fig. 1. Echocardiographic findings of pulmonary embolism in the parasternal long-axis (A) and short-axis (B) views.

Abnormal Finding	Description
Right ventricular dilatation	The ratio of the right ventricular end-diastolic area to left ventricular end-diastolic area exceeds the upper limit of normal (>0.6 on parasternal long-axis views and >0.9 on apical four-chamber views)
Septal flattening and paradoxical septal motion	The interventricular septum bulges toward the left ventricle
Reduced respiratory variability of the dilated inferior vena cava	Subcostal view, diameter >2 cm with <50% respiratory variability; indirect sign of increased central venous pressure
Pulmonary artery dilation	Main pulmonary artery >2.5 cm on parasternal short-axis views; indirect sign of pulmonary hypertension
Tricuspid regurgitation jet velocity >2.6 m/s	Direct evidence of pulmonary hypertension
Right ventricular regional systolic wall motion abnormalities	Hypokinesis of the free wall but preserved apical kinesis

Table 1. Abnormal echocardiographic findings in patients with pulmonary embolism

3. Computed tomography assessment of right ventricular dysfunction

Contrast-enhanced pulmonary CT angiography is increasingly used for first-line imaging in patients suspected of PE. This method allows the direct visualization of emboli, as well as providing information regarding the status of the right heart. Several methods have been suggested for the quantitative assessment of RV dysfunction by CT.

3.1 Computed tomography findings of right ventricular dysfunction

3.1.1 RV dilation (RV/LV ratio)

Similar to echocardiography, contrast-enhanced CT allows assessment of the right-to-left ventricular ratio. RV and LV diameters are assessed on each single image at the plane of maximal visualization of the ventricular cavities, usually at the mitral valve plane for LV and the tricuspid valve level for RV, between the inner surface endocardial border of the free wall and the surface of the interventricular septum (Fig. 2).

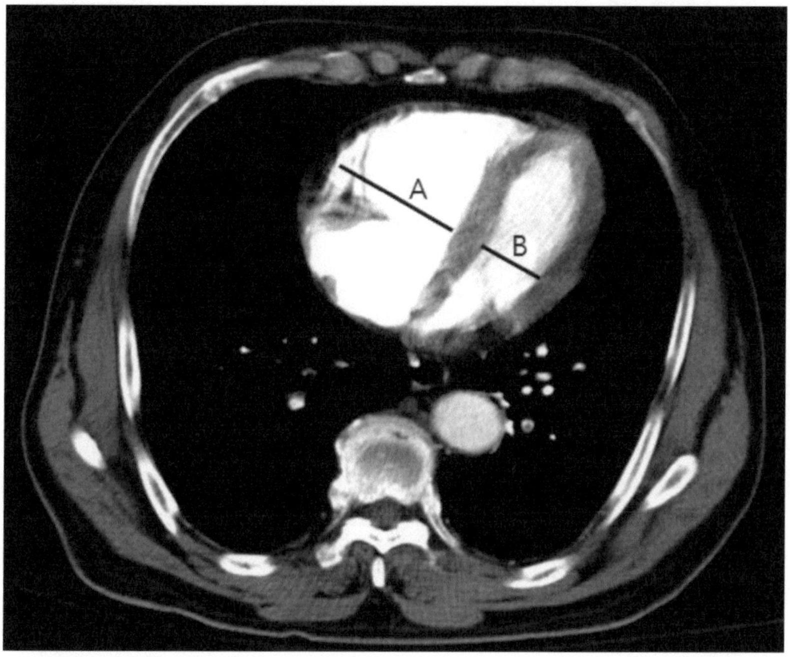

Fig. 2. Transverse contrast-enhanced CT scan showing maximum minor axis measurements of the right ventricle (A) and left ventricle (B). RV/LV ratio = 2

The RV/LV minor axis ratio is widely accepted as a measure of RV dilatation on CT, however, the cut-off values of RV/LV ratio used for RV dysfunction vary among reports. Ghuysen et al suggested an RV/LV ratio >1.5 indicates a severe episode of PE (Ghuysen et al., 2005), Araoz et al suggested an RV/LV ratio >1 was associated with a 3.6-fold increased risk of admission to the intensive care unit (Araoz et al., 2003), and in another study, the same threshold was shown to be a significant risk factor for mortality within 3 months, with an RV/LV ratio ≤1.0 having a PPV of 10.1% (95% CI: 2.9%, 17.4%) and an NPV of 100% (95% CI: 94.3%, 100%) for an uneventful outcome (van der Meer et al., 2005). An RV/LV ratio >0.9 on reconstructed CT four-chamber views has been associated with a poorer prognosis in patients with PE (Schoepf et al., 2004), with an NPV of 92.3% and a PPV of 15.6% for 30-day mortality, and a hazard ratio for predicting 30-day mortality of 5.17 (95% CI, 1.63 - 16.35; P=0.005).

Concerns have arisen regarding whether non-gated CT may be inaccurate in measuring ventricular chamber size because the images are acquired in different phases of the cardiac cycle. However ECG-gated CT scan is not always available, and is time-consuming. Thus, a ECG-gated CT scan is impractical in an emergency situation. In addition, recent findings have indicated that the benefits from a separate ECG-gated CT scan for the evaluation of RV ventricular diameter are minimal and do not justify its routine clinical use instead of the standard measurements of the minor axis (Lu et al., 2009).

Although most studies have indicated that CT assessments of RV dilatation contribute to the risk stratification of patients with PE, two recent meta-analyses have found that CT findings of RV dilatation have limited prognostic importance for mortality among patients with non-high-risk PE (Coutance et al., 2011; Sanchez et al., 2008), and that the greatest value of this method appears to be the identification of low-risk patients based on the lack of RV dilatation. These analyses suggested that measurements made on the four-chamber view are more reliable than traditional measurements made on the minor axis. However, most of these studies were of retrospective design and in small numbers of patients with generally undefined clinical presentations. Hence, any conclusions about the usefulness of this marker must be treated with some caution, although future large clinical studies and standardized definitions of RV dilatation will be required in this patient subset.

3.1.2 Interventricular septal straightening/bowing

If RV afterload suddenly increases, the interventricular septum, which normally bows toward the RV, may shift toward the LV because of its confinement within the pericardium. This phenomenon is readily visible on helical CT pulmonary angiography as straightening or bowing of the interventricular septum.

Leftward bowing of the interventricular septum on CT has been related to severe PA obstruction (Fig. 3). This bowing was found to strongly predict admission to the intensive care unit for PE, but was not associated with in-hospital mortality (Araoz et al., 2003). Thus, this sign is likely not an indicator of outcome and is not specific for PE (van der Meer et al., 2005). This bowing has also been observed in patients with chronic pulmonary artery hypertension, although, in the latter condition, the RV wall is usually thickened (>6 mm), whereas, in acute PE, the RV wall thickness is usually normal.

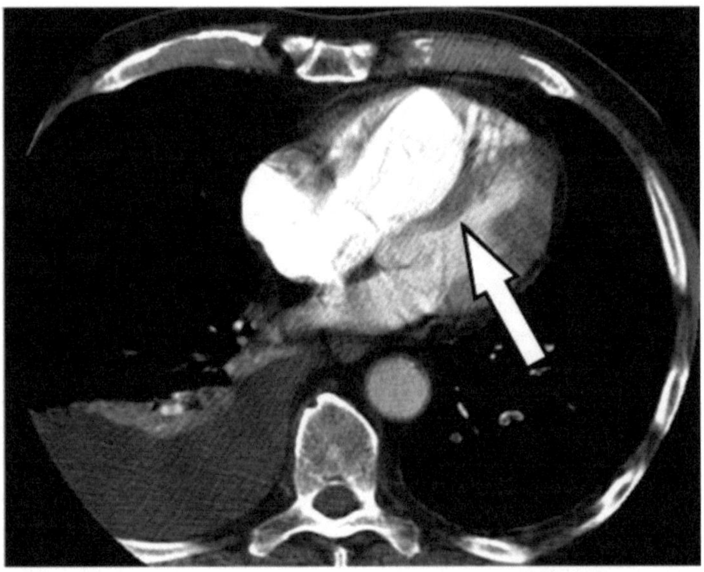

Fig. 3. Ventricular septal bowing (arrow) into the left ventricular lumen

3.1.3 Obstruction index

The PA obstruction index, or the percentage of vascular obstruction of the pulmonary arterial tree caused by PE, may be calculated as Σ (n × d) expressed as percentage vascular obstruction ([Σ (n × d)/40] × 100), where n is the value of the proximal clot site that equals the number of segmental branches arising distally, and d is the degree of obstruction, with partial obstruction scored as 1 and complete obstruction as 2. Values for n range from a minimum of 1 (obstruction of one segment) to a maximum of 20 (obstruction of both right and left pulmonary arteries) (Qanadli et al., 2001). With this scoring system, the maximum obstruction score is 40 (thrombus completely obstructing the pulmonary trunk), which corresponds to a 100% obstruction index. Using a cutoff of 60%, 83% of the patients with an index >60% died, whereas 98% of patients with a lower index remained alive (Wu et al., 2004). Patients with an obstruction index ≥ 40% were found to be at an 11.2-fold (95% CI: 1.3, 93.6) increased risk of dying from PE (van der Meer et al., 2005). However this index may not be practical for routine application without the aid of radiologists.
Another obstruction index, the pulmonary embolism severity index (PESI), was developed to estimate 30-day mortality in patients with acute PE. This index has also been used to identify patients with a low mortality risk who may be suitable for outpatient management of acute PE (Aujesky et al., 2007). The PESI contains 11 differently weighted baseline clinical parameters and is relatively complicated to administer and score. A simplified version of the PESI (sPESI) was therefore developed for ease of application. The sPESI showed similar prognostic accuracy and clinical utility as the PESI, although its use made it easier to identify patients at low-risk of adverse outcomes (Jimenez et al., 2010) (Table 2).

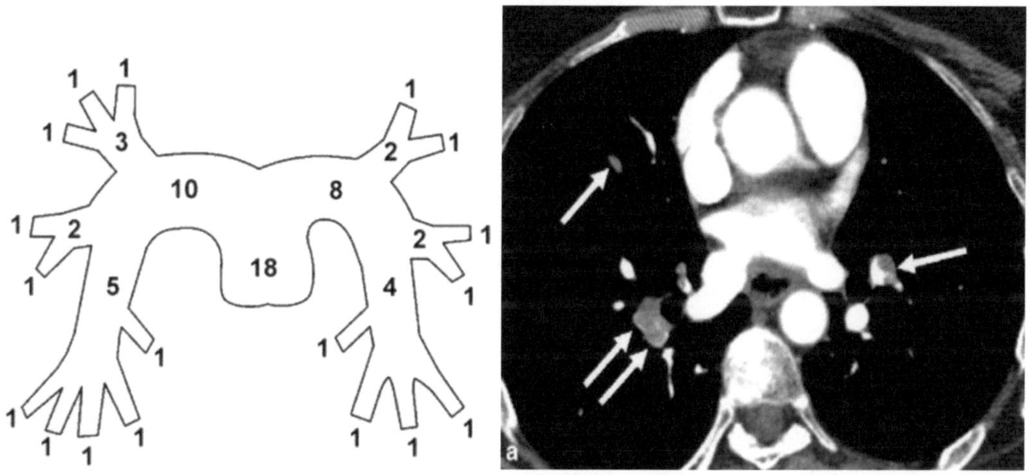

Fig. 4. Transverse contrast-enhanced chest computed tomographic scan showing pulmonary emboli (arrows) in both main pulmonary arteries (PAs). This patient had a PA obstruction index of 55%

3.1.4 Pulmonary artery diameter measurement

A pulmonary artery (PA) diameter greater than 30 mm indicates a PA pressure greater than 20 mmHg (Kuriyama et al., 1984). Moreover, the diameter of the central PA has been significantly correlated with the severity of PE (Collomb et al., 2003). In other studies, however, the diameter of the main PA and the ratio of the diameters of the main PA and the

Variable	Score PESI [a]	sPESI [b]
Age > 80 y	Age in years	1
Male sex	+10	
History of cancer	+30	1
History of heart failure	+10	1 [c]
History of chronic lung disease	+10	
Pulse ≥110 beats/min	+20	1
Systolic blood pressure <100 mmHg	+30	1
Respiratory rate ≥30 breaths/min	+20	
Temperature <36°C	+20	
Altered mental status	+60	
SaO2 < 90%	+20	1

[a] The total point score for each patient is calculated as the sum the patient's age in years and the points for each predictor when present.
Scores corresponding to risk classes include: 65 or less, class I; 66 to 85, class II; 86 to 105, class III; 106 to 125, class IV; and more than 125, class V. Patients in risk classes I and II are defined as being at low risk.
[b]The total point score for each patient is calculated as the sum of the points. Scores correspond to the following risk classes: 0, low risk; 1 or more, high risk.
[c] The variables were combined into a single category of chronic cardiopulmonary disease.

Table 2. Original and simplified pulmonary embolism severity index (PESI)

aorta were not indicators of mortality or severity of acute PE (Araoz et al., 2003; van der Meer et al., 2005).

3.1.5 Saddle pulmonary embolism

Saddle PE is defined as a visible thromboembolus stradding the bifurcation of the main PA (Fig. 5). Saddle PE occurs at frequency of (5.2%) in all patients with PE (Pruszczyk et al., 2003). Such proximal thrombus may be regarded unstable, large clot burden in the PA, and "in-transit" embolus, which can fragment spontaneously or secondary to treatment and obstruct multiple, distal pulmonary arteries (Pruszczyk et al., 2003).

Debate has been going on regarding the size of the clot and prognosis. Some studies suggest that simple distinction of saddle versus non-saddle PE by CT findings was associated with death within 1 year (OR 7.4, 95% CI 1.7-31.5) and may provide a straight forward method for risk stratification (Yusuf et al., 2010). Whereas other studies found that saddle PE was not associated with mortality rate and may not necessitate aggressive medical management (Ryu et al., 2007; Musani, 2010). Therefore the prognosis value of saddle PE is not well established.

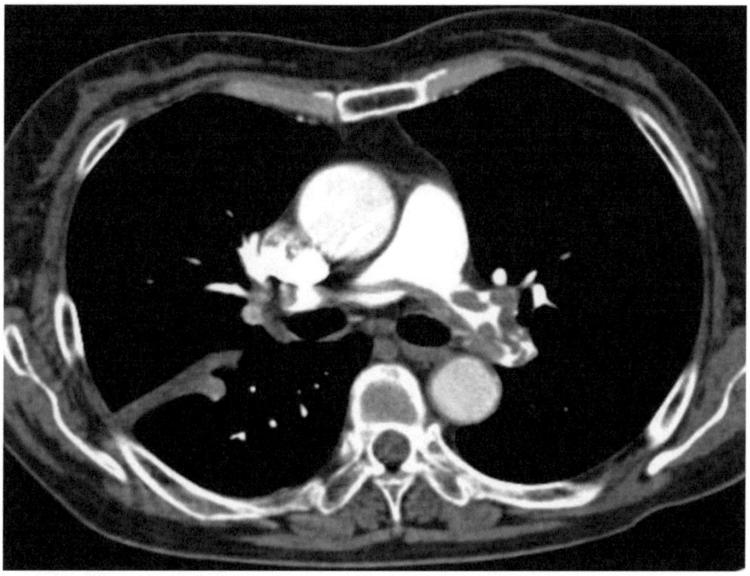

Fig. 5. Saddle pulmonary embolism.

4. Dual E CT

Physiologic changes in patients with acute PE, such as RV overload, may be more closely related to the extent of the pulmonary perfusion defect than to the burden of intravascular emboli. Several studies have reported that the extent of the pulmonary perfusion defect, as assessed by perfusion scintigraphy or SPECT, is an important risk factor for recurrence of pulmonary embolism and RV dysfunction (Wolfe et al., 1994; Palla et al., 2010). However, CT angiography has shown better performance than perfusion scintigraphy or SPECT in the initial diagnosis of pulmonary embolism, since the former has several advantages, including high spatial resolution, rapid scanning time and easy availability.

Recent advances in CT technology have included dual-energy CT (DECT), using two tubes (dual-source CT) or a single tube with a rapid kVp switching technique. As iodine has unique spectral properties and X-ray absorption characteristics at higher and lower photon energies (e.g., 140-kVp and 80-kVp), iodine map images can be generated using DECT angiography (DECTA). These images may represent the regional perfusion status of lung parenchyma and showed good correlation with scintigraphic findings in patients with PE (Pontana et al., 2008; Thieme et al., 2008). Weighted-average 120-kVp equivalent CT angiography obtained from DECTA can be used for the direct visualization of a thromboembolism and for the evaluation of CT signs of RV dysfunction, similar to standard CT angiography. That is, information about regional lung perfusion status, as well as the burden of intravascular emboli and right-sided heart failure, can be evaluated by single scanning DECT.

RV dysfunction is predictive of a poor prognosis in patients with acute PE. On CT angiography images, RV/LV diameter ratio is a reliable marker of RV dysfunction, with higher RV/LV diameter ratios related to poor clinical outcomes (Quiroz et al., 2004; Schoepf et al., 2004; van der Meer et al., 2005). Furthermore, the extent of perfusion defect on DECTA has been correlated with RV/LV diameter ratio (Zhang et al., 2009; Chae et al., 2010; Bauer et al., 2011). A novel dual energy perfusion defect score has been proposed, in which the degree of lung perfusion in each segment is graded on a 3-point scale (0, normal perfusion; 1, moderately reduced perfusion, 2, profoundly reduced or absent perfusion), with the perfusion defect score calculated as $\sum(n \cdot d)/40x100$, where n is the number of segments and d is the degree of the perfusion defect (Chae et al., 2010). The perfusion defect score has shown good correlation with RV/LV diameter ratio ($r = 0.69$, $p < 0.001$). In addition, the numbers of lobes with pulmonary perfusion defects on iodine images of DECTA correlated well with RV/LV diameter ratio ($r = 0.66$, $p < 0.05$), whereas the number of lobes with PE on CT angiography did not ($p > 0.05$). Quantification of the area of pulmonary perfusion defect on iodine images showed that an pulmonary perfusion defect over 215.4 ml or a relative volume over 9.9% was related to an RV/LV diameter ratio > 1 (Bauer et al., 2011). These results therefore indicate that pulmonary perfusion defect size may be a surrogate marker for RV dysfunction (Fig. 6, Fig. 7). Readmission and death due to PE were observed only in patients with a relative perfusion defect size >5% of total lung volume, but not in any patient with a relative perfusion defect < 5% (Bauer, Frellesen et al. 2011). Patients with a relative perfusion defect >5% also showed lower median survival with increased relative hazard ratio for death than those with a relative perfusion defect <5%. These results indicate that pulmonary perfusion defect size may be prognostic in patients with PE.

The status of the pulmonary microvasculature is important in evaluating disease severity and prognosis in patients with PE. Although ventilation/perfusion scintigraphy was used to assess the pulmonary nomenclature, multi-detector CT angiography has replaced scintigraphy in the evaluation of these patients, since CT has higher spatial resolution and shorter acquisition time. Recently developed advanced CT techniques, including DECT, permits the evaluation of pulmonary perfusion status without significant additional radiation dose. Therefore, DECTA may become a leading imaging tool, both for detecting emboli and for risk stratification regarding of regional pulmonary perfusion status in patients with PE.

5. The role of chest computed tomography as an alternative to echocardiography

Retrospective studies have shown that multidetector chest CT and echocardiography yield similar prognostic data (Sanchez et al., 2008). While CT provides information on RV dilatation only, echocardiography also provides some information on contractility, e.g., septal or RV hypo- or dyskinesia. However, echocardiography is not always available in emergency settings and has limitations, including poor RV image quality and lack of a universal definition of RV dysfunction. Indeed, this method has limited sensitivity and negative findings on echocardiography do not exclude a diagnosis of PE (Miniati et al., 2001). In contrast, CT pulmonary angiography allows direct visualization of clots, as well as providing information on the status of the right heart and other adjacent organs. This tool is available around the clock at most institutions and has become the first-line test for patients suspected of having PE. PE may be diagnosed and its risk stratified at the same time. Of course, CT has several limitations, including an inability to assess RV function in real time and the lack of universally accepted criteria. Confirmation of these findings in further, prospective studies may make multidetector-row chest CT a reasonable alternative to echocardiography for diagnosing RV dysfunction. Imaging techniques are constantly being improved in the diagnostic workup of patients with suspected PE. Thus, CT has the potential to become the link between diagnostic and risk stratification strategies in this setting.

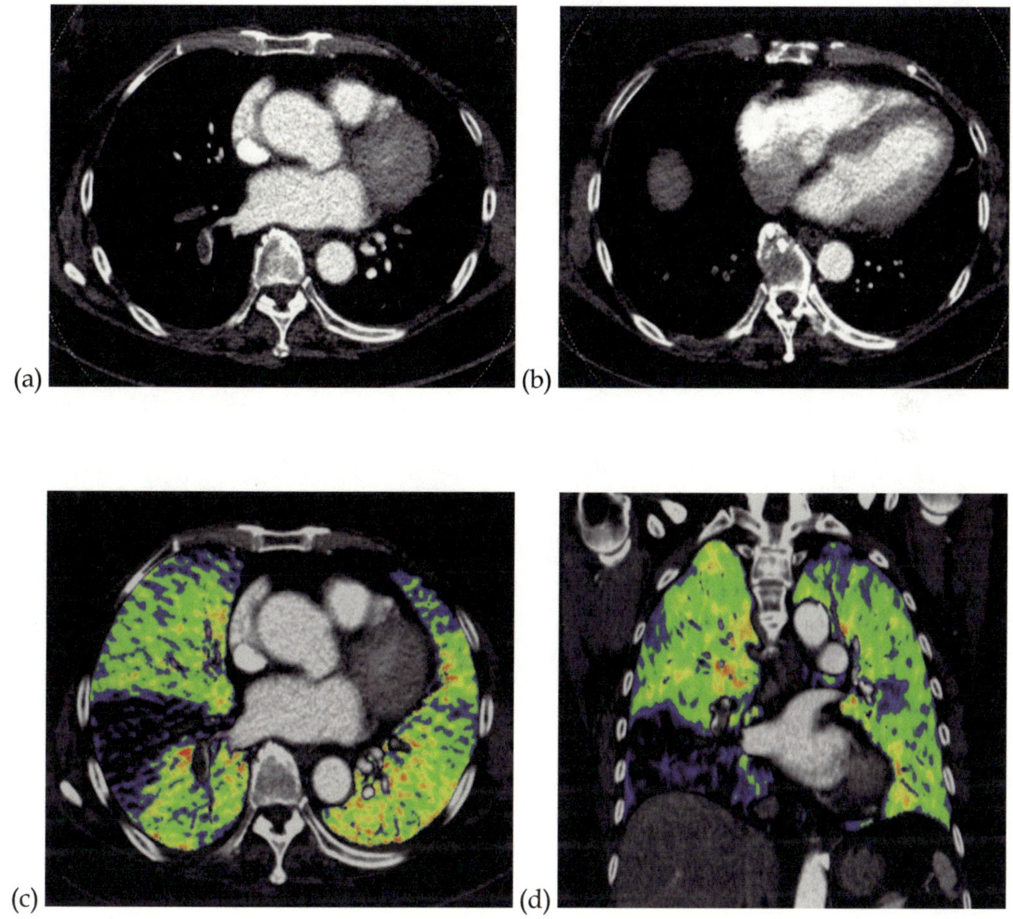

Fig. 6. Pulmonary embolism without right ventricular dysfunction. (a) Dual-energy CT angiography (DECTA) shows filling defect in segmental branches of pulmonary arteries in right lower lobe. (b) DECTA shows normal ranged diameters of ventricles (RV/LV ratio < 1). (c & d) Lung iodine images show wedge shaped pulmonary perfusion defect in right lower lobe lateral basal segment where emboli completely occludes pulmonary artery. However, the posterior basal segment of right lower lobe shows normal perfusion status, because emboli partly occlude corresponding pulmonary artery. The relative volume of pulmonary perfusion defect was 8.3% and perfusion defect score was 10.

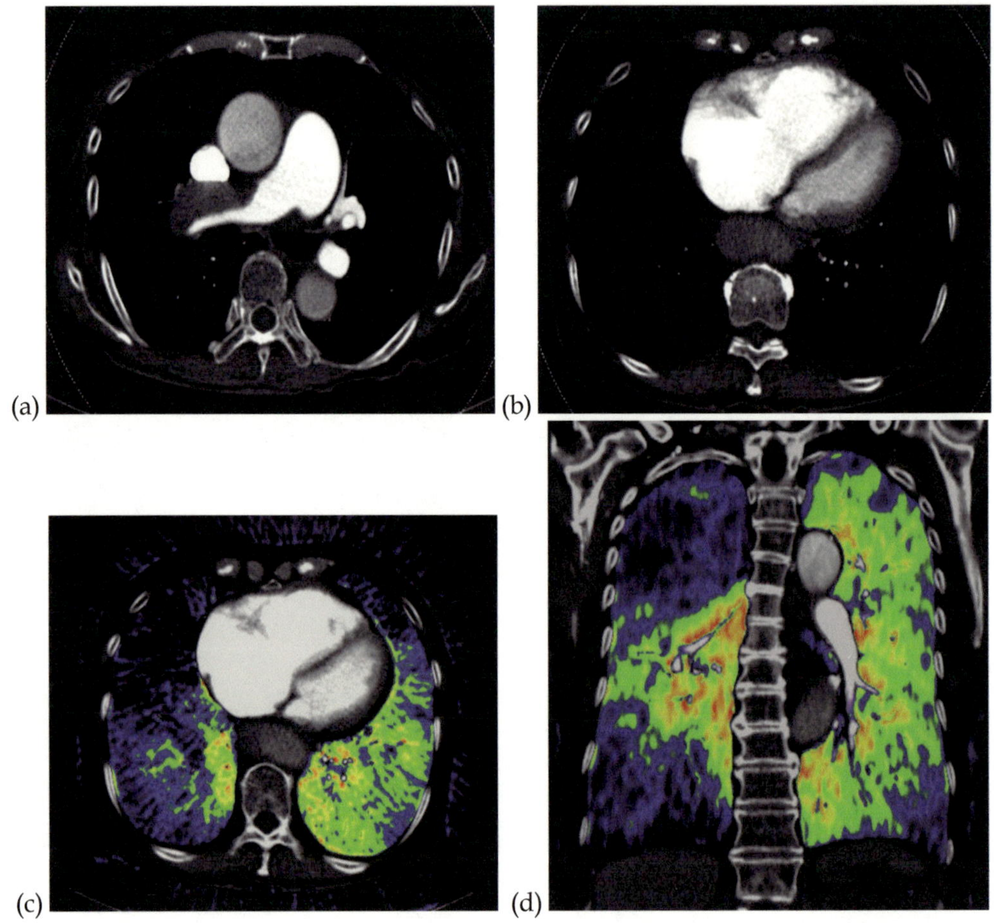

Fig. 7. Pulmonary embolism with right ventricular dysfunction. (a) Dual-energy CT angiography (DECTA) shows filling defect in right main pulmonary artery. (b) DECTA shows enlarged right ventricle (RV/LV ratio > 1). (c & d) Lung iodine images show perfusion defect in right lung except superior segment and posterior basal segment of right lower lobe. Multifocal wedge shaped perfusion defect in also noted in subpleural portion of left lung. The relative volume of pulmonary perfusion defect was 47.8% and perfusion defect score was 52.5.

6. Conclusion

This chapter focused on the prognostic value of RV dysfunction as measured by chest CT in patients with hemodynamically stable PE. Although echocardiographic assessment of RV dysfunction is a generally accepted imaging modality, the lack of a clear echocardiographic definition of RV dysfunction, and the poor RV images, reduces its diagnostic capabilities. RV dysfunction assessed by CT, including RV enlargement, RV/LV ratio, interventricular septal bowing, pulmonary obstruction score, and pulmonary perfusion defect have been associated with poor patient outcomes. Risk stratification of patients with stable PE based on chest CT findings may comparable in results to echocardiography and may be useful.

7. References

Araoz, P. A., Gotway, M. B., Trowbridge, R. L., Bailey, R. A., Auerbach, A. D., Reddy, G. P., et al. (2003). Helical CT pulmonary angiography predictors of in-hospital morbidity and mortality in patients with acute pulmonary embolism, *J Thorac Imaging* Vol. 18 (4): 207-216.

Aujesky, D., Perrier, A., Roy, P. M., Stone, R. A., Cornuz, J., Meyer, G., et al. (2007). Validation of a clinical prognostic model to identify low-risk patients with pulmonary embolism, *J Intern Med* Vol. 261 (6): 597-604.

Bauer, R. W., Frellesen, C., Renker, M., Schell, B., Lehnert, T, Ackermann, H., et al. (2011). Dual energy CT pulmonary blood volume assessment in acute pulmonary embolism - correlation with D-dimer level, right heart strain and clinical outcome, *Eur Radiol* Vol. 21 (9): 1914-1921.

Chae, E. J., Seo, J. B., Jang, Y. M., Krauss, B., Lee, C. W., Lee, H. J., et al. (2010). Dual-energy CT for assessment of the severity of acute pulmonary embolism: pulmonary perfusion defect score compared with CT angiographic obstruction score and right ventricular/left ventricular diameter ratio. *AJR Am J Roentgenol* Vol. 194 (3): 604-610.

Collomb, D., Paramelle, P. J., Calaque, O., Bosson, J. L., Vanzetto, G., Barnoud, D., et al. (2003). Severity assessment of acute pulmonary embolism: evaluation using helical CT, *Eur Radiol* Vol. 13 (7): 1508-1514.

Coutance, G., Cauderlier, E., Ehtisham, J., Hamon, M., & Hamon, M. (2011). The prognostic value of markers of right ventricular dysfunction in pulmonary embolism: a meta-analysis, *Crit Care* Vol. 15 (2): R103.

Fremont, B., Pacouret, G., Jacobi, D., Puglisi, R., Charbonnier, B., & de Labriolle, A. (2008). Prognostic value of echocardiographic right/left ventricular end-diastolic diameter ratio in patients with acute pulmonary embolism: results from a monocenter registry of 1,416 patients, *Chest* Vol. 133 (2): 358-362.

Ghaye, B., Ghuysen, A., Willems, V., Lambermont, B., Gerard, P., D'Orio, V., et al. (2006). Severe pulmonary embolism:pulmonary artery clot load scores and cardiovascular parameters as predictors of mortality, *Radiology* Vol. 239 (3): 884-891.

Ghuysen, A., Ghaye, B., Willems, V., Lambermont, B., Gerard, P., Dondelinger, R. F., et al. (2005). Computed tomographic pulmonary angiography and prognostic significance in patients with acute pulmonary embolism, *Thorax* Vol. 60 (11): 956-961.

Goldhaber, S. Z., & Elliott, C. G. (2003). Acute pulmonary embolism: part II: risk stratification, treatment, and prevention, *Circulation* Vol. 108 (23): 2834-2838.

Goldhaber, S. Z., Visani, L., & De Rosa, M. (1999). Acute pulmonary embolism: clinical outcomes in the International Cooperative Pulmonary Embolism Registry (ICOPER), *Lancet* Vol. 353 (9162): 1386-1389.

Goldhaber, S. Z. (2002). Echocardiography in the management of pulmonary embolism, *Ann Intern Med* Vol. 136 (9): 691–700

Grifoni, S., Olivotto, I., Cecchini, P., Pieralli, F., Camaiti, A., Santoro, G., et al. (2000). Short-term clinical outcome of patients with acute pulmonary embolism, normal blood pressure, and echocardiographic right ventricular dysfunction, *Circulation* Vol. 101 (24): 2817-2822.

Jimenez D., Escobar C., Marti D., Diaz G., Vidal R., Taboada D., et al. (2007). Prognostic value of transthoracic echocardiography in hemodynamically stable patients with acute symptomatic pulmonary embolism, *Arch Bronconeumol* Vol. 43 (9): 490-494

Jimenez, D., Aujesky, D., Moores, L., Gomez, V., Lobo, J. L., Uresandi, F., et al. (2010). Simplification of the pulmonary embolism severity index for prognostication in patients with acute symptomatic pulmonary embolism, *Arch Intern Med* Vol. 170 (15): 1383-1389.

Konstantinides, S. (2005). Pulmonary embolism: impact of right ventricular dysfunction, *Curr Opin Cardiol* Vol. 20 (6): 496-501.

Konstantinides, S. V. (2008). Massive pulmonary embolism: what level of aggression?, *Semin Respir Crit Care Med* Vol. 29 (1): 47-55.

Kreit, J. W. (2004). The impact of right ventricular dysfunction on the prognosis and therapy of normotensive patients with pulmonary embolism, *Chest* Vol. 125 (4): 1539-1545.

Kucher, N., Rossi, E., De Rosa, M., & Goldhaber, S. Z. (2005). Prognostic role of echocardiography among patients with acute pulmonary embolism and a systolic arterial pressure of 90 mm Hg or higher, *Arch Intern Med* Vol. 165 (15): 1777-1781.

Kuriyama, K., Gamsu, G., Stern, R. G., Cann, C. E., Herfkens, R. J., & Brundage, B. H. (1984). CT-determined pulmonary artery diameters in predicting pulmonary hypertension, *Invest Radiol* Vol. 19 (1): 16-22.

Lu, M. T., Cai, T., Ersoy, H., Whitmore, A. G., Levit, N. A., Goldhaber, S. Z., et al. (2009). Comparison of ECG-gated versus non-gated CT ventricular measurements in thirty patients with acute pulmonary embolism, *Int J Cardiovasc Imaging* Vol. 25 (1): 101-107.

Musani M.H. (2010). Asymptomatic saddle pulmonary embolism: case report and literature review, *Clin Appl Thromb Hemost.*

McConnell M.V., Solomon S.D., Rayan M.E., Come P.C., Goldhaber S.Z., Lee R.T. (1996). Regional right ventricular dysfunction detected by echocardiography in acute pulmonary embolism, *Am J Cardiol.* Vol. 78 (4): 469-73.

Miniati, M., Monti, S., Pratali, L., Di Ricco, G., Marini, C., Formichi, B., et al. (2001). Value of transthoracic echocardiography in the diagnosis of pulmonary embolism: results of a prospective study in unselected patients, *Am J Med* Vol. 110 (7): 528-535.

Palla, A., Ribas, C., Rossi, G., Pepe, P., Marconi, L. & Prandoni, P. (2010). The clinical course of pulmonary embolism patients anticoagulated for 1 year: results of a prospective, observational, cohort study. *J Thromb Haemost* Vol. 8 (1): 68-74.

Pontana, F., Faivre, J. B., Remy-Jardin, M., Flohr, T., Schmidt, B., Tacelli N., et al. (2008). Lung perfusion with dual-energy multidetector-row CT (MDCT): feasibility for the evaluation of acute pulmonary embolism in 117 consecutive patients. *Acad Radiol* Vol. 15 (12): 1494-1504.

Pruszczyk P., Pacho R., Ciurzynski M., Burakowska B., Tomkowski W., Bochowicz A., et al., et al. (2003). Short term clinical outcome of acute saddle pulmonary embolism, *Heart* Vol. 89 (3): 335-336.

Qanadli, S. D., El Hajjam, M., Vieillard-Baron, A., Joseph, T., Mesurolle, B., Oliva, V. L., et al. (2001). New CT index to quantify arterial obstruction in pulmonary embolism: comparison with angiographic index and echocardiography, *AJR Am J Roentgenol* Vol. 176 (6): 1415-1420.

Quiroz, R., Kucher, N., Schoepf, U. J., Kipfmueller, F., Solomon, S.D., Costello, P., et al. (2004). Right ventricular enlargement on chest computed tomography: prognostic role in acute pulmonary embolism. *Circulation* Vol. 109 (20): 2401-2404.

Ribeiro, A., Lindmarker, P., Juhlin-Dannfelt, A., Johnsson, H., & Jorfeldt, L. (1997). Echocardiography Doppler in pulmonary embolism: right ventricular dysfunction as a predictor of mortality rate, *Am Heart J* Vol. 134 (3): 479-487.

Ryu J.H., Pellikka P.A., Froehling D.A., Peters S.G., Aughenbaugh G.L. (2007). Saddle pulmonary embolism diagnosed by CT angiography: frequency, clinical features and outcome, *Respir Med* Vol. 101 (7): 1537-1542.

Sanchez, O., Trinquart, L., Colombet, I., Durieux, P., Huisman, M. V., Chatellier, G., et al. (2008). Prognostic value of right ventricular dysfunction in patients with haemodynamically stable pulmonary embolism: a systematic review, *Eur Heart J* Vol. 29 (12): 1569-1577.

Schoepf, U. J., & Costello, P. (2004). CT angiography for diagnosis of pulmonary embolism: state of the art, *Radiology* Vol. 230 (2): 329-337.

Schoepf, U. J., Kucher, N., Kipfmueller, F., Quiroz, R., Costello, P., & Goldhaber, S. Z. (2004). Right ventricular enlargement on chest computed tomography: a predictor of early death in acute pulmonary embolism, *Circulation* Vol. 110 (20): 3276-3280.

ten Wolde, M., Sohne, M., Quak, E., Mac Gillavry, M. R., & Buller, H. R. (2004). Prognostic value of echocardiographically assessed right ventricular dysfunction in patients with pulmonary embolism, *Arch Intern Med* Vol. 164 (15): 1685-1689.

Thieme, S. F., Becker, C. R., Hacker, M., Nikolaou, K., Reiser, M. F., & Johnson, T. R. (2008). Dual energy CT for the assessment of lung perfusion--correlation to scintigraphy. *Eur J Radiol* Vol. 68 (3): 369-374.

Torbicki, A., Galie, N., Covezzoli, A., Rossi, E., De Rosa, M., & Goldhaber, S. Z. (2003). Right heart thrombi in pulmonary embolism: results from the International Cooperative Pulmonary Embolism Registry, *J Am Coll Cardiol* Vol. 41 (12): 2245-2251.

Torbicki, A., Perrier, A., Konstantinides, S., Agnelli, G., Galie, N., Pruszczyk, P., et al. (2008). Guidelines on the diagnosis and management of acute pulmonary embolism: the Task Force for the Diagnosis and Management of Acute Pulmonary Embolism of the European Society of Cardiology (ESC), *Eur Heart J* Vol. 29 (18): 2276-2315.

van der Meer, R. W., Pattynama, P. M., van Strijen, M. J., van den Berg-Huijsmans, A. A., Hartmann, I. J., Putter, H., et al. (2005). Right ventricular dysfunction and pulmonary obstruction index at helical CT: prediction of clinical outcome during 3-month follow-up in patients with acute pulmonary embolism, *Radiology* Vol. 235 (3): 798-803.

Wu, A. S., Pezzullo, J. A., Cronan, J. J., Hou, D. D., & Mayo-Smith, W. W. (2004). CT pulmonary angiography: quantification of pulmonary embolus as a predictor of patient outcome--initial experience, *Radiology* Vol. 230 (3): 831-835.

Wolfe, M. W., Lee, R. T., Feldstein, M. L., Parker, J. A., Come, P. C., & Goldhaber, S. Z. (1994). Prognostic significance of right ventricular hypokinesis and perfusion lung scan defects in pulmonary embolism. *Am Heart J* Vol. 127 (5): 1371-1375.

Zhang, L. J., Yang, G. F., Zhao, Y. E., Zhou, C. S., & Lu, G M. (2009). Detection of pulmonary embolism using dual-energy computed tomography and correlation with cardiovascular measurements: a preliminary study. *Acta Radiol* Vol. 50 (8): 892-901.

9

Quantitative Ventilation/Perfusion Tomography: The Foremost Technique for Pulmonary Embolism Diagnosis

Marika Bajc and Jonas Jögi
Department of Clinical Physiology
Lund University and Skåne University Hospital, Lund
Sweden

1. Introduction

The value of perfusion scintigraphy in the detection of pulmonary embolism (PE) was demonstrated as early as 1964 by Wagner et al. PE causes perfusion defects that conform to the anatomical distribution of the pulmonary vascular bed. Perfusion defects in acute PE are therefore of sub-segmental, segmental or lobar character. Ventilation is normally preserved in these areas and the observed wedge shaped mismatch between ventilation and perfusion is typical for PE. Planar ventilation/perfusion scintigraphy (V/P scan) was until the 1990s the method of choice for studying patients with suspected PE. However, the large Prospective Investigation of Pulmonary Embolism Diagnosis (PIOPED I), showed a high number of non-diagnostic examinations (65%) with V/P scan and the probabilistic interpretation criteria were confusing to the clinicians (Gray et al., 1993; The PIOPED Investigators, 1990). Planar imaging has become obsolete, particularly when the issue is identification and quantification of focal or regional aberration of organ function.
The advantage of three dimensional tomography over planar imaging for PE detection had already been shown in 1983 in a study on dogs (Osborne et al., 1983). Furthermore, Magnussen et al. (1999) used a computerized model of PE to highlight the advantage of SPECT over planar imaging in the assessment of the size and location of perfusion defects. Using a dual head camera, Palmer et al. (2001), developed a fast and efficient method for ventilation/perfusion tomography (V/P SPECT) for clinical practice with total acquisition time of only 20 minutes. Moreover, they developed an algorithm to calculate the quotient between ventilation and perfusion and to present it as $V/P_{quotient}$ images. This facilitated PE diagnosis and the quantification of PE extension, which led to the use of the term quantitative V/P SPECT. Using a porcine model, Bajc et al. validated V/P SPECT for diagnosis of PE and confirmed the superior value of tomography over planar imaging with excellent interobserver agreement of defects down to the sub-segmental level (Bajc et al., 2002b).
The objective of this chapter is to acquaint readers with the latest methodological approach of V/P SPECT in the diagnosis of PE, in accordance with the new guidelines of the European Association of Nuclear Medicine (Bajc et al., 2009a, b). In this chapter we also discuss the value of V/P SPECT in the follow up after acute PE and in the diagnosis of other cardiopulmonary diseases.

Efficient and effective diagnostics for PE and other diseases should meet the following basic requirements:

- Fast procedure and prompt availability of results
- Feasibility for all patients
- High diagnostic accuracy and few non-diagnostic reports
- Low radiation dose
- Utility for selection of treatment strategy
- Suitability for follow up and research

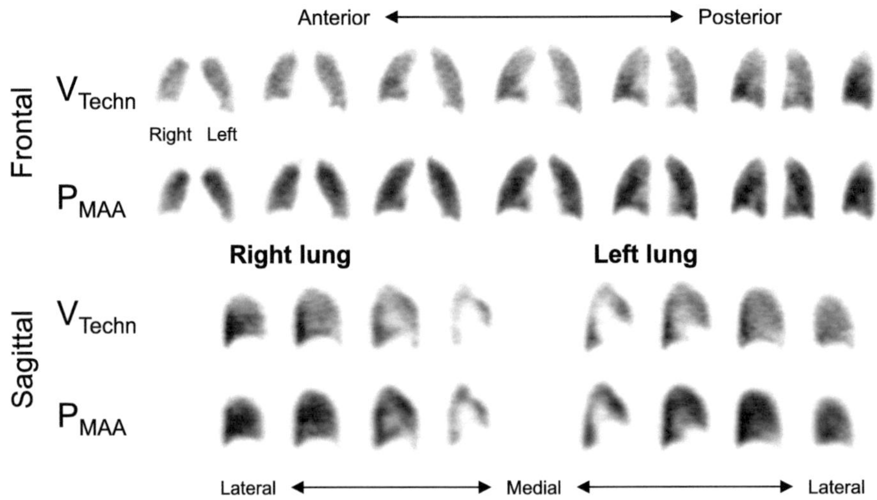

Fig. 1. V/P SPECT images of a patient with normal ventilation (V) and perfusion (P). Techn = Technegas, MAA = Macroaggregated albumin

2. Ventilation and perfusion imaging

In healthy patients, regional ventilation and perfusion match each other to optimize gas exchange (Fig 1). In diseased patients, changes in distribution of ventilation or perfusion or both are common. Vascular occlusive diseases, like PE, cause perfusion defects in conformity with pulmonary circulation while ventilation stays intact in these areas. This disconcordant ventilation/perfusion pattern, so called mismatch, provides the basis for PE diagnosis. Ventilation might be disturbed in acute PE due to bronchial constriction (Giuntini, 2001) but perfusion defects are usually observable in other areas (Fig 2a).
Ventilation commonly shows disturbances in lung diseases like pneumonia, tumours and obstructive diseases. Such perfusion patterns are essential to recognize as they provide additional specificity and significance to observed conditions.

2.1 Ventilation

For the ventilation study, gases may be used as they are distributed strictly according to regional ventilation. The gas that is used for V/P SPECT is metastable 81-krypton (81mKr). Its short half life, 13 s, implies that it disappears from the alveoli by decay at a much faster rate than by exhalation. Therefore, after a few minutes of breathing the test gas, the alveolar

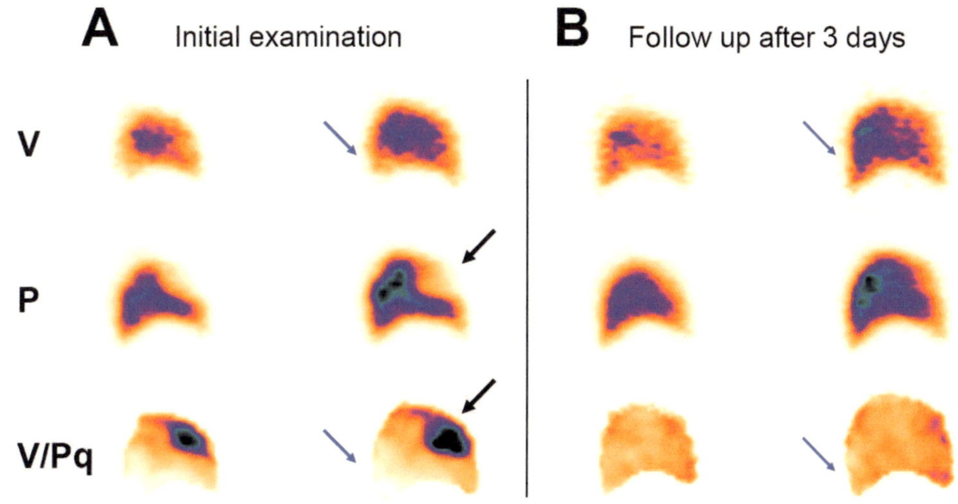

Fig. 2. A patient with acute PE. Sagittal ventilation (V), perfusion (P) and V/P quotient (V/Pq) images of the right lung. **A)** At the initial examination, segmental perfusion defects are seen (arrow). The V/P mismatch is clearly delineated on V/P quotient images which improves visualization. Reduced ventilation is observed in posterior parts of the lung, where perfusion is preserved (blue arrows). **B)** Normalization of ventilation (blue arrows and perfusion is seen already after three days.

concentration will reflect alveolar ventilation. Ventilation is performed during continuous breathing of this gas. 81mKr has higher gamma energy than 99m-Technetium (99mTc) (191 compared to 140 keV) allowing simultaneous imaging of ventilation and perfusion. 81mKr is diluted from a rubidium generator that has a half life of 4.6 h. Its availability is limited and it is too expensive for general use.

Routinely in clinical practice, inhalation of a radio-aerosol is used for ventilation scintigraphy. Aerosol particles are liquid or solid. The size of the particles is of critical importance. Particles larger than 2 µm are deposited in large airways. Smaller particles are deposited by sedimentation and diffusion in small airways and alveoli. Particles smaller than 1 µm, are mainly deposited in alveoli by diffusion. Aerosol deposition is modified by flow pattern. High flow rates at forced breathing patterns and turbulent flow enhances particle deposition in airways and increases the likelihood of hot spots formation on ventilation images, particularly in Chronic Obstructive Pulmonary Disease (COPD).

Diethylenetriaminepentaacetic acid labeled with technetium, 99mTc-DTPA, is the most common agent used for ventilation scintigraphy. It is soluble in water and the size of the molecule is 492 Dalton. The average size of particles after nebulization is at best 1.3 to 1.8 µm. Due to the water solubility, particle size tends to increase during inhalation and to agglutinate in cases of bronchial obstruction where there are turbulent flows; this leads to the creation of hot spots. Because of the water solubility, 99mTc-DTPA particles also diffuse through the alveolo-capillary membrane to the blood. In a healthy patient, clearance of 99mTc-DTPA occurs with a half life of about 70 minutes. Increased clearance, leading to a shorter half life is observed where there is alveolar inflammation for any reason, such as alveolitis of an allergic or toxic nature and even in smokers. Clearance of 99mTc-DTPA can for diagnostic purposes be measured at a routinely performed V/P SPECT.

Technegas is a newer solid aerosol with extremely small carbon particles, 0.005-0.2 μm, labeled with 99mTc which are generated in a high temperature furnace. The small particle size implies that they are distributed in the lungs almost like a gas and are deposited in alveoli by diffusion (James et al., 1992). Technegas provides images which are equivalent to those with 81mKr. Technegas significantly reduces problems of central airway deposition and peripheral hotspots. Patients routinely admitted for V/P SPECT and a group of patients with known COPD were recently studied with both 99mTc-DTPA and Technegas showing superiority of the latter (Jögi et al., 2010). Unevenness of radiotracer deposition and degree of central deposition were significantly reduced with Technegas, particularly in the obstructive patients (Fig 3). In some patients, mismatched perfusion defects were only identified using Technegas because the significant peripheral unevenness of 99mTc-DTPA obscured mismatch. PE might have been overlooked in COPD patients using 99mTc-DTPA. In a few patients, 99mTc-DTPA yielded images of very poor quality. Technegas is therefore recommended as the superior radio-aerosol, particularly in patients with obstructive lung disease. A further advantage of Technegas is that relatively few breaths are sufficient to achieve an adequate amount of activity in the lungs.

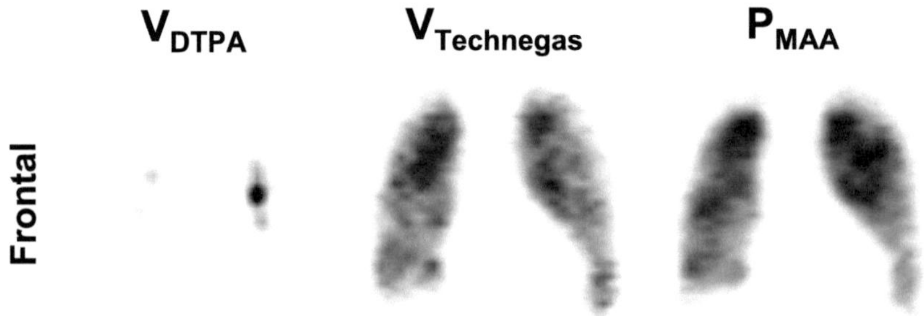

Fig. 3. Comparison between 99mTc-DTPA and Technegas ventilation studies in a patient with COPD.

2.2 Perfusion

Perfusion scintigraphy involves an intravenous injection of radio-labeled macro-aggregates of albumin (MAA), sized 15-100 μm, which cause microembolization of pulmonary capillaries and pre-capillary arterioles in amounts reflecting regional perfusion. At least 60 000 particles are required to obtain a representative activity distribution (Heck & Duley, 1974). Routinely, about 400 000 particles are injected. As there are over 280 billion pulmonary capillaries and 300 million pre-capillary arterioles, only a very small fraction of the pulmonary bed will be obstructed. A preparation of 100 000-200 000 particles is recommended for patients with known pulmonary hypertension or after a single lung transplant. Degradation of MAA results in its elimination from the lung within a few hours.

2.3 Acquisition

To perform V/P SPECT takes only one hour from referral to report (Bajc et al., 2004; Palmer et al., 2001). The ventilation study starts with inhalation of 25-30 megabecquerel (MBq) Technegas, usually 2-3 breaths. Immediately after ventilation SPECT, a dose of 100-120 MBq 99mTc-MAA is given intravenously for perfusion imaging.

During the examination, the supine patient carefully maintains the position between ventilation and perfusion acquisitions. Immobilization for only 20 minutes is well tolerated by nearly all patients. Examination in supine position is comfortable even for critically ill patients. It is also more convenient for the staff. It is noteworthy that V/P SPECT can be performed in all patients, since there is no contraindication related to age, radiation, contrast media or co-morbidity.

2.4 Reconstruction and calculation of V/P quotient images

Iterative OSEM is essential for SPECT reconstruction. Ventilation activity is subtracted from perfusion images. A valuable parameter in clinical SPECT is the Ventilation/Perfusion quotient, $V/P_{quotient}$ (Bajc et al., 2004; Palmer et al., 2001). $V/P_{quotient}$ is calculated after normalization of ventilation counts to perfusion counts. Hot spot removal is important, especially when 99mTc-DTPA is used.

2.5 Presentation of V/P SPECT

V/P SPECT images are usually presented in frontal, sagittal and transversal projections, available in any modern system. The slices must be accurately aligned so that ventilation and perfusion slices match each other for correct comparison. Therefore, it is crucial to achieve this acquisition in one session with maintained body position. This is also a prerequisite for the calculation of $V/P_{quotient}$ images, which greatly facilitates identification of ventilation/perfusion mismatches typical of PE as well as other patterns characteristic of other pulmonary diseases.
Volume rendered images, such as "Maximum Intensity Projection" are available with almost all SPECT systems, allowing rotating 3D views. This function is another valuable option, particularly for quantification and follow-up of PE patients.

3. Interpretation

According to the new European guidelines, the holistic interpretation of lung SPECT is recommended (Bajc et al., 2009b). The clinician can only benefit from reports, which clearly express the presence or absence of PE. This goal was not achieved with previous probabilistic reporting methods according to PIOPED or modified PIOPED. Large V/P SPECT studies show that this is achievable if all patterns are considered, where these combine ventilation and perfusion. Conclusive reports were given in 97 to 99 % of studies.
Holistic interpretation of V/P SPECT should be based upon: a) Clinical pre-test probability and b) the application of criteria for interpreting V/P patterns to distinguish between patterns indicative of PE and other diseases.

3.1 Criteria for acute PE according the european guidelines

In accordance with the guidelines of the European Association of Nuclear Medicine (Bajc et al., 2009a, b), PE is reported if there is:

- V/P mismatch of at least one segment or two sub-segments that conforms to the pulmonary vascular anatomy.

No PE is reported if there is:

- normal perfusion pattern conforming to the anatomic boundaries of the lungs,
- matched or reversed mismatch V/P defects of any size, shape or number in the absence of mismatch

- mismatch that does not have a lobar, segmental or sub-segmental pattern

Non-diagnostic for PE is reported if there are:

- Multiple V/P abnormalities not typical of specific diseases.

The fundamental point is that lobar, segmental or sub-segmental V/P mismatch serves as the basis for confirming a diagnosis of PE among patients with suspected PE. Howarth et al. state that: "at least 0.5 of a segment of ventilation/perfusion mismatch is considered diagnostic of PE" (Howarth et al., 2006). This simplified criterion gave the highest combined sensitivity and specificity, observer reproducibility and fewest indeterminate results. In PE, a mismatch has its base along the pleura and conforms to known sub-segmental and segmental vascular anatomy (Miniati et al., 1996). Applying these principles of interpretation, recent V/P SPECT studies of more than 3000 cases showed a negative predictive value of 97-99 %, a sensitivity of 96-99%, and a specificity of 91-98% for PE diagnosis (Bajc et al., 2008; Leblanc et al., 2007; Lemb & Pohlabeln, 2001; Miniati et al., 1996; Reinartz et al., 2004). The rate of non-diagnostic findings was 1-3%. V/P SPECT yields ventilation and perfusion images in exactly the same projections, facilitating recognition of mismatch. This is of particular importance in the middle lobe and lingula where mismatch may be overlooked if the lung is not accurately delineated by its ventilation images (Meignan, 2002).

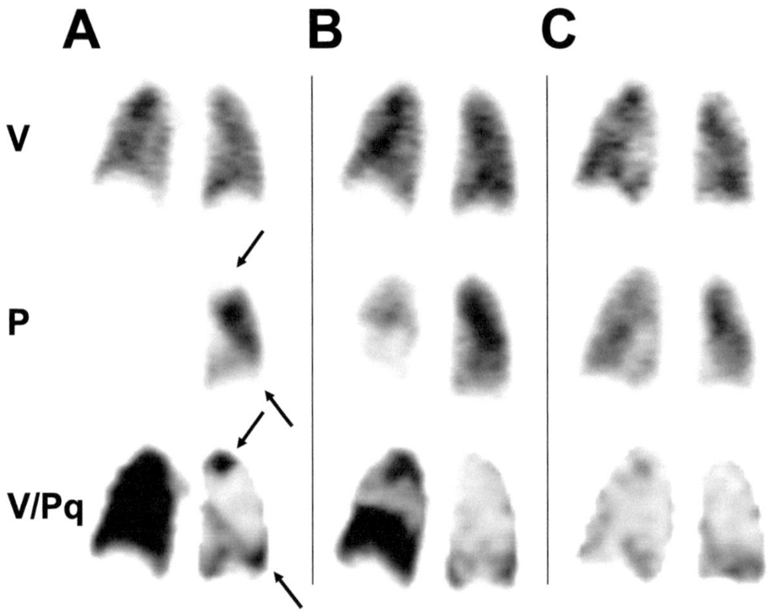

Fig. 4. Patient with massive PE. A) Absent perfusion is seen in the right lung and sub-segmental perfusion defects are seen in the left lung (arrows). **B)** After approximately one week of anticoagulant therapy. **C)** The day after thrombolysis.

Furthermore, V/P SPECT allows quantification of PE extension which is a prerequisite for individual treatment of PE. As suggested by Olsson et al., the number of segments and sub-segments indicating PE are counted and expressed in % of the total lung parenchyma (Olsson et al., 2006). Moreover, areas with ventilation abnormalities were recognized

allowing estimation of the degree of total lung malfunction. A segmental reduction or a sub-segmental total deficiency of function is attributed 1 point, a segmental total deficiency, 2 points. Each lung comprises according to our charts 9 segments, representing 18 points. Mismatch defects are expressed as mismatch points, which after division by 36 give the fraction of the lung that is embolised. Regions with ventilation or perfusion defects are totalled in order to estimate the reduction in overall lung function.
The study showed that patients with up to 40 % PE could be safely treated at home if ventilation abnormalities engaged less than 20 % of the lung. Since 2004, the Skåne University Hospital, Lund, has successfully treated more than 2000 patients with PE and about 60 % of these patients were treated at home.

3.2 Diagnosis of pulmonary embolism

In PE, an embolus blocks the blood flow, causing a perfusion defect, while ventilation remains normal because there is no corresponding blockage in the airway. To characterize the pattern of perfusion defects is crucial. Perfusion defects due to blockage of a pulmonary artery should reflect the branching of pulmonary circulation and its classical segmental anatomy. A segmental defect is wedge shaped with its base on the pleura.
On V/P SPECT images, it is relatively easy to identify segmental and sub-segmental patterns of perfusion defects. Figure 4a shows multiple perfusion defects in acute stage in a female patient with chest pains, who had fainted outside the hospital. Applying quantification on V/P SPECT images, extension of PE was estimated to be ca 60%. The patient was treated first with heparin for a week. However, Follow up showed limited regression (Fig 4b). As brain hemorrhage was excluded, thrombolysis was administered. The following day perfusion was normalized (Fig 4c).
Figure 2 shows sagittal slices of right lung of a patient studied for acute breathlessness. A segmental perfusion defect was well delineated, in perfusion and $V/P_{quotient}$ images (Fig 2a). Moreover, it was possible to see broncho-constriction in the posterior part of the lung (blue arrow). The extension of perfusion defect was estimated at 10% and ventilation defect 25%. Three days later nearly complete resolution of the embolus was observed, as well as normalization of the ventilation (Fig 2b).
In planar images, the identification of a solitary segmental perfusion defect within middle lobe and lingula is often impossible or, at best, difficult. With tomographic images these changes are well delineated.
It is important to be aware that mismatch findings not having segmental character do not usually represent PE. Non segmental mismatch means that perfusion defects do not conform to segmental anatomy and are caused by other diseases. This is observed in patients with heart failure (Jögi et al., 2008), pneumonia, mediastinal adenopathy, post radiation therapy etc. Total absence of perfusion in one lung without any other region of mismatch is often caused by pathology other than PE, such as a central tumour or abscess.

3.3 Follow up

Follow up is a frequently overlooked aspect of diagnostic strategies although it is essential both for clinical and scientific reasons. The follow up is necessary to assess the effect of treatment, especially to see the effect of anticoagulant therapy (Fig 4b) and in these cases to be able to adjust therapy or, if necessary, continue with thrombolysis (Fig 4c).

Moreover follow up is important

- To assess the need for prolonged oral anticoagulation beyond 6 months, where there are extensive remnants of PE.
- To allow differentiation between new and old PE, where a recurrence of PE is suspected.
- To explain physical incapacity after PE in case of permanently impaired lung function.
- To evaluate and compare drugs and treatment strategies.
- To identify patients with remaining perfusion defects after treatment as these could be particularly susceptible to developing pulmonary hypertension

For follow up, V/P SPECT is the only suitable method for the following reasons:

- Detection of all emboli requires that the whole lung is examined with a sensitive method.
- The cumulative radiation dose is a central issue when the indication for PE is relative
- V/P SPECT is the only method which enables functional impairment to be determined due to increased dead space from non-perfused lung units and increased pulmonary vascular resistance due to a reduced vascular bed.

To be able to study the efficacy of treatment, in individual patients the same method should be used both for diagnosis and follow up. This is a further strong argument in favour of V/P SPECT as the primary diagnostic method for PE.

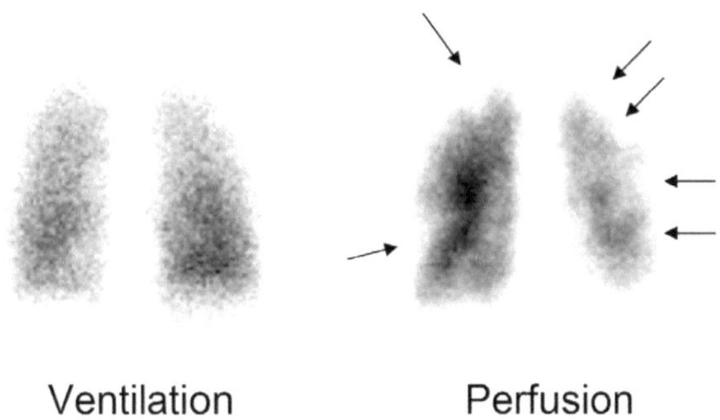

Fig. 5. Patient with chronic PE. Frontal slices. Multiple perfusion defects are seen (arrows). MDCT was normal.

3.4 Chronic pulmonary embolism

Chronic PE is a progressive disease that develops in about 5 % of patients, even after treatment (Begic et al., 2011; Pengo et al., 2004), after an acute episode of PE . However, it often has an insidious onset. It might lead to pulmonary hypertension, right heart failure and arrhythmia, which are frequent causes of death. The value of ventilation/perfusion scintigraphy is well established. It has recently been confirmed in a head to head comparison between MDCT and planar scintigraphy with pulmonary angiography as reference. Among patients with pulmonary hypertension, scintigraphy had a sensitivity of 96-97% and specificity of 90 %, while MDCT had a sensitivity of 51% (Tunariu et al., 2007). The conclusion was that ventilation/perfusion scintigraphy "has a higher sensitivity than MDCT as well as very good specificity in detecting chronic pulmonary thromboembolic disease as a potentially curable cause of pulmonary hypertension". Scintigraphic features of chronic PE vary. Figure 5 illustrates a case of multiple perfusion defects which are similar to acute PE. MDCT was

normal. In some patients mismatch without clear segmental or sub-segmental pattern is observed. Peripheral zones of the lung lack perfusion. The centre of the lung is hyperperfused. The lung appears significantly smaller on perfusion images compared to ventilation and the $V/P_{quotient}$ images show mismatch along the lung periphery (Fig 6).
In recent guidelines for the diagnosis and treatment of pulmonary hypertension it is stated that "ventilation/perfusion scan remains the screening method of choice for chronic pulmonary hypertension" (Galie et al., 2009). It was also pointed out that pulmonary veno-occlusive disease is a rare but important differential diagnosis.

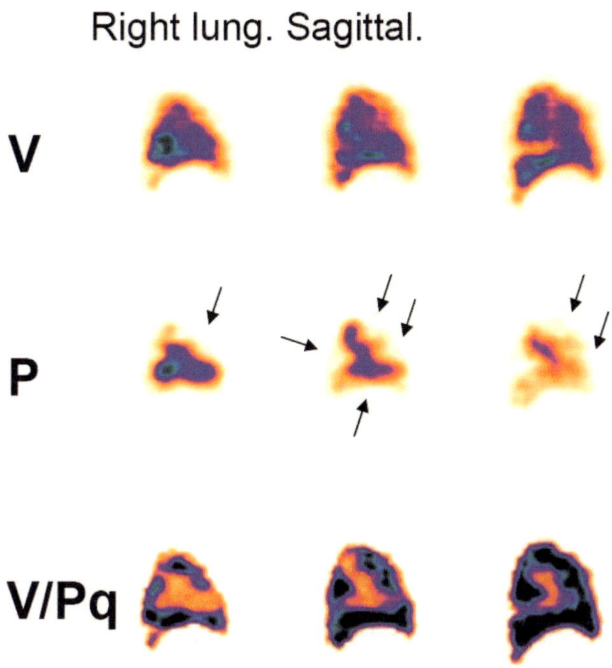

Fig. 6. Patient with pulmonary hypertension caused by chronic PE. Peripheral zones of the lung lack perfusion (arrows). The centre of the lung is hyperperfused .$V/P_{quotient}$ images shows mismatch along the lung periphery.

4. Sensitivity and specificity of V/P SPECT and other methodological considerations

In a clinical study, 53 % more mismatch points were identified with V/P SPECT compared to planar technique (Bajc et al., 2004). Similar results have been found by others (Gutte et al., 2010; Reinartz et al., 2001). SPECT eliminates superimposed structures, clarifying segmental and sub-segmental nature of perfusion defects caused by PE.
The value of V/P SPECT is further confirmed in clinical studies (Bajc et al., 2008; Gutte et al., 2009; Leblanc et al., 2007; Lemb & Pohlabeln, 2001). V/P SPECT is today the recommended method for clinical diagnosis, follow up and research (Bajc et al., 2009b).
Powell reported that sensitivity and specificity of CT for central PE are about 90% (Powell & Muller, 2003). Perrier et al. found in a broad clinical material that CT had a sensitivity of 70% for PE and a specificity of 91 % (Perrier et al., 2001). They concluded: "clinical CT should not

be used alone for suspected PE but could replace angiography in combined strategies that include ultrasonography and lung scanning". Likewise, van Strijen et al. found in a multicentre prospective study that sensitivity of CT was 69% while specificity was 84% and "concluded that the overall sensitivity of spiral CT is too low to endorse its use as the sole test to exclude PE" and that "this holds true even if one limits the discussion to patients with larger PE in segmental or larger pulmonary artery branches" (Van Strijen et al., 2005). Our experience supports this view. Also, CT as a second procedure following scintigraphy has limited value (van Strijen et al., 2003). Multislice CT seems to improve resolution but sensitivity for small PE appears not to be improved (Stein et al., 2006).

A problem associated with limited sensitivity of CT and incomplete coverage of the total lung is that the degree of embolism and lung function deficiency cannot be quantified. Quantification is important for treatment selection.

In spite of excellent diagnostic qualities of V/P SPECT and documented low sensitivity of CT, the latter method is often recommended. A high number of non-diagnostic scintigraphies were reported in the PIOPED study (65%) (1990). This is still used as an argument against lung scintigraphy. In PIOPED, scintigraphy was performed with inferior technique and inflexible sub-optimal interpretation criteria. Even with planar scintigraphy, a reduction in the number of non-diagnostic reports to 10% can be achieved with adequate acquisition and a holistic interpretation strategy (Bajc et al., 2002a). With V/P SPECT, this number is further reduced to between 1 and 4%, as found in several studies (Bajc et al., 2008; Leblanc et al., 2007; Lemb & Pohlabeln, 2001).

Some practitioners hold that sub-segmental emboli are of little importance for otherwise healthy people and may be left untreated and, as a consequence, are prepared to accept less sensitive methods for PE diagnosis. However, small emboli are important because they 1) may be a first and only sign of silent deep venous thrombosis, 2) may precede larger emboli 3) if not diagnosed and/or untreated, further episodes may lead to chronic PE and pulmonary hypertension (Fig. 6). 4) form a threat to patients with limited cardio-pulmonary reserve, 5) are clinically essential for quantification, which is necessary to scientifically establish appropriate treatment protocols. Thus, each embolus is relevant, irrespective of size. Sub-segmental emboli should not be left untreated without further scientific evidence.

5. Selection of therapeutic strategy

Management of PE was previously confined to in-hospital therapy, using anticoagulation, heparin injections followed by oral anticoagulants for extended periods of time.

About 20 % to 55 % of patients with deep venous thrombosis have concomitant PE, which is usually not diagnosed because symptoms of PE are absent. Outpatient treatment of patients with deep venous thrombosis, which is perceived as a safe routine, implies that many patients with PE are treated at home. Home treatment of patients with diagnosed PE has been suggested (Kovacs et al., 2000) but in order to determine the appropriateness of the treatment on an individual basis, the extension of PE obviously need to be estimated. Whilst patients with limited extension of PE may be treated at home, intermediate cases and patients with co-morbidity may need in-hospital treatment. Those with very extensive PE may require thrombolysis, necessitating inpatient treatment.

Obviously, quantification requires studies of the whole lung with methods allowing identification of large and small emboli. V/P SPECT is the ideal method for this purpose as segmental and sub-segmental emboli can be both detected with a high degree of sensitivity and quantified in terms of mismatch points. In a prospective study Olsson et al. studied 102 out-patients with a moderate degree of PE (up to 40%) (Olsson et al., 2006). After only 5 days, embolism diminished by 44 % on average. There was no tromboembolic mortality in the trial. Later follow up indicated that PE had not recurred in patients showing resolution after 5 days. Since 2004, more than 1000 patients, of Skåne University Hospital, Lund, with up to 50% extension of PE have been treated as out-patients. After this positive experience, out-patient treatment is now perceived as a safe routine in patients who have been selected on the basis of V/P SPECT and relevant clinical information.

6. Additional findings

PE is a condition known for its non-specific symptoms. Medical imaging, such as V/P SPECT, is therefore necessary to confirm or exclude the diagnosis among patients with suspected PE. The majority of patients that are examined with V/P SPECT, due to the initial assumption of PE, will not have PE. It is therefore important that any alternative diagnoses, which could explain the patients' symptoms, are identified and provided to the referring physician. Possible alternative diagnoses include pneumonia, heart failure, pleural fluid, malignancy and chronic obstructive pulmonary disease (COPD) (Richman et al., 2004). Another important aspect is that these conditions sometimes coexist and that they also elevate the risk of PE (Elliott et al., 2000). V/P SPECT can be employed to identify other diagnoses than PE.

6.1 Chronic obstructive pulmonary disease

COPD is a major cause of both morbidity and mortality globally (Mannino et al., 2006). It is one of the few diseases that continues to rise in numbers in many countries. COPD is an inflammatory disease characterized by airflow limitation that is not fully reversible (Celli & MacNee, 2004). The airflow limitation is caused by a combination of airway obstruction and parenchymal destruction (emphysema). The pulmonary changes in COPD lead to inhomogeneous regional ventilation. V/P SPECT is sufficiently sensitive as a method to identify the functional changes in COPD. In comparison with DTPA aerosols, Technegas penetrates the lung periphery better (Jögi et al., 2010), which is especially important in COPD (exemplified in Fig 3). Technegas ventilation imaging has been shown to visualise the early changes of COPD before they can be observed with high resolution CT (HRCT) (Yokoe et al., 2006). As COPD initially affects the airways, the ventilation defects are commonly more prominent than those of perfusion. Perfusion within the lungs also becomes abnormal as the lungs attempt to adapt the regional blood flow to ventilation to preserve an efficient gas exchange. Often this adaptation is incomplete and perfused but non-ventilated areas (low V/P ratio) occur, i.e. reverse mismatch (Gottschalk et al., 1993). With progressive disease, concurrent destruction of airways and blood vessels takes place and matched defects with absence of both ventilation and perfusion are seen. Vascular remodeling in COPD may lead to regions with elevated V/P ratios. Garg et al. (1983) found that the degree of abnormality on aerosol ventilation images significantly correlated to pulmonary function tests. In a recent paper, which evaluated the role of V/P SPECT in patients with COPD, it was shown that V/P SPECT correlated significantly both to traditional lung function tests as well as the extent of emphysema as measured with HRCT (Jögi et al., 2011). It was also shown that V/P SPECT could be used to characterize the severity of COPD. Pulmonary embolism and heart failure are common comorbidities with overlapping symptoms that complicate the manifestation of COPD. The prevalence of PE in patients hospitalized with exacerbation has been reported to be as high as 25% but is generally under-diagnosed (Mispelaere et al., 2002; Tillie-Leblond et al., 2006). In patients with stable COPD, PE accounts for 10% of deaths (Schonhofer & Kohler, 1998). The prevalence of heart failure among patients with stable COPD has been reported to be about 20% and even higher in patients with exacerbation (Rizkallah et al., 2009; Rutten et al., 2006). The previous finding of the PIOPED study that V/P scintigraphy cannot be used to diagnose PE among patients with pathology of ventilation is an outdated belief (1990). Figure 7 shows extensive PE in a patient with COPD. This heavy smoker had a short history of progressive dyspnea. V/P SPECT showed uneven ventilation and perfusion with a pattern that is typical for COPD. Moreover, extensive perfusion defects were seen in areas with preserved ventilation. V/P quotient images could be used to quantify the extent of PE to approximately 70% of the lung parenchyma.

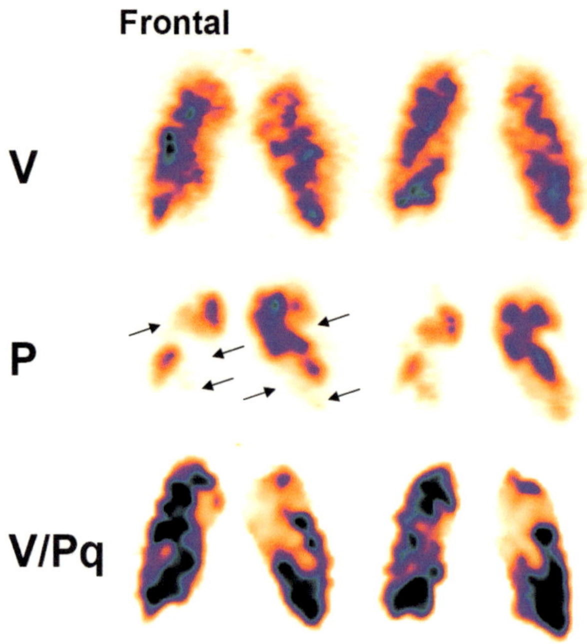

Fig. 7. Patient with severe COPD and chronic PE. Frontal slices; ventilation is very uneven in the whole lung. In addition, multiple perfusion defects are seen in ventilated areas. Mismatches are highlighted in $V/P_{quotient}$ images.

6.2 Heart failure

Left heart failure is a complex clinical syndrome that can result from any cardiac disorder that affects the ability of the left ventricle to function as a pump. When the left chamber is unable to meet the functional demands of the body, symptoms such as dyspnea and fatigue, as well as signs of pulmonary fluid retention appear. In patients with heart failure the risk of developing venous thromboembolic disease, including PE, is elevated (Anderson & Spencer, 2003). As early as the 1960s, Friedman and Braunwald, West and others demonstrated that patients with mitral valve disease and left heart failure showed an inversion or "cephalization" of the normal dependent distribution of blood flow (Friedman & Braunwald, 1966; West et al., 1964). The inverted distribution of blood flow to non-dependent lung zones seen in heart failure has been correlated to elevated pulmonary venous pressure, interstitial oedema, alveolar space flooding and, when longstanding, perivascular fibrosis (Mohsenifar et al., 1989; Pistolesi et al., 1988). Ventilation is not affected to the same degree as perfusion and mismatch in the dependent lung is therefore common. This mismatch, however, is not of a segmental character. V/P SPECT can therefore identify patients with congestive heart failure. In a study of 247 patients examined with V/P SPECT for suspected PE, we found that 15% of the patients had signs of heart failure, sometimes in combination with PE (Jögi et al., 2008). Figure 8 shows a patient who suffered from increasing breathlessness. V/P SPECT was performed to exclude PE. V/P SPECT in supine position identified redistribution of ventilation and perfusion towards ventral regions (Fig 8a). Perfusion is more affected than ventilation and mismatch is therefore observed. This is, however, non-segmental and the diagnosis was therefore reported as heart failure and not PE. After 12 days of anticongestive treatment, the patient had improved clinically and the follow-up V/P SPECT (Fig 8b) showed complete normalization of both ventilation and perfusion.

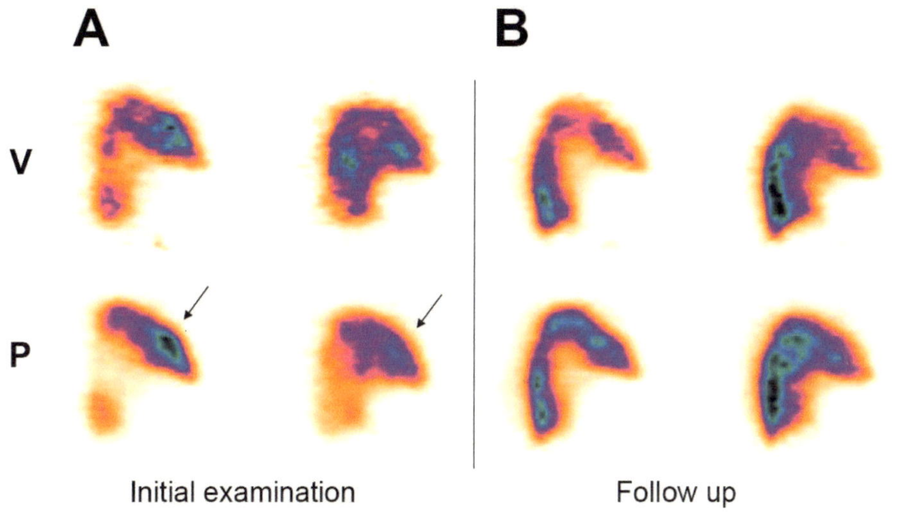

Fig. 8. Patient with acute heart failure. A) In the supine patient, perfusion is redistributed to anterior parts of the lung. Ventilation is also affected but not to the same degree, which causes non-segmental perfusion defects. **B)**. Follow up after 12 days of anticongestive treatment

6.3 Pneumonia

Pneumonia is an inflammatory condition of the lung parenchyma, especially affecting the alveoli. There are both infectious and non-infectious causes. The pneumonic regions of the lung become non-ventilated although the blood flow is often maintained to some extent. This can cause shunting and lead to hypoxemia. As the ventilation defect often exceeds the perfusion defect, reverse mismatch is a common finding (Carvalho & Lavender, 1989). In a study by Li et al. (1994) reverse mismatch represented pneumonia in 81% of the cases. In severe cases both ventilation and perfusion are reduced or abolished and matched defects are then frequently found (Li et al., 1994). Another sign of pneumonia that often has been described is the "stripe sign" (Sostman & Gottschalk, 1982, 1992). The "stripe sign" refers to the observation of a stripe of a relatively well preserved perfusion adjacent to the pleural surface, by contrast with the more pronounced perfusion defects within the pneumonic lesion. This distinguishes pneumonia from the segmental perfusion defects found in PE. The enhanced performance of V/P SPECT compared to planar imaging has facilitated the detection of the stripe sign (Pace & Goris, 1998).

Hampson as well as the ICOPER study illustrated that the risk of PE is increased in patients with pneumonia or other coexisting diseases (Elliott et al., 2000; Hampson, 1995). In the ICOPER study, 17% of 2000 patients with confirmed PE had infiltrates on chest X-ray. Pneumonia has also been shown to be a common finding in patients with autopsy proven PE (Mandelli et al., 1997).

7. Radiation exposure

The doses of 30 MBq and 120 MBq for ventilation and perfusion, respectively, allows excellent V/P SPECT quality at an effective radiation dose of 1.8 mSv (ICRP, 1998). The absorbed dose to the breasts with V/P SPECT is 0.8 mGy (ICRP, 1998). Estimation of exposure is relatively easy when short-lived radio-isotopes are used in nuclear medicine. In contrast, for X-ray technologies this is much more difficult because of a number of factors, such as differences in equipment and the size of the exposed fields. According to ICRP, the average effective dose for 4–16-detector MDCT is 5.4 mSv (Valentin, 2007). Notably, this information was based on computed rather than measured dose data. Hurwitz et al. reported for a current adult PE protocol with 64-detector MDCT a measured effective dose of 19.9±1.38 mSv (Hurwitz et al., 2007). These authors point out that the actual measured dose is about 50% higher than the computed dose. The absorbed dose to the breasts was 35–42 mGy. Absorbed radiation dose to the breast for a single-slice CT study was 20–50 mGy and 30– 50% greater with a four-slice CT. In a very recent study, Hurwitz et al. (Hurwitz et al., 2009) studied radiation dose-saving protocols. Phantoms of women were exposed to MDCT protocols with automatic current modulation, lower tube voltage and bismuth shields over the chest. In the case of a medium sized female patient when automatic current modulation was applied at 140 kVp, breast doses were estimated at 62 mGy and this reduced to 33 mGy when bismuth shields were added. At 120 kVp the doses were 44 mGy without shields and 20 mGy with shields. Some limitations of the study were discussed. No phantom with significant subcutaneous fat was studied. The authors were not able to directly assess the effect of increased noise for the diagnosis of PE. Dose-saving protocols are promising.

8. Conclusions

The superiority of V/P SPECT over other imaging techniques in the diagnosis of PE has been well demonstrated. The examination is without contraindication and can be performed in 99% of patients with suspected PE. V/P SPECT makes it possible to quantify the extent of perfusion loss, so that PE treatment can be better adapted to the needs of individual patients. By using V/P SPECT, it is also possible to diagnose other cardiopulmonary conditions.

Because of the very low radiation exposure, it is an ideal method for evaluating treatment and follow up. Low radiation doses are particularly important for women in the reproductive period and during pregnancy.

The above mentioned advantages of V/P SPECT for studying PE lead to the conclusion that it is the only suitable technique both for follow-up in patients with PE as well as for validation of treatment therapies. Moreover, it is an essential tool for research.

9. References

Anderson, F.A., Jr., and Spencer, F.A. (2003). Risk factors for venous thromboembolism. *Circulation*, Vol. 107, No. 23 Suppl 1, (2003), pp. I9-16

Bajc, M., Albrechtsson, U., Olsson, C.G., Olsson, B., and Jonson, B. (2002a). Comparison of ventilation/perfusion scintigraphy and helical CT for diagnosis of pulmonary embolism; strategy using clinical data and ancillary findings. *Clin Physiol Funct Imaging*, Vol. 22, No. 6, (2002a), pp. 392-397

Bajc, M., Bitzen, U., Olsson, B., Perez de Sa, V., Palmer, J., and Jonson, B. (2002b). Lung ventilation/perfusion SPECT in the artificially embolized pig. *J Nucl Med*, Vol. 43, No. 5, (2002b), pp. 640-647

Bajc, M., Neilly, J.B., Miniati, M., Schuemichen, C., Meignan, M., and Jonson, B. (2009a). EANM guidelines for ventilation/perfusion scintigraphy : Part 1. Pulmonary imaging with ventilation/perfusion single photon emission tomography. *Eur J Nucl Med Mol Imaging*, Vol. 36, No. 8, (2009a), pp. 1356-1370

Bajc, M., Neilly, J.B., Miniati, M., Schuemichen, C., Meignan, M., and Jonson, B. (2009b). EANM guidelines for ventilation/perfusion scintigraphy : Part 2. Algorithms and clinical considerations for diagnosis of pulmonary emboli with V/P(SPECT) and MDCT. *Eur J Nucl Med Mol Imaging*, Vol. 36, No. 9, (2009b), pp. 1528-1538

Bajc, M., Olsson, B., Palmer, J., and Jonson, B. (2008). Ventilation/Perfusion SPECT for diagnostics of pulmonary embolism in clinical practice. *Journal of internal medicine*, Vol. 264, No. 4, (2008), pp. 379-387

Bajc, M., Olsson, C.G., Olsson, B., Palmer, J., and Jonson, B. (2004). Diagnostic evaluation of planar and tomographic ventilation/perfusion lung images in patients with suspected pulmonary emboli. *Clin Physiol Funct Imaging*, Vol. 24, No. 5, (2004), pp. 249-256

Begic, A., Jögi, J., Hadziredzepovic, A., Kucukalic-Selimovic, E., Begovic-Hadzimuratovic, S., and Bajc, M. (2011). Tomographic ventilation/perfusion lung scintigraphy in the monitoring of the effect of treatment in pulmonary embolism: serial follow-up over a 6-month period. *Nucl Med Commun*, Vol. 32, No. 6, (2011), pp. 508-514

Carvalho, P., and Lavender, J.P. (1989). The incidence and etiology of the ventilation/perfusion reverse mismatch defect. *Clin Nucl Med*, Vol. 14, No. 8, (1989), pp. 571-576

Celli, B.R., and MacNee, W. (2004). Standards for the diagnosis and treatment of patients with COPD: a summary of the ATS/ERS position paper. *Eur Respir J*, Vol. 23, No. 6, (2004), pp. 932-946

Elliott, C.G., Goldhaber, S.Z., Visani, L., and DeRosa, M. (2000). Chest radiographs in acute pulmonary embolism. Results from the International Cooperative Pulmonary Embolism Registry. *Chest*, Vol. 118, No. 1, (2000), pp. 33-38

Friedman, W.F., and Braunwald, E. (1966). Alterations in regional pulmonary blood flow in mitral valve disease studied by radioisotope scanning. A simple nontraumatic technique for estimation of left atrial pressure. *Circulation*, Vol. 34, No. 3, (1966), pp. 363-376

Galie, N., Hoeper, M.M., Humbert, M., Torbicki, A., Vachiery, J.L., Barbera, J.A., Beghetti, M., Corris, P., Gaine, S., Gibbs, J.S., *et al.* (2009). Guidelines for the diagnosis and treatment of pulmonary hypertension: the Task Force for the Diagnosis and Treatment of Pulmonary Hypertension of the European Society of Cardiology (ESC) and the European Respiratory Society (ERS), endorsed by the International Society of Heart and Lung Transplantation (ISHLT). *Eur Heart J*, Vol. 30, No. 20, (2009), pp. 2493-2537

Garg, A., Gopinath, P.G., Pande, J.N., and Guleria, J.S. (1983). Role of radio-aerosol and perfusion lung imaging in early detection of chronic obstructive lung disease. *Eur J Nucl Med*, Vol. 8, No. 4, (1983), pp. 167-171

Giuntini, C. (2001). Ventilation/perfusion scan and dead space in pulmonary embolism: are they useful for the diagnosis? *Q J Nucl Med*, Vol. 45, No. 4, (2001), pp. 281-286

Gottschalk, A., Sostman, H.D., Coleman, R.E., Juni, J.E., Thrall, J., McKusick, K.A., Froelich, J.W., and Alavi, A. (1993). Ventilation-perfusion scintigraphy in the PIOPED study. Part II. Evaluation of the scintigraphic criteria and interpretations. *J Nucl Med*, Vol. 34, No. 7, (1993), pp. 1119-1126

Gray, H.W., McKillop, J.H., and Bessent, R.G. (1993). Lung scan reports: interpretation by clinicians. *Nucl Med Commun*, Vol. 14, No. 11, (1993), pp. 989-994

Gutte, H., Mortensen, J., Jensen, C.V., Johnbeck, C.B., von der Recke, P., Petersen, C.L., Kjaergaard, J., Kristoffersen, U.S., and Kjaer, A. (2009). Detection of Pulmonary Embolism with Combined Ventilation-Perfusion SPECT and Low-Dose CT: Head-to-Head Comparison with Multidetector CT Angiography. *J Nucl Med*, Vol. 50, (2009), pp. 1987-1992

Gutte, H., Mortensen, J., Jensen, C.V., von der Recke, P., Petersen, C.L., Kristoffersen, U.S., and Kjaer, A. (2010). Comparison of V/Q SPECT and planar V/Q lung scintigraphy in diagnosing acute pulmonary embolism. *Nucl Med Commun*, Vol. 31, No. 1, (2010), pp. 82-86

Hampson, N.B. (1995). Pulmonary embolism: difficulties in the clinical diagnosis. *Semin Respir Infect*, Vol. 10, No. 3, (1995), pp. 123-130

Heck, L.L., and Duley, J.W., Jr. (1974). Statistical considerations in lung imaging with 99mTc albumin particles. *Radiology*, Vol. 113, No. 3, (1974), pp. 675-679

Howarth, D.M., Booker, J.A., and Voutnis, D.D. (2006). Diagnosis of pulmonary embolus using ventilation/perfusion lung scintigraphy: more than 0.5 segment of ventilation/perfusion mismatch is sufficient. *Intern Med J*, Vol. 36, No. 5, (2006), pp. 281-288

Hurwitz, L.M., Reiman, R.E., Yoshizumi, T.T., Goodman, P.C., Toncheva, G., Nguyen, G., and Lowry, C. (2007). Radiation dose from contemporary cardiothoracic multidetector CT protocols with an anthropomorphic female phantom: implications for cancer induction. *Radiology*, Vol. 245, No. 3, (2007), pp. 742-750

Hurwitz, L.M., Yoshizumi, T.T., Goodman, P.C., Nelson, R.C., Toncheva, G., Nguyen, G.B., Lowry, C., and Anderson-Evans, C. (2009). Radiation dose savings for adult pulmonary embolus 64-MDCT using bismuth breast shields, lower peak kilovoltage, and automatic tube current modulation. *AJR Am J Roentgenol*, Vol. 192, No. 1, (2009), pp. 244-253

ICRP (1998). Radiation dose to patients from radiopharmaceuticals (addendum 2 to ICRP publication 53). *Ann ICRP*, Vol. 28, No. 3, (1998), pp. 1-126

James, J.M., Lloyd, J.J., Leahy, B.C., Church, S., Hardy, C.C., Shields, R.A., Prescott, M.C., and Testa, H.J. (1992). 99Tcm-Technegas and krypton-81m ventilation scintigraphy: a comparison in known respiratory disease. *Br J Radiol*, Vol. 65, No. 780, (1992), pp. 1075-1082

Jögi, J., Ekberg, M., Jonson, B., Bozovic, G., and Bajc, M. (2011). Ventilation/perfusion SPECT in chronic obstructive pulmonary disease: an evaluation by reference to symptoms, spirometric lung function and emphysema, as assessed with HRCT. *Eur J Nucl Med Mol Imaging*, Vol. 38, No. 7, (2011), pp. 1344-1352

Jögi, J., Jonson, B., Ekberg, M., and Bajc, M. (2010). Ventilation-perfusion SPECT with 99mTc-DTPA versus Technegas: a head-to-head study in obstructive and nonobstructive disease. *J Nucl Med*, Vol. 51, No. 5, (2010), pp. 735-741

Jögi, J., Palmer, J., Jonson, B., and Bajc, M. (2008). Heart failure diagnostics based on ventilation/perfusion single photon emission computed tomography pattern and quantitative perfusion gradients. *Nucl Med Commun*, Vol. 29, No. 8, (2008), pp. 666-673

Kovacs, M.J., Anderson, D., Morrow, B., Gray, L., Touchie, D., and Wells, P.S. (2000). Outpatient treatment of pulmonary embolism with dalteparin. *Thromb Haemost*, Vol. 83, No. 2, (2000), pp. 209-211

Leblanc, M., Leveillee, F., and Turcotte, E. (2007). Prospective evaluation of the negative predictive value of V/Q SPECT using 99mTc-Technegas. *Nucl Med Commun*, Vol. 28, No. 8, (2007), pp. 667-672

Lemb, M., and Pohlabeln, H. (2001). Pulmonary thromboembolism: a retrospective study on the examination of 991 patients by ventilation/perfusion SPECT using Technegas. *Nuklearmedizin*, Vol. 40, No. 6, (2001), pp. 179-186

Li, D.J., Stewart, I., Miles, K.A., and Wraight, E.P. (1994). Scintigraphic appearances in patients with pulmonary infection and lung scintigrams of intermediate or low probability for pulmonary embolism. *Clin Nucl Med*, Vol. 19, No. 12, (1994), pp. 1091-1093

Magnussen, J.S., Chicco, P., Palmer, A.W., Bush, V., Mackey, D.W., Storey, G., Magee, M., Bautovich, G., and Van der Wall, H. (1999). Single-photon emission tomography of a computerised model of pulmonary embolism. *Eur J Nucl Med*, Vol. 26, No. 11, (1999), pp. 1430-1438

Mandelli, V., Schmid, C., Zogno, C., and Morpurgo, M. (1997). "False negatives" and "false positives" in acute pulmonary embolism: a clinical-postmortem comparison. *Cardiologia*, Vol. 42, No. 2, (1997), pp. 205-210

Mannino, D.M., Watt, G., Hole, D., Gillis, C., Hart, C., McConnachie, A., Davey Smith, G., Upton, M., Hawthorne, V., Sin, D.D., *et al.* (2006). The natural history of chronic obstructive pulmonary disease. *Eur Respir J*, Vol. 27, No. 3, (2006), pp. 627-643

Meignan, M.A. (2002). Lung ventilation/perfusion SPECT: the right technique for hard times. *J Nucl Med*, Vol. 43, No. 5, (2002), pp. 648-651

Miniati, M., Pistolesi, M., Marini, C., Di Ricco, G., Formichi, B., Prediletto, R., Allescia, G., Tonelli, L., Sostman, H.D., and Giuntini, C. (1996). Value of perfusion lung scan in the diagnosis of pulmonary embolism: results of the Prospective Investigative Study of Acute Pulmonary Embolism Diagnosis (PISA-PED). *Am J Respir Crit Care Med*, Vol. 154, No. 5, (1996), pp. 1387-1393

Mispelaere, D., Glerant, J.C., Audebert, M., Remond, A., Sevestre-Pietri, M.A., and Jounieaux, V. (2002). [Pulmonary embolism and sibilant types of chronic obstructive pulmonary disease decompensations]. *Rev Mal Respir*, Vol. 19, No. 4, (2002), pp. 415-423

Mohsenifar, Z., Amin, D.K., and Shah, P.K. (1989). Regional distribution of lung perfusion and ventilation in patients with chronic congestive heart failure and its relationship to cardiopulmonary hemodynamics. *Am Heart J*, Vol. 117, No. 4, (1989), pp. 887-891

Olsson, C.G., Bitzen, U., Olsson, B., Magnusson, P., Carlsson, M.S., Jonson, B., and Bajc, M. (2006). Outpatient tinzaparin therapy in pulmonary embolism quantified with ventilation/perfusion scintigraphy. *Med Sci Monit*, Vol. 12, No. 2, (2006), pp. PI9-13

Osborne, D.R., Jaszczak, R.J., Greer, K., Roggli, V., Lischko, M., and Coleman, R.E. (1983). Detection of pulmonary emboli in dogs: comparison of single photon emission computed tomography, gamma camera imaging, and angiography. *Radiology*, Vol. 146, No. 2, (1983), pp. 493-497

Pace, W.M., and Goris, M.L. (1998). Pulmonary SPECT imaging and the stripe sign. *J Nucl Med*, Vol. 39, No. 4, (1998), pp. 721-723

Palmer, J., Bitzen, U., Jonson, B., and Bajc, M. (2001). Comprehensive ventilation/perfusion SPECT. *J Nucl Med*, Vol. 42, No. 8, (2001), pp. 1288-1294

Pengo, V., Lensing, A.W., Prins, M.H., Marchiori, A., Davidson, B.L., Tiozzo, F., Albanese, P., Biasiolo, A., Pegoraro, C., Iliceto, S., *et al.* (2004). Incidence of chronic thromboembolic pulmonary hypertension after pulmonary embolism. *N Engl J Med*, Vol. 350, No. 22, (2004), pp. 2257-2264

Perrier, A., Howarth, N., Didier, D., Loubeyre, P., Unger, P.F., de Moerloose, P., Slosman, D., Junod, A., and Bounameaux, H. (2001). Performance of helical computed tomography in unselected outpatients with suspected pulmonary embolism. *Ann Intern Med*, Vol. 135, No. 2, (2001), pp. 88-97

Pistolesi, M., Miniati, M., Bonsignore, M., Andreotti, F., Di Ricco, G., Marini, C., Rindi, M., Biagini, A., Milne, E.N., and Giuntini, C. (1988). Factors affecting regional pulmonary blood flow in chronic ischemic heart disease. *J Thorac Imaging*, Vol. 3, No. 3, (1988), pp. 65-72

Powell, T., and Muller, N.L. (2003). Imaging of acute pulmonary thromboembolism: should spiral computed tomography replace the ventilation-perfusion scan? *Clin Chest Med*, Vol. 24, No. 1, (2003), pp. 29-38, v

Reinartz, P., Schirp, U., Zimny, M., Sabri, O., Nowak, B., Schafer, W., Cremerius, U., and Bull, U. (2001). Optimizing ventilation-perfusion lung scintigraphy: parting with planar imaging. *Nuklearmedizin*, Vol. 40, No. 2, (2001), pp. 38-43

Reinartz, P., Wildberger, J.E., Schaefer, W., Nowak, B., Mahnken, A.H., and Buell, U. (2004). Tomographic imaging in the diagnosis of pulmonary embolism: a comparison between V/Q lung scintigraphy in SPECT technique and multislice spiral CT. *J Nucl Med*, Vol. 45, No. 9, (2004), pp. 1501-1508

Richman, P.B., Courtney, D.M., Friese, J., Matthews, J., Field, A., Petri, R., and Kline, J.A. (2004). Prevalence and significance of nonthromboembolic findings on chest computed tomography angiography performed to rule out pulmonary embolism: a multicenter study of 1,025 emergency department patients. *Acad Emerg Med*, Vol. 11, No. 6, (2004), pp. 642-647

Rizkallah, J., Man, S.F., and Sin, D.D. (2009). Prevalence of pulmonary embolism in acute exacerbations of COPD: a systematic review and metaanalysis. *Chest*, Vol. 135, No. 3, (2009), pp. 786-793

Rutten, F.H., Cramer, M.J., Lammers, J.W., Grobbee, D.E., and Hoes, A.W. (2006). Heart failure and chronic obstructive pulmonary disease: An ignored combination? *Eur J Heart Fail*, Vol. 8, No. 7, (2006), pp. 706-711

Schonhofer, B., and Kohler, D. (1998). Prevalence of deep-vein thrombosis of the leg in patients with acute exacerbation of chronic obstructive pulmonary disease. *Respiration*, Vol. 65, No. 3, (1998), pp. 173-177

Sostman, H.D., and Gottschalk, A. (1982). The stripe sign: a new sign for diagnosis of nonembolic defects on pulmonary perfusion scintigraphy. *Radiology*, Vol. 142, No. 3, (1982), pp. 737-741

Sostman, H.D., and Gottschalk, A. (1992). Prospective validation of the stripe sign in ventilation-perfusion scintigraphy. *Radiology*, Vol. 184, No. 2, (1992), pp. 455-459

Stein, P.D., Fowler, S.E., Goodman, L.R., Gottschalk, A., Hales, C.A., Hull, R.D., Leeper, K.V., Jr., Popovich, J., Jr., Quinn, D.A., Sos, T.A., *et al.* (2006). Multidetector computed tomography for acute pulmonary embolism. *N Engl J Med*, Vol. 354, No. 22, (2006), pp. 2317-2327

The PIOPED Investigators (1990). Value of the ventilation/perfusion scan in acute pulmonary embolism. Results of the prospective investigation of pulmonary embolism diagnosis (PIOPED). . *Jama*, Vol. 263, No. 20, (1990), pp. 2753-2759

Tillie-Leblond, I., Marquette, C.H., Perez, T., Scherpereel, A., Zanetti, C., Tonnel, A.B., and Remy-Jardin, M. (2006). Pulmonary embolism in patients with unexplained exacerbation of chronic obstructive pulmonary disease: prevalence and risk factors. *Ann Intern Med*, Vol. 144, No. 6, (2006), pp. 390-396

Tunariu, N., Gibbs, S.J., Win, Z., Gin-Sing, W., Graham, A., Gishen, P., and Al-Nahhas, A. (2007). Ventilation-perfusion scintigraphy is more sensitive than multidetector CTPA in detecting chronic thromboembolic pulmonary disease as a treatable cause of pulmonary hypertension. *J Nucl Med*, Vol. 48, No. 5, (2007), pp. 680-684

Wagner, H.N., Jr., Sabiston, D.C., Jr., McAfee, J.G., Tow, D., and Stern, H.S. (1964). Diagnosis of Massive Pulmonary Embolism in Man by Radioisotope Scanning. *N Engl J Med*, Vol. 271, (1964), pp. 377-384

Valentin, J. (2007). Managing patient dose in multi-detector computed tomography(MDCT). ICRP Publication 102. *Ann ICRP*, Vol. 37, No. 1, (2007), pp. 1-79, iii

van Strijen, M.J., de Monye, W., Kieft, G.J., Pattynama, P.M., Huisman, M.V., Smith, S.J., and Bloem, J.L. (2003). Diagnosis of pulmonary embolism with spiral CT as a second procedure following scintigraphy. *Eur Radiol*, Vol. 13, No. 7, (2003), pp. 1501-1507

Van Strijen, M.J., De Monye, W., Kieft, G.J., Pattynama, P.M., Prins, M.H., and Huisman, M.V. (2005). Accuracy of single-detector spiral CT in the diagnosis of pulmonary embolism: a prospective multicenter cohort study of consecutive patients with abnormal perfusion scintigraphy. *J Thromb Haemost*, Vol. 3, No. 1, (2005), pp. 17-25

West, J.B., Dollery, C.T., and Heard, B.E. (1964). Increased Vascular Resistance in the Lower Zone of the Lung Caused by Perivascular Oedema. *Lancet*, Vol. 284, (1964), pp. 181-183

Yokoe, K., Satoh, K., Yamamoto, Y., Nishiyama, Y., Asakura, H., Haba, R., and Ohkawa, M. (2006). Usefulness of 99mTc-Technegas and 133Xe dynamic SPECT in ventilatory impairment. *Nucl Med Commun*, Vol. 27, No. 11, (2006), pp. 887-892

10

Dual Source, Dual Energy Computed Tomography in Pulmonary Embolism

Yan'E Zhao[1], Long Jiang Zhang[1], Guang Ming Lu[1],
Kevin P. Gibbs[2] and U. Joseph Schoepf[2]
[1]*Department of Medical Imaging, Jinling Hospital, Clinical School of Medical College, Nanjing University, Nanjing, Jiangsu Province*
[2]*Department of Radiology and Radiological Science Medical University of South Carolina, Ashley River Tower*
[1]*China*
[2]*USA*

1. Introduction

More than 650,000 cases of pulmonary embolism (PE) are reported each year, resulting in an estimated 300,000 annual fatalities. This level of occurrence ranks PE as the third leading cause of death in the USA [Laack TA, 2004; Tapson VF, 2008]. Multidetector CT (MDCT) pulmonary angiography has now largely replaced ventilation/perfusion scintigraphy and conventional pulmonary angiography for the evaluation of possible PE [Patel S,2003]. In 2007, MDCT pulmonary angiography was accepted as the reference standard for diagnosis of acute PE [Remy-Jardin M,2007]. However, conventional MDCT pulmonary angiography only provides morphological information and its ability to assess subsegmental pulmonary arteries is variable: sensitivities range from 37%-96%. The ability to assess subsegmental pulmonary arteries has increased with advances in MDCT technology.

In the past, various CT techniques have been developed to evaluate the assessment of lung perfusion in patients with suspected PE. (1) Dynamic multi-section electron beam CT [Schoepf UJ,2000]. This perfusion-based CT technique had a scanning volume of 7.6 cm, required a long patient breathhold, and delivered a high additional radiation dose to the patient. (2) Color-coding the density of lung parenchyma in contrast-enhanced CTA [Wildberger JE,2001]. This technique is of limited use when lung diseases, such as ground-glass opacities (e.g., in pulmonary edema or pneumonia) were present. (3) A subtraction CTA technique of whole-thorax multi-detector CT scans acquired before and after intravenous contrast within a single breathhold. This technique was limited by a longer breathhold time, misregistration artifacts because of the mismatched unenhanced and contrast-enhanced scans, and additional radiation dose caused by the fact that an additional unenhanced scan had to be performed to assess the iodine distribution in the lung [Wildberger JE,2005].

Recently, DECT with different dual energy CT hardware (dual source CT and rapid kV switching technique) became available to simultaneously provide the functional and morphological information, overcoming the limitations of the above-mentioned CT

perfusion techniques. Iodine, shows a proportionally larger increase of CT values with decreasing X-ray tube voltage compared to other materials, e.g., to soft tissue, iodinated contrast medium enhanced DECT provides the opportunity to assess pulmonary parenchyma iodine maps (i.e., lung perfusion). Compared with the previously developed CT perfusion techniques, DECT technique eliminates registration problems and allows selective visualization of iodine distribution with high spatial resolution and no additional radiation exposure to the patient compared with the conventional CT pulmonary angiography technique.
This chapter will present the techniques, scanning and contrast medium injection protocols, image postprocessing and image interpretation, clinical applications and radiation dose of dual source, dual energy CT pulmonary angiography.

2. Techniques

Recent generations of MDCTs are able to acquire dual-energy data by applying two X-ray tubes and two corresponding detectors at different kVp and mA settings simultaneously in a dual-source CT (Siemens Healthcare), by ultra-fast kVp switching in a single source CT (GE Healthcare) or by compartmentalization of detected X-ray photons into energy bins by the detectors of a single-source CT operating at constant kVp and mA settings (Philips Healthcare). The dual-source CT scanner is composed of two x-ray tubes and two corresponding detectors. The two acquisition systems are mounted on the rotating gantry with an angular offset of 90°/95° with regard to their kilovoltage and milliamperage settings. For dual-energy CT acquisition, the tube voltages are set at high energy (140 kVp) for tube A and low energy (80 kVp) for tube B. The rapid kilovoltage switching technique from GE Healthcare uses a single x-ray source. A generator electronically switches rapidly the tube energies from low energy (80 kVp) to high energy (140 kVp) and back again to acquire dual-energy images. Each exposure takes about 0.5 msec.

3. Scanning injection protocols

3.1 Scanning protocols

The protocol aims to display both the pulmonary arteries and lung perfusion from a single contrast-enhanced CT scan. Various scanning protocols with dual source dual energy CT scanners have been proposed in the literature [Fink C, 2008], but currently there are few published protocols for CT systems of other vendors **[Thieme SF, 2009]**. The scan protocols recommended for dual-energy lung perfusion scans by dual-source CT（Siemens）are presented in Table 1. Patients should be centrally placed in the scanner to ensure that the entire pulmonary parenchyma is covered by the smaller field-of-view of the second tube detector array (the field-of-view of the second tube detector array is 260 mm or 330mm) when dual source CT was used.

3.2 Contrast Medium injection protocols

High-concentration iodine-based contrast material is recommended for DECT scans to improve the differentiation of iodine by the dual-energy post-processing algorithm. As mentioned above in the section of scanning protocols, thoracic DECT scans should be acquired in the caudo-cranial direction so that the chaser bolus is being injected by the time

	Siemens Definition	Siemens Definition Flash
Scan mode	Spiral dual energy	Spiral dual energy
Scan area	Diaphragm to lung apex	Diaphragm to lung apex
Scan direction	Caudo-cranial/cranio-caudal	Caudo-cranial/cranio-caudal
Scan time(s)(for 300 mm length)	10	9
Tube voltage A/B (kVp)	140/80	100/140Sn (tin filter)
Tube current A/B (quality ref. mAs)	51/213	89/76
Dose modulation	CARE Dose 4D	CARE Dose 4D
CTDIvol (mGy)	6	7.3
Rotation time (s)	0.33	0.28
Pitch	0.7	0.55
Slice collimation (mm)	1.2	0.6
Acquisition (mm)	14x1.2	128x0.6
DE composition factor	0.3	0.6
Reconstruction kernel	D30f	D30f

Table 1. Scan protocols recommended for a dual-energy lung perfusion scan on the currently available dual-source CT systems (Siemens Healthcare)

the scan reached the upper chest to avoid streak artifacts due to highly concentrated contrast material in the subclavian vein or superior vena cava. In order to acquire both pulmonary arteries and lung perfusion in an optimal scan, the scan delay should be a little longer (e.g.4-7s) to allow the contrast material to pass into the lung parenchyma. Bolus tracking should be used for timing with the region of interest placed in the pulmonary artery trunk. There was no significant difference in pulmonary artery enhancement between test bolus and automatic bolus tracking in previously performed studies **[Geyer LL, 2011]**. Therefore, automatic bolus tracking is recommended because it is operator friendly and independent. The patient should be instructed to hold his breath at mild inspiration to avoid excessive influx of non-enhanced blood from the inferior vena cava. Contrast injection protocol of dual source dual-energy CT pulmonary angiography is seen in Table 2.

	Iodine concentration 300mg I ml^{-1}	Iodine concentration 370mg I ml^{-1}	Iodine concentration 400mg I ml^{-1}
Contrast media volume (ml kg^{-1})	1.5	1.2	1.1
Contrast media flow rate (ml s^{-1})	4	4	4
Bolus timing	Bolus tracking	Bolus tracking	Bolus tracking
Bolus tracking threshold(HU)	100	100	100
ROI position	Pulmonary trunk	Pulmonary trunk	Pulmonary trunk
Scan deldy(s)	6	6	7
Saline flush volume(ml)	40	40	60
Saline injection rate(ml s^{-1})	4	4	4
Needle size(G)	18	18	18
Injection site	Antecubital vein	Antecubital vein	Antecubital vein

Table 2. Contrast injection protocol of dual-energy pulmonary CT angiography

4. Image post-processing and image interpretation

4.1 Image post-processing

From the raw spiral projection data of both tubes, images were automatically reconstructed to three separate image sets: 80 kVp, 140 kVp and average weighted virtual 120 kVp images with 80:140 kVp linear weighting of 0.3 (i.e. 30% image information from the 80 kVp image and 70% information from the 140 kVp image). For each image set, the slice thickness was 0.75 mm and interval was 0.50 mm. The only currently commercially available software (syngo DE Lung PBV by Siemens HealthCare) for DECT lung perfusion image analysis is part of the dual energy post-processing software package available for the Siemens syngo MultiModality Workplace. For the calculation of iodine distribution in the lung parenchyma, the application class is designed for iodine extraction, and the material parameters for iodine extraction are as follows: -1,000 HU for air at 80 kVp, -1,000 Hounsfield unit (HU) for air at 140 kVp, 60 HU for soft tissue at 80 kVp, 54 HU for soft tissue at 140 kVp, 2 for relative contrast enhancement, -960 HU for minimum value, -200~-300 HU for maximum value, and 4 for range (Figure 1A).The lung parenchyma is color coded using gray scale 16-bit or hot metal 16-bit color coding (default setting) with different optional color scales available. The software enables a multiplanar view of the lung parenchyma image. The software also enables users to set a mixing ratio between a non color-coded virtual 120 kV dataset and color-coded lung parenchyma. This mixing ratio can be fluently set between 0% showing a anatomy image and 100% showing a blood flow image (BFI) images where only the color-coded, segmented lung parenchyma is displayed. Windowing functionality for the original and color-coded dataset, basic measurement tools, and a few dual-energy-specific measurements are also available. The fused images are obtained by mixing the anatomy image and BFI images with different ratios. The fused images are used for visualization of CT pulmonary angiography and the lung perfusion.

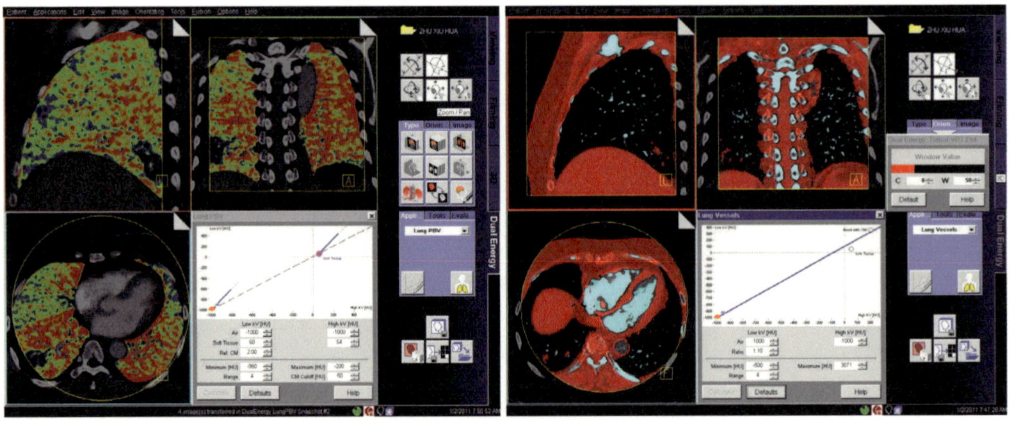

A B

Fig. 1. Parameter settings of the postprocessing software for dual energy CT pulmonary angiography
A) Parameter settings of Lung Pulmonary Blood Volume (PBV) software; B) Parameter settings of Lung Vessels software

The Lung Vessels application was developed to discriminate non-enhancing subsegmental pulmonary arteries from enhancing ones by using dual energy iodine extraction data. This technique had a high negative predictive value being important for exclusion of segmental PE. In the Lung Vessels application, results are displayed as color-coded multi planar reformatted data and a 3D volume rendered dataset, where vessels with high iodine content are color-coded blue and soft tissue or vessels with low or no iodine content due to PE are color-coded red. The material parameters for iodine extraction of Lung Vessels are as follows: -1,000 HU for air at 80 kVp, -1,000 Hounsfield unit (HU) for air at 140 kVp, 60 HU for soft tissue at 80 kVp, 54 HU for soft tissue at 140 kVp, 1.1 for relative contrast enhancement, -500 HU for minimum value, 3071 HU for maximum value, and 4 for range (Figure 1B).

4.2 BFI image interpretation

It is very important to recognize the normal findings or artifacts at DECT lung perfusion. Normal pulmonary BFI images were defined as showing homogeneous perfusion in the normal range (color-coded yellow-green or blue) with dependent symmetric lung iodine distribution (Figure 2). Dependent lung perfusion at DECT refers to relatively low contrast enhancement in the ventral regions (color coded yellow-green) and relatively higher enhancement in the dorsal regions (color coded blue -black) with the patient in the supine position (Figure 3).

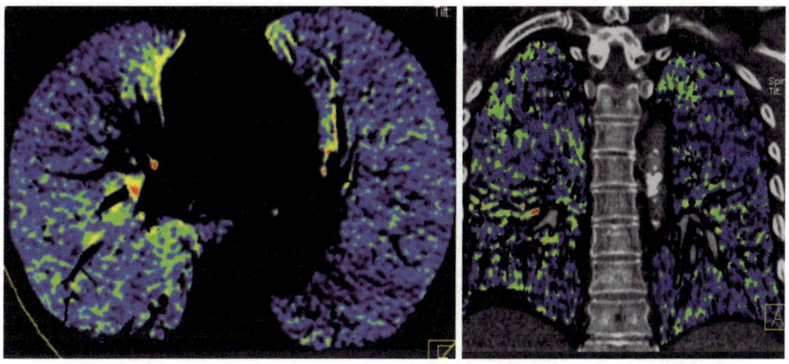

A B

Fig. 2. Normal pulmonary blood flow imaging
A) Axial BFI image and B) coronal fused image show homogeneous blood flow distribution in both lungs

In the analysis of BFI images, sources of pitfall should be kept in mind to avoid misdiagnoses. When interpreting BFI images, these pitfalls can relate to artifacts from contrast material, diaphragmatic or cardiac motion, pulmonary pathology and the occlusive degree of pulmonary arteries.

Streak and beam-hardening effects resulting from high-concentration contrast agent in the thoracic veins and right cardiac chambers can commonly cause heterogeneous artifacts in BFI images (Figure 4); these artifacts must be considered when an unexpected contrast enhancement defect is noted adjacent to an area of high contrast enhancement. In this setting, the perfusion defect may appear band-like and be mostly in both upper lobes. Optimization of contrast medium injection parameters, including the use of a saline chaser, can reduce the beam-hardening artifact, improve the image quality of DECT and increase diagnostic confidence. Nance JW Jr et al [,Nance JW Jr,2011] reported that iomeprol 400 at 4 mL/s (an IDR of 1.6 g I/s) resulted in superior quality CTPA and perfusion map images compared with the protocols using a lower concentration or delivery rate.

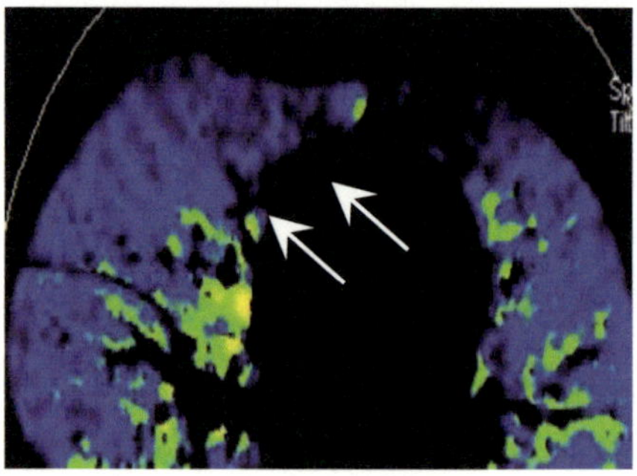

Fig. 3. Gravity-dependent lung perfusion states
A normal pulmonary BFI image obtained in one patient in the supine position shows relatively low pulmonary contrast enhancement anteriorly (arrows) and relatively high contrast enhancement in more dependent lung portions

Diaphragmatic or cardiac motion can cause apparent lower areas of lung contrast enhancement in the lung parenchyma adjacent to the diaphragm or cardiac chambers (Figure 5). In this setting, the perfusion defect is crescent-shaped; blurring or double lines adjacent to the diaphragm or heart border can be seen on images obtained with lung windows or mediastinal windows. Patients should hold their breath while scanning to reduce the diaphragm motion artifacts. A potential method to improve image quality in the vicinity of the cardiac chambers might be to synchronize data acquisition with electrocardiographic tracing, a technological development currently exclusively available for myocardial "perfusion" analysis **[Pontana F,2008]**; however, such methodology could also potentially introduce stair-step or misregistration artifacts and requires further study. Normal physiological gravity dependent variation in pulmonary "perfusion" should also be recognized **[Zhang LJ,2009(Eur Rdiol)/2009(Acta Radio)].**

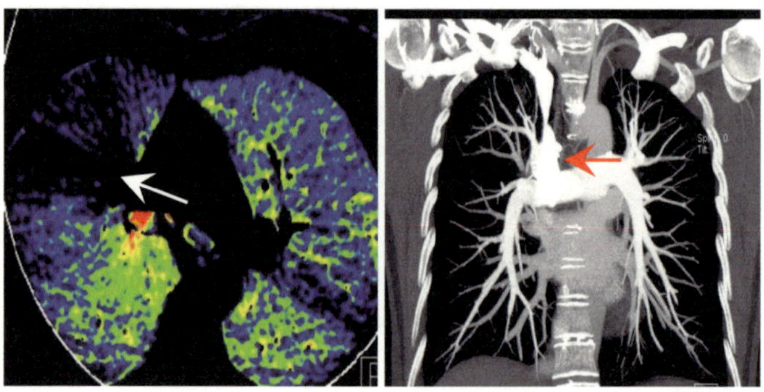

A B

Fig. 4. Pseudo-high perfusion due to dense contrast material in the superior vena cava
A) An axial BFI image shows radiating pseudo-high perfusion and pseudo-iodine defect adjacent to the superior vena cava (white arrow) due to streak artifact from high concentration contrast material. B) Coronal maximum intensity projection image shows a higher opacity of superior vena cava (red arrow) than pulmonary artery

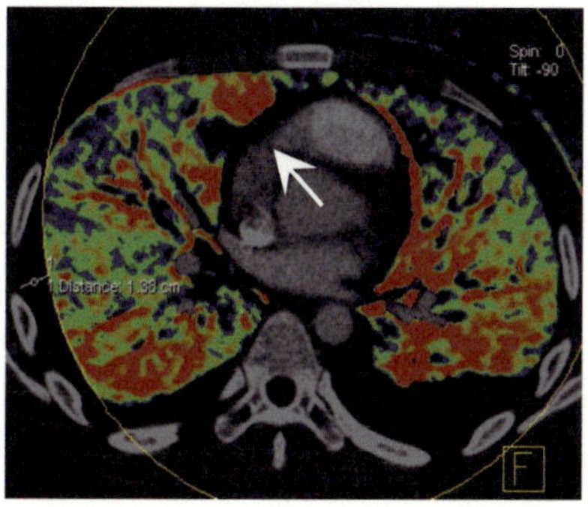

Fig. 5. Cardiac motion artifact
Crescent-shaped perfusion defect is seen in the lung parenchyma adjacent to the cardiac chambers (white arrow)

In addition, the anatomy CT images should be evaluated for pulmonary pathology, such as emphysema (Figure 6), tumors invading or compressing the pulmonary arteries (Figure 7) and pulmonary consolidation (Figure 8), all of which will result in contrast enhancement defects in BFI images. The occlusive degree of pulmonary arteries will affect perfusion defects at BFI and result in the false-negatives (Figure 9). But, misdiagnosis resulting from these factors is rare when BFI images are interpreted in conjunction with CTPA, which can reliably detect the lobar and segmental emboli. Nevertheless, small peripheral pulmonary emboli causing minimal contrast enhancement defect alterations can be overlooked even when state-of-the-art MDCT scanners are employed. Also, the considerable reduction in the pulmonary capillary bed often seen in the elderly or patients with emphysema can cause diffuse decreased pulmonary "perfusion" **[Boroto K, 2008].**

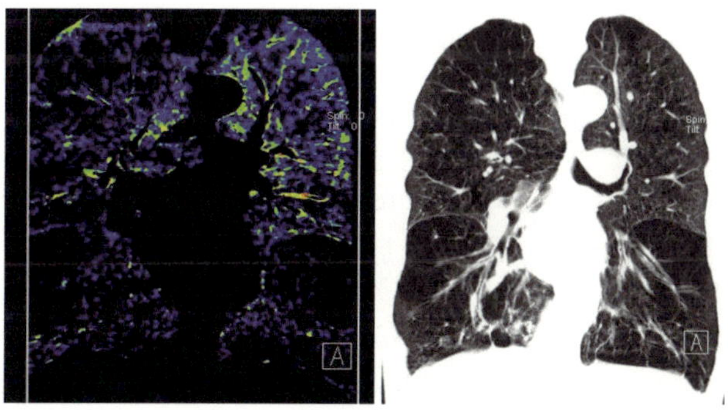

A B

Fig. 6. Contrast defect in the BFI image caused by emphysema
A) A coronal BFI image shows heterogeneous contrast enhancement in both lungs caused by the emphysema that is readily seen at coronal reformatted multiplanar reformation viewed with lung windows (B)

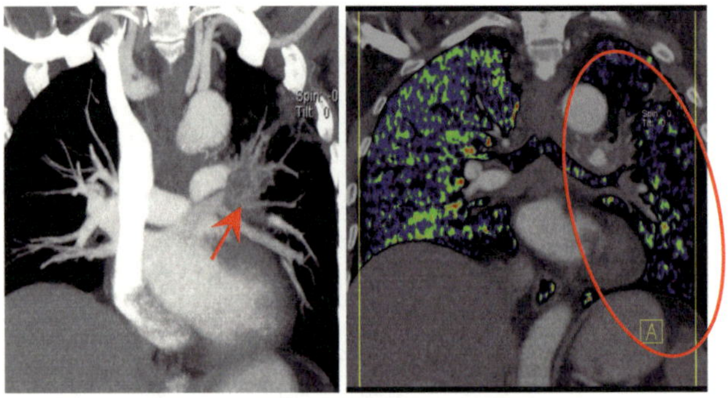

A B

Fig. 7. Contrast defect in the pulmonary blood volume image caused by lung carcinoma
A) A coronal MIP image shows a left lung hilar carcinoma invading the left pulmonary lobar arteries (red arrow), resulting in diffuse decreased contrast enhancement of the left lung (red circle)at the corresponding coronal BFI image fused with the CT angiogram (B)

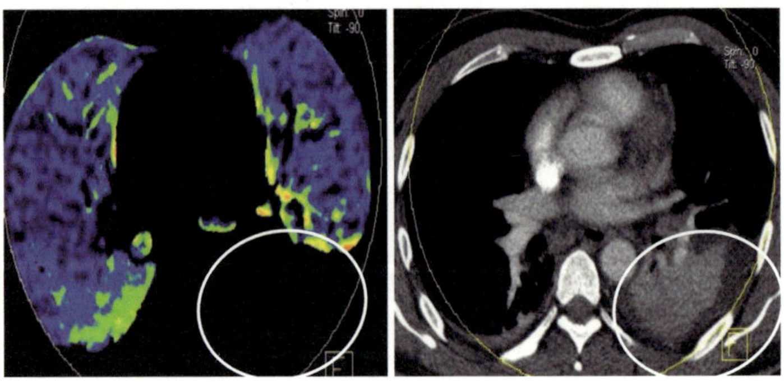

A B

Fig. 8. Contrast enhancement defect in the pulmonary blood volume image caused by lung consolidation
A) Axial BFI image shows a contrast enhancement defect in the left lower lobe (white circle);
B) The corresponding axial CT image clearly shows pulmonary consolidation in the corresponding left lower lung lobe (white circle)

5. Clinical applications

5.1 Acute PE detection

Perfusion defects that are consistent with acute PE include those that are peripherally located, wedge-shaped, and in a segmental or lobar distribution (Figure 10). All other perfusion defects, such as patchy or band-like defects without segmental distribution, or complete loss of color-coding (indicating lack of air-containing voxels due to consolidation), were considered to be inconsistent with PE. For the Lung Vessels application, color-coded red PAs was regarded as positive for PE (Figure 11), while color-coded red soft tissue around PAs was discarded.

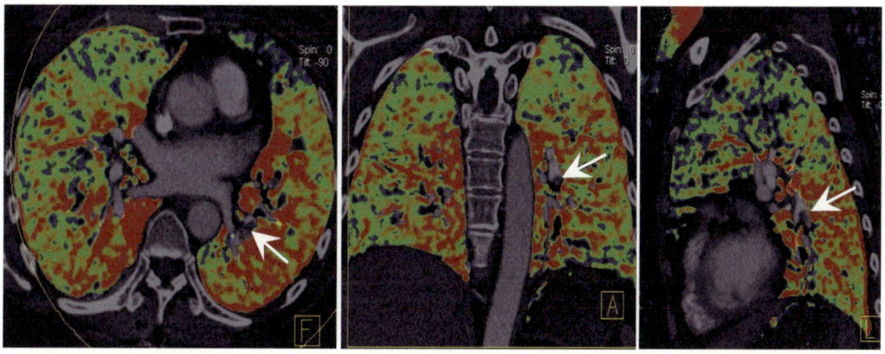

A B C

Fig. 9. Negative BFI image in one patient with left lower pulmonary artery embolus
A) axial, B) coronal, and C) sagittal fused images show normal findings with non-occlusive PE(white arrow) and result in the false-negatives

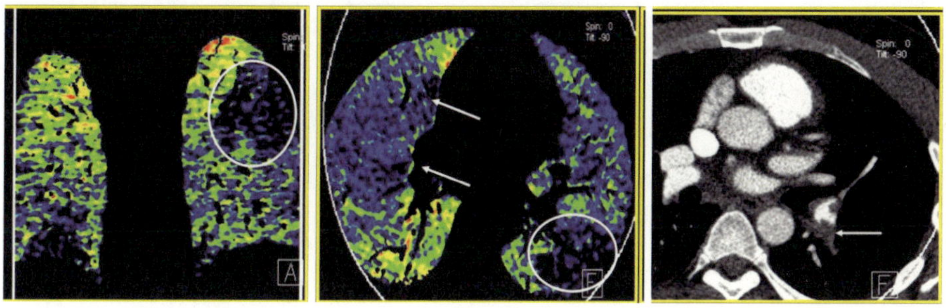

A B C

Fig. 10. Acute PE in a 24-year-old man
A) Coronal and B) Axial BFI images show a wedge-shaped perfusion defect in the left lung lower lobe dorsal segment (white circle). Pseudo-high contrast enhancement is seen in the anterior portion of the right middle lung anterior to the normal pulmonary contrast enhancement seen in the right middle lobe more posteriorly (arrows). C) Axial contrast-enhanced CT image shows a corresponding occlusive filling defect representing pulmonary emboli in the left lower lobe segmental pulmonary arteries (arrow), and non-occlusive emboli elsewhere

Several studies have examined DECT for the detection of PE. Fink et al **[Fink C, 2008]** reported that both sensitivity and specificity of DECT for the assessment of PE were 100% on a per patient basis. On a per segment basis, the sensitivity and specificity ranged from 60%-66.7% and from 99.5%-99.8%; CTPA was used in this study as the standard of reference in 24 patients with suspected PE, 4 of whom actually had PE. With scintigraphy as the standard of reference, Thieme et al **[Thieme SF ,2008]** reported 75% sensitivity and 80% specificity on a per patient basis and 83% sensitivity and 99% specificity on a per segment basis in a small group of patients with DECT. A group of 117 patients was examined by Pontana et al **[Pontana F, 2008]** to investigate the accuracy of DECT in the depiction of perfusion defects in patients with acute PE, concluding that simultaneous information on the presence of endoluminal thrombus and lung perfusion impairment can be obtained with

DECT. In an experimental study by Zhang et al **[Zhang LJ ,2009],** conventional CTPA identified pulmonary emboli in only 12 and the absence of emboli in 18 pulmonary lobes, corresponding to a sensitivity and specificity of 67% and 100%. In contrast, DECT and BFI each correctly identified pulmonary emboli in 16 of 18 pulmonary lobes and reported the absence of emboli in 11 of 12 lobes, corresponding to sensitivity and specificity of 89% and 92% for detecting pulmonary emboli. Thus, pulmonary CTA and DECT lung perfusion have complimentary roles in the diagnosis of PE and DECT lung perfusion images increase the sensitivity for detection of PE (Figure 12), particular for tiny peripheral emboli **[**Lu GM **,2010].** It can be presumed that a simultaneous detection of a clot in a pulmonary artery in the pulmonary CTA and of a corresponding perfusion defect in DECT lung perfusion indicate an occlusive PE.

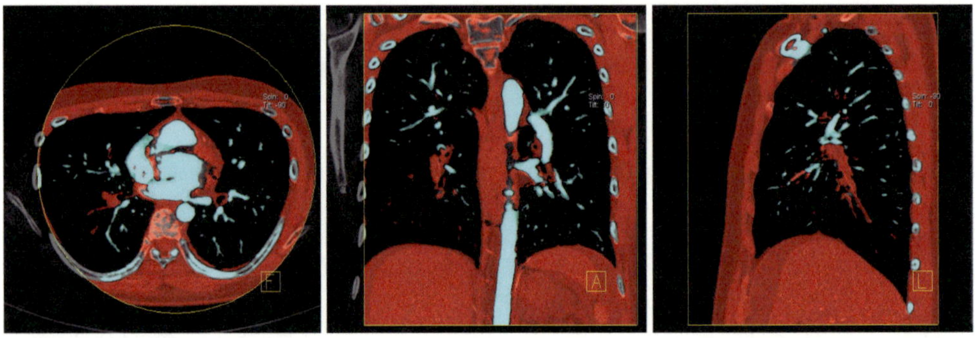

A B C

Fig. 11. Acute pulmonary embolism in one 17-year-old man
A) axial, B) coronal, and C) right sagittal lung vessel images show the pulmonary emboli in the right lower pulmonary artery color coded as red

Furthermore, pulmonary CTA and DECT lung perfusion could assist in the detection of pulmonary emboli that are not evident by conventional MDCT pulmonary angiography. Thieme **et al [Thieme SF ,2008] found** that corresponding perfusion defects were observed in DECT and scintigraphy in two patients in whom there was no evidence of intravascular clots in angiographic CT images. They proposed that the observed pulmonary perfusion defects probably corresponded to segments of prior embolism with re-perfused, segmental vessels and residual peripheral thrombosed vessels that were too small to visualize in CTPA. The same assumption was also made in the study by Po**ntana et al [Pontana F, 2008],** in which four subsegmental perfusion defects were depicted by BFI images, whereas endoluminal thrombi were not visualised in the corresponding arteries by CTPA. **Zhang et al [Lu GM ,2010]** also found a similar so-called false-positive DECT result in one patient with chronic PE in the pulmonary images of BFI. In another patient undergoing anticoagulant therapy, the conventional CTPA performed initially did not visualize abnormal findings. However, the magnified view of the targeted pulmonary arteries corresponding to contrast enhancement defect in the BFI images showed a subtle subsegmental filling defect. These findings indicate that CTPA might not be an adequate gold standard to detect all PE, especially for the small peripheral emboli or chronic PE. However, this does not mean to deny the mainstay role of MDCT in the evaluation of pulmonary emboli. The detection of small emboli is of clinical importance because even small emboli require treatment to prevent chronic PE and pulmonary artery hypertension in several clinical scenarios in patients with a small embolus and inadequate cardiopulmonary reserve; in patients who have a small embolus and coexisting acute deep venous thrombosis; and in patients with recurrent small emboli possibly owing to thrombophilia **[Remy-JardinM, 2007].** Certainly, the significance of small emboli needs further study.

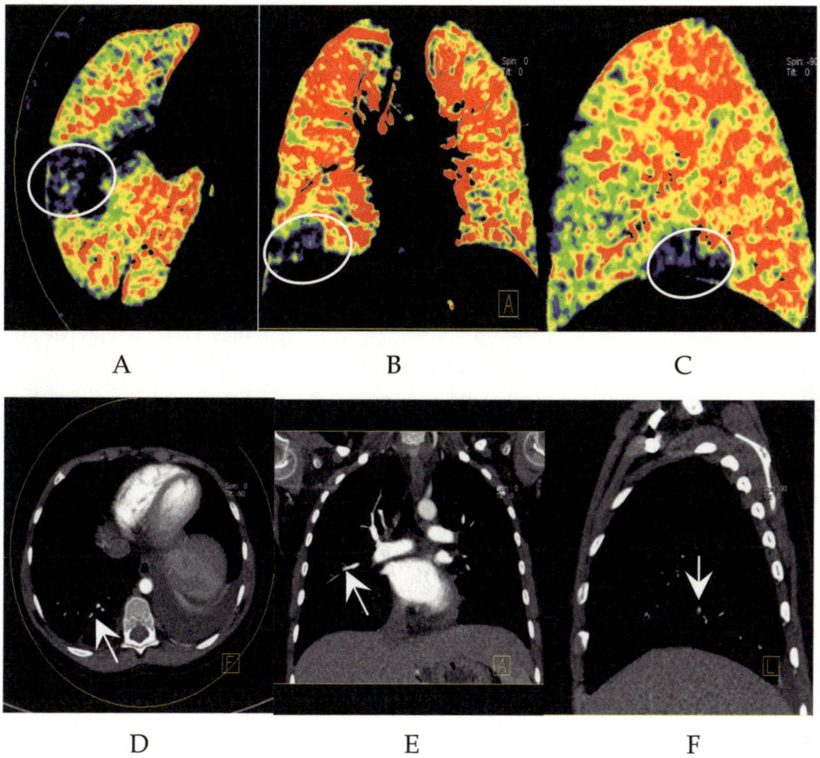

Fig. 12. Tiny peripheral emboli in right lower pulmonary artery
A) Axial, B) coronal, and C) left sagittal BFI images show a wedge-shaped perfusion defect in the right lung lower lobe dorsal segment (white circle); D) Axial, E) coronal, F) left sagittal contrast-enhanced CT image shows no filling defect in the corresponding right lower pulmonary artery (white arrow)

5.2 Evaluation of PE severity

In patients with acute PE, rapid risk assessment is critical because high-risk patients may benefit from life-saving thrombolytic therapy or invasive therapies, including catheter-guided thrombosuction or thrombectomy **[Dogan H, 2007].** Right heart strain (RHS) has been shown to be independently predictive of 30-day mortality. In addition to use as a CT marker of RHS, the ratio between the size of the right ventricle (RV) and left ventricle (LV) has demonstrated a significant positive correlation with severity of PE and mortality **[Ghaye B, 2006]**. Chae et al. **[Chae EJ , 2010]** and Zhang et al **[Zhang LJ, 2099(Acta Radio)]** reported good correlation between RV/LV diameter ratio with a novel self-defined dual energy perfusion score or the number of pulmonary segments with perfusion defects, respectively.

Recently, Bauer RW et al [Bauer RW, 2011] reported patients with RHS had significantly higher perfusion defect (PD) size than patients without RHS and confirm that PD size can be seen as marker for RHS. Bauer RWet al [Bauer RW, 2011] also reported that looking at the incidence of readmission and death due to PE demonstrated these major hard endpoints only in patients with a relative PD size of >5% of the total lung volume, whereas no such event was recorded for patients with <5% RelPD (relatively to the total lung volume, RelPD). Median survival time, however, was significantly lower for patients with >5% RelPD at an increased relative hazard ratio for death compared to patients with <5% RelPD or the control group without PE. Thus, PD size might even be an additional instrument for prognostic evaluation in PE itself.

6. Chronic PE

DECT pulmonary angiography can also allow for the depiction of perfusion defects in patients with chronic PE or patients with chronic thrombembolic pulmonary hypertension (CTEPH). A typical imaging characteristic of chronic PE can be mosaic patterns of lung attenuation, that is, areas of ground-glass attenuation mixed with areas of normal lung attenuation, suggesting a redistribution of blood flow.

These perfusion defects in BFI beyond chronic clots, similar to what is achievable for acute PE, and these changes closely mirror the mosaic attenuation pattern which is very suggestive of blood flow redistribution in CTEPH. Mosaic attenuation can sometimes be subtle, and BFI appears to accentuate regional differences in parenchymal attenuation, which become very conspicuous when displayed as a color map. In CTEPH, DECT can identify matched defects (i.e., occluded pulmonary arteries to lobe and negligible residual blood flow), mismatched defects (i.e., occluded lobar artery and demonstrable residual blood flow), and normal lung regions (i.e., unobstructed pulmonary arteries with demonstrable normal or increased flow). Perhaps of most interest are areas of mismatch where there is blood supply maintained beyond the occluded pulmonary arteries [2].

7. Radiation dose

There are concerns about radiation dose of DECT pulmonary angiography. For a DECT pulmonary angiography variable dose length product (DLP) have been reported (range, 143-302 mGy*cm) [Schenzle JC, 2010; Zhang LJ, 2009; Thieme SF, 2010] depending on the acquisition parameters, especially on the mAs settings. This value is lower than the published DLP of chest CT for PE (882 mGy*cm) and similar to the previously published DLP of routine chest CT (411 mGy * cm). Pontana et al **[Pontana F , 2008]** reported that the mean DLP of DECT pulmonary angiography for PE is 280 mGy *cm, corresponding to an average effective patient dose of about 5 mSv. Kang et al [Kang MJ, 2010] reported that the mean DLP of DECT with the PE protocol was 376 mGy*cm. All reported values for pulmonary DECT imaging are substantially lower than the reference value of 650 mGy*cm from the European guidelines on quality criteria for CT. Thus, even if the dose of DECT of the thorax can be a little bit higher than the dose values reported for a standard, single-source, single-energy thoracic CT, the above-mentioned benefits of DECT of the lung in patients with suspected PE seem to justify the moderate increase in the overall radiation dose. It is the only technique allowing for a direct comparison of CT angiograms acquired at different energies in the same patient, at the same time point after the injection of the contrast medium, and within strictly similar hemodynamic conditions.

8. Conclusion

DECT can provide both anatomical and iodine mapping information of the whole lungs in a single contrast-enhanced CT scan. After recognition of some artifacts in DECT pulmonary angiography, this technology has the capacity to improve the detection and severity evaluation of acute and chronic PE through comprehensive analysis of BFI and CT pulmonary angiography obtained during a single contrast-enhanced chest CT scan in a dual-energy mode. DECT pulmonary angiography can be used as a one-stop-shop technique for the evaluation of PE.

9. Acknowledgement

Long Jiang Zhang received the grant from the Peak of six major talents of Jiangsu Province Grant (No. WSW-122 for L.J. Z.).
Guang Ming Lu received the grant from the Natural Science Foundation of Jiangsu Province of China (No. BK2009316 for G.M.L.).

10. References

Boroto K, et al. (2008). Thoracic applications of dual-source CT technology. Eur J Radiol 68(3):375–84.

Bauer RW, et al. (2011). Dual energy CT pulmonary blood volume assessment in acute pulmonary embolism - correlation with D-dimer level, right heart strain and clinical outcome. Eur Radiol 21(9): 1914-1921.

Chae EJ, et al. (2010) .Dual-energy CT for assessment of the severity of acute pulmonary embolism: pulmonary perfusion defect score compared with CT angiographic obstruction score and right ventricular/left ventricular diameter ratio. Am J Roentgenol 194(3):604–610.

Dogan H, et al. (2007). Right ventricular function in patients with acute pulmonary embolism: analysis with electrocardiography-synchronized multi-detector row CT. Radiology 242(1):78-84.

Fink C, et al. (2008) Dual-energy CT angiography of the lung in patients with suspected pulmonary embolism: Initial results. Rofo 180(10):879-883.

Geyer LL, et al. (2011). Imaging of acute pulmonary embolism using a dual energy CT system with rapid kVp switching: Initial results. Eur J Radiol Mar 18. [Epub ahead of print]

Ghaye B, et al. (2006). Severe pulmonary embolism: pulmonary artery clot load scores and cardiovascular parameters as predictors of mortality. Radiology ;239(3):884-91.

Kang MJ, et al. (2010) Dual-energy CT: clinical applications in various pulmonary diseases. Radiographyics 30(3):685-698.

Lu GM, et al. (2010). Dual-energy computed tomography in pulmonary embolism. Brit J Radiol 83(992):707–718.

Laack TA & Goyal DG. (2004). Pulmonary embolism: an unsuspected killer. Emerg Med Clin North Am 22:961–983.

Nance JW Jr, et al. (2011). Optimization of contrast material delivery for dual-energy computed tomography pulmonary angiography in patients with suspected pulmonary embolism. Invest Radiol May 13. [Epub ahead of print].

Pontana F, et al. (2008). Lung perfusion with dual-energy multidetector-row CT (MDCT): feasibility for the evaluation of acute pulmonary embolism in 117 consecutive patients. Acad Radiol 15(12):1494–1504.

Patel S, et al. (2003). Pulmonary embolism: optimization of small pulmonary artery visualization at multidetector row CT. Radiology 227(2):455–460.

Remy-Jardin M, et al. (2007). Management of suspected acute pulmonary embolism in the era of CT angiography: a statement from the Fleischner Society. Radiology 245(2):315–29.

Schoepf UJ, et al. (2000). Pulmonary embolism: comprehensive diagnosis by using electron-beam CT for detection of emboli and assessment of pulmonary blood flow. Radiology 217(3):693–700.

Schenzle JC, et al. (2010). Dual energy CT of the chest—How about the dose? Invest Radiol 45(6): 64-71.

Thieme SF, et al. (2010). Dual-energy lung perfusion computed tomography: a novel pulmonary functional imaging method. Semin Ultrasound CT MR 31(4):301-308.

Thieme SF, et al. (2008). Dual energy CT for the assessment of lung perfusion—correlation to scintigraphy. Eur J Radiol 68(3):369–74.

Tapson VF. (2008). Acute pulmonary embolism. N Engl J Med 358(10):1037–1052.

Thieme SF, et al. (2009). Dual-energy CT for the assessment of contrast material distribution in the pulmonary parenchyma. AJR Am J Roentgenol ;193(1):144-149.

Wildberger JE, et al. (2001). Multi-slice CT for visualization of pulmonary embolism using perfusion weighted color maps. Rofo 173(4):289–294.

Wildberger JE,et al. (2005). Multislice computed tomography perfusion imaging for visualization of acute pulmonary embolism: animal experience. Eur Radiol 15(7):1378–1386

Zhang LJ, et al. (2009). Detection of pulmonary embolism by dual energy CT:correlation with perfusion scintigraphy and histopathological findings in rabbits. Eur Radiol 19(12): 2844–2854.

Zhang LJ, et al. (2009). Detection of pulmonary embolism using dual-energy computed tomography and correlation with cardiovascular measurements: a preliminary study. Acta Radiol 50(8):892–901

Zhang LJ, et al. (2009). Detection of pulmonary embolism by dual energy CT: an experimental study in rabbits. Radiology 252(1):61–70.

11

Numerical Analysis of the Mechanical Properties of a Vena Cava Filter

Kazuto Takashima[1,2], Koji Mori[3], Kiyoshi Yoshinaka[4] and Toshiharu Mukai[2]
[1]*Kyushu Institute of Technology*
[2]*RIKEN*
[3]*Yamaguchi University*
[4]*National Institute of Advanced Industrial Science and Technology*
Japan

1. Introduction

When anticoagulants are contraindicated for the venous thromboembolism therapy and thromboembolism recurs, a vena cava filter is inserted percutaneously into a major vein in order to prevent blood clots from entering the lungs (Ando & Kuribayashi, 2000; Streiff, 2000) (Fig. 1). The inferior vena cava filter is a mesh structure designed to capture blood clots while not impeding blood flow. This filter is inserted using an introducer catheter from either the femoral or jugular vein and is fixed by a hook attached to the tip of a wire. Several filters have been designed to lyse captured clots.

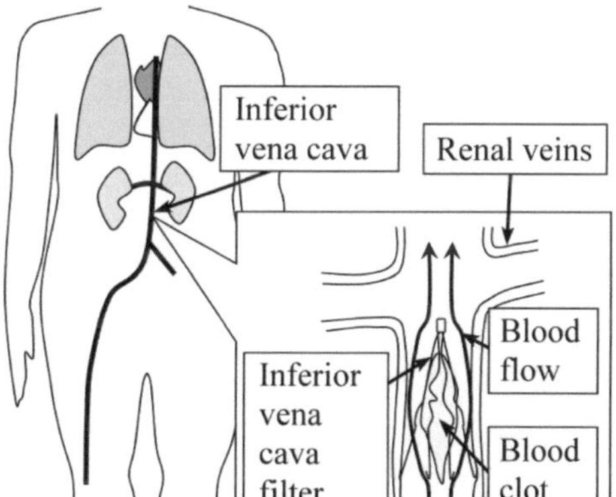

Fig. 1. Placement of the inferior vena cava filter.

Ideally, the filter should capture blood clots efficiently while not impeding the blood flow. Moreover, the filter should not move in the blood vessel after deployment and should pass smoothly through the slim introducer catheter. Although insertion appears to be a safe and effective method by which to prevent the recurrence of pulmonary embolism, patients in whom the filter has become tilted may experience pulmonary embolism recurrence because of a decrease in the thrombus-trapping performance of the filter (Nara et al., 1995; Rogers et al., 1998). In order to satisfy these requirements, several types of filters, such as permanent, temporary, and retrievable filters, have been proposed. For example, several types of vena cava filters, such as Greenfield filter, Vena Tech filter, Bird's nest filter, Simon-Nitinol filter, TrapEase filter, Günther tulip filter, Antheor filter, Neuhaus protect filter, and Recovery-Nitinol filter, have been developed (Ando & Kuribayashi, 2000; Boston Scientific, 2007; Greenfield et al., 1990, 1991; Kinney et al., 1997; Nara et al., 1995; Rogers et al., 1998; Streiff, 2000; Swaminathan et al., 2006). However, there are few quantitative data on the mechanical properties of these filters. In particular, although Swaminathan reported the blood clot capturing efficiency from the viewpoint of computational fluid dynamics (Swaminathan et al., 2006), there are few quantitative data concerning, for example, the ease of filter delivery.

Therefore, in the present study, we evaluated through numerical analysis the mechanical properties of a Greenfield filter deployed into a vein. In particular, since the filter expands rapidly, the surgeon cannot perceive the expanding motion or the transition of the contact force applied to the blood vessel wall. Therefore, a complete understanding of the mechanical properties of the filters must be determined on not only input from doctors but also on the results of numerical analysis regarding the expansion. These methods are expected to be useful for analyzing the structure of filters and may help to guide the design of new filters.

Based on the above considerations, we herein evaluate by numerical analysis the dynamic motion of a deployed filter using the evaluation standard of the incline and misalignment between the filter and the blood vessel. First, we evaluated whether the filter tilts when the catheter tilts or is misaligned or when the filter cannot expand. Second, we evaluated the migration of the deployed filter under a constant force.

2. Methods

Catheters and guidewires are used in the treatment of infarctions and aneurysms. In a previous study, in order to make intravascular treatment safer, we developed a computer-based surgical simulation system in order to simulate a catheter placed inside blood vessels for treatment of the brain (Takashima et al., 2006, 2007b, 2009). In the present study, we applied the simulation methods for the guidewire to the inferior vena cava filter because both the guidewire and the inferior vena cava filter are flexible structures. Using a similar model, we can easily combine the filter model with our catheter simulator. Actually, a catheter simulator has been developed as a training environment for inferior vena cava filter placement (Hahn et al., 1998). Ease of percutaneous filter delivery provides numerous advantages to both doctors and patients, including improved operational efficiency and reduced cost. Therefore, it is important that the filter be easy to use in combination with a catheter.

2.1 Filter model

In the present study, we used a Greenfield filter (GF) constructed of titanium (Fig. 2) (Ando & Kuribayashi, 2000; Boston Scientific, 2007; Greenfield et al., 1990, 1991; Kinney et al., 1997; Nara et al., 1995; Rogers et al., 1998; Streiff, 2000; Swaminathan et al., 2006). This permanent filter is commonly used in Japan. The GF is constructed of either titanium or stainless steel and come in various shapes. The GF used herein is cone-shaped and consists of six wires connected to a head. The diameter of the wires is 0.45 mm (Swaminathan et al., 2006), and each leg has a "zigzag" pattern. The bottom diameter of the cone is 38 mm (Greenfield et al.,

1991). The total length of the GF is 47 mm (Greenfield et al., 1991). We used a head without a hole and determined the diameter ($2R_h$) and length (L_h) of the head by measurement. The over-the-wire filter has a head with a small hole and inserted over the guidewire to optimize the alignment of the filter with the inferior vena cava (Kinney et al., 1997).

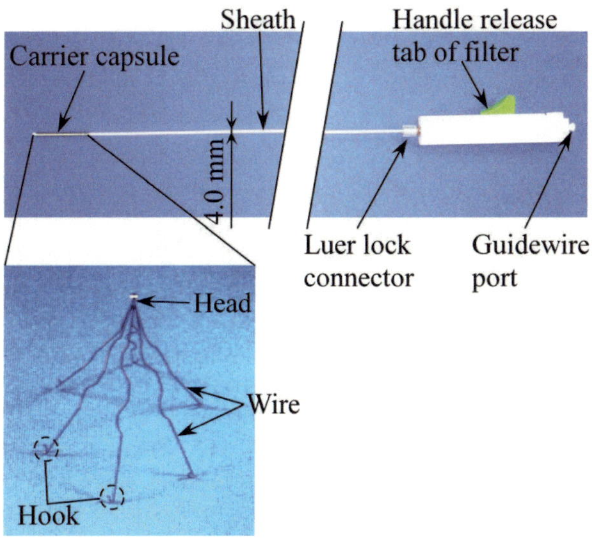

Fig. 2. The Greenfield inferior vena cava filter.

This model of the filter is constructed with viscoelastic springs and n segments for the dynamic deformation of a flexible structure. The viscoelastic springs express the bending and torsional stiffness of the wire. The motion of the filter model is represented by the Newton-Euler equations of motion as follows:

$$\boldsymbol{M}(\boldsymbol{q})\ddot{\boldsymbol{q}} + \boldsymbol{V}(\boldsymbol{q},\dot{\boldsymbol{q}}) = \sum_{i}^{n} \boldsymbol{J}_{\mathrm{r}}^{\mathrm{T}}(\boldsymbol{q})\boldsymbol{F}_{\mathrm{i}} - \boldsymbol{K}(\boldsymbol{q} - \boldsymbol{q}_{\mathrm{o}}) - D_{\mathrm{w}}\dot{\boldsymbol{q}} \tag{1}$$

where $\boldsymbol{q}$ is the joint displacement vector, $\boldsymbol{q}_o$ is the joint displacement vector when no load is applied, $\boldsymbol{M}(\boldsymbol{q})$ is the inertia matrix, $\boldsymbol{V}(\boldsymbol{q},\dot{\boldsymbol{q}})$ is the centrifugal force (Coriolis force), $\boldsymbol{F}_i$ is contact force vector of each segment (i), and $\boldsymbol{K}$ and D_w are elastic and viscous coefficients of a mobile joint, respectively. The second and third terms of the right-hand side in this equation correspond to the viscoelastic forces of a mobile joint. The head and the wire of the filter consist of one and three segments (diameter: $2R_w$, length: L_w), respectively. Each segment of the wire has a mobile joint in the center. The elastic coefficient of the mobile joint ($\boldsymbol{K}$) with respect to bending resistance (K_{wx}) and torsional resistance (K_{wz}) are approximated as follows (Yamamura et al., 2003):

$$K_{wx} = E_w I_x / L_w \tag{2}$$

$$K_{wz} = G_w I_p / L_w \tag{3}$$

where E_w and G_w are Young's modulus and the modulus of transverse elasticity of the wire of the filter, respectively, I_x and I_p are the area moment of inertia and the polar moment of inertia of area, respectively. In the present study, since the wire is a rod (radius: R_w), K_{wx} and I_p are expressed as follows:

$$K_{wx} = \pi E_w R_w{}^4 / L_w \quad (4)$$

$$I_p = 2I_x \quad (5)$$

Assuming an isotropic material, G_w is expressed using Poisson's ratio (ν) as follows:

$$G_w = E_w / 2(1+\nu) \quad (6)$$

In the present study, $\nu = 0.3$ (Petrini et al., 2005).

The parameters and dimensions of the filter model are shown in Table 1 and Fig. 3, respectively. In this table, subscripts w and h indicate the parameters of the wire and the head, respectively. Here, K_{wx} and K_{wz} are obtained by substituting R_w and E_w in Table 1 into Eqs. (2) and (3). Assuming a fixed joint, the values of the joints between the wire and the head are 100 times as large as those obtained using Eqs. (2) and (3). The recurved hook is set at an angle of 80° (Greenfield et al., 1991). The actual leg hook consists of a twisted and complicated structure in order to avoid migration of the filter after deployment or penetration of the vein (Greenfield et al., 1990, 1991) (Fig. 2). However, since the penetration of the vein was not evaluated in the present study, the bending number of the hook is one. The change of the bending angle is equal to the change of q_o, as shown in Eq. (1). In a manner similar to the catheter simulator (Takashima et al., 2006, 2007b, 2009), the viscous term for each movable joint was considered in terms of D_w. Since we cannot measure the exact values, we assumed D_w to be smaller than K_{wx} and K_{wz}. We neglected the "zigzag" pattern and the slight flare of the wire. In the design of the titanium GF, the addition of a slight flare to the legs was made in order to facilitate discharge from the carrier without leg crossing, particularly from the jugular direction where the legs discharge first (Greenfield et al., 1990).

R_w (mm)	0.225
R_h (mm)	0.875
E_w (GPa)	22
Density (g/cm^3)	5.3
D_w (N·m·s/rad)	0.005
L_w (mm)	4, 43
L_h (mm)	2
n	25

Table 1. Parameters of the filter model used in simulation.

2.2 Blood vessel model

The vessel is a circular elastic cylinder defined by a centerline and a radius (R_v). The centerlines are represented by numerical data. The position of the centerline of the vessel is constant. The contact forces between the filter and the vessel are calculated according to the stiffness and the friction of the vessel wall. The friction force are derived from the fixation of the hook. Moreover, the diameter of the blood vessel ($2R_v$) is assumed to be 20 mm, which is similar to Swaminathan (Swaminathan et al., 2006). In the instructions for the use of the GF (Boston Scientific, 2007), the maximum diameter of the inferior vena into which the filter can be deployed is 28 mm.

The simulation models used in the present study are shown in Fig. 4. The centerline of the blood vessel is along the z-axis.

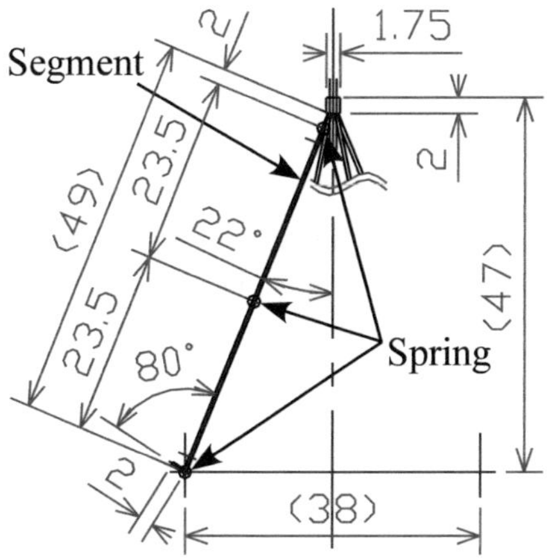

Fig. 3. Dimensions of the filter model (unit: mm).

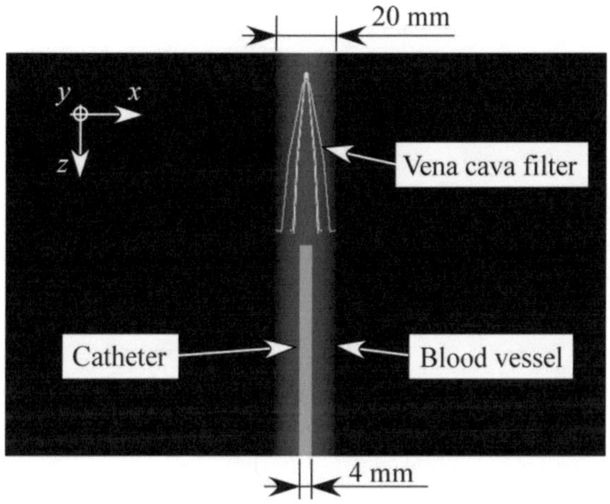

Fig. 4. Simulation model (vena cava filter, catheter, and blood vessel).

2.3 Calculation of contact force

In order to determine whether contact occurs between the filter and the vessel, the distances between the joints and the tip of the filter model ($\boldsymbol{p}_i$) and the centerline of the vessel, were calculated. Considering the clearance of the filter and the blood vessel, we calculated the contact force according to the distance. Here, $\boldsymbol{F}_i$ is decomposed into three components along the centerline of the blood vessel (f_{ti}), the normal direction to the centerline (f_{ni}), and the circumferential direction of the cross-section (f_{ri}). f_{ni} is expressed as follows:

$$f_{ni} = -K_v(|\boldsymbol{l}_i| + R_w - R_v)^{3/2}\, \boldsymbol{l}_i / |\boldsymbol{l}_i| \quad (7)$$

where K_v is the elastic coefficient of vessel deformation and $\boldsymbol{l}_i$ is the distance vector between each joint and nearest point on the central curve of the blood vessel.

In our previous studies (Takashima et al., 2006, 2007b), we assumed that the frictional force is opposite the direction of motion. In other words, the model includes only dynamic friction, and there is no friction when the model does not move. However, the titanium GF has an improved hook design and does not move at the contact position (Greenfield et al., 1990, 1991). As a preliminary test, we measured the resistance force that occurs when the head of a commercial GF is pushed and pulled in acryl and silicon rubber tubing (inner diameter: 20 mm). The maximum resistance force is summarized in Table 2. In this table, when the GF is pulled, the force acts in the direction of blood flow after deployment (along the -z-axis in Fig. 4). Since the mass of the GF is 0.3 g (measured value), this resistance force is very large. Moreover, the resistance force in the silicon rubber tubing changed according to the direction of the applied force because of the hook biting into the wall of the tubing. Therefore, taking the bite of the hook into consideration, we approximated the constraint force of the tip of the wire on the blood vessel wall as follows.

1. After the tip of the wire contacts the blood vessel wall, the contact point ($\boldsymbol{r}_i$) is calculated.
2. The expression $\boldsymbol{k}_i = \boldsymbol{p}_i - \boldsymbol{r}_i$ is decomposed into the components along the surface of the blood vessel wall ($\boldsymbol{k}_{ti}$ and $\boldsymbol{k}_{ri}$ are the components along the centerline and in the circumferential direction of the cross-section, respectively). Using a constant (K_f), the contact force is calculated as follows:

$$\boldsymbol{f}_{ti} = -K_f \boldsymbol{k}_{ti} \tag{8}$$

$$\boldsymbol{f}_{ri} = -K_f \boldsymbol{k}_{ri} \tag{9}$$

where $\boldsymbol{r}_i$ is calculated whenever the contact condition is changed. In the present study, we calculated the conditions without the constrained force approximated by Eqs. (8) and (9). The actual condition may lie somewhere between the conditions with and without the constraint force.

Tubing material	Push (N)	Pull (N)
Acryl	0.4	0.2
Silicon rubber	0.4	1.4

Table 2. Friction force required to move the Greenfield filter in acryl and silicon rubber tubing.

The parameters for simulation are summarized in Table 3. The value of K_v (= 32 N/mm$^{3/2}$) was determined from the experimental results using a porcine aorta (Takashima et al., 2007a). Moreover, along the surface of the blood vessel wall, we assumed that K_f = 32 N/mm. As shown in Fig. 4, the filter model was initially inserted into the introducer catheter model. The inner diameter of the catheter model is 12 Fr. The catheter model is fixed along the z-axis at $z > 0$ and is assumed to be a rigid tube. In the catheter, the contact force is calculated with respect to the catheter, and we approximated K_v as 20,000 N/mm$^{3/2}$, because the catheter is more rigid than a blood vessel. There is no friction in the catheter. Using these models, the position and the configuration of the filter were calculated in order to model the deployment of a GF inside a blood vessel and the existence of the GF for a fixed time under a constant force.

R_v (mm)	10
K_v(N/mm$^{3/2}$)	32
K_f (N/mm)	32

Table 3. Parameters of the vessel model used in the simulation.

2.4 Simulation procedure

The simulation procedure is as follows (Fig. 5).

1. The filter model is initially inserted into the introducer catheter model (12 Fr) (Fig. 5, left).
2. The filter is moved axially and is freed from the catheter (Fig. 5, center). The filter model is made to contact the blood vessel wall for 10 s (Fig. 5, right).
3. Assuming the blood flow and gravity, the filter inside the blood vessel is applied for a fixed time (60 s) under a constant force along the z-axis.

The GF is deployed with the head downstream. Therefore, the direction in the introducer catheter changes according to the insertion site (from the femoral vein or the jugular vein). In the present study, we inserted the catheter from the femoral vein.

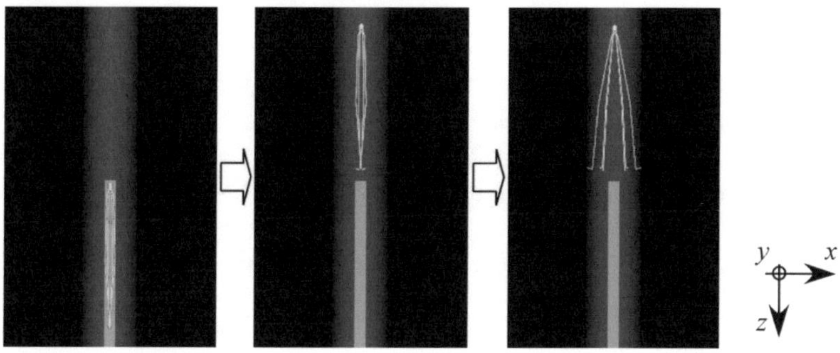

Fig. 5. Insertion procedure.

When large clots occlude the filter, the effects of the filter wires and the head on the flow would be negligible in comparison with the effects of the large particles because the wires are thin and the head is behind the blood clot. Moreover, since the pulsatility of the blood flow in the inferior vena cava is relatively low and is a low-pressure system, we assumed a constant, time-averaged flow (Swaminathan et al., 2006). Under the above assumptions, we calculated the drag (D) generated by the blood flow considering a ball (diameter, d) in a uniform flow, as follows (Tagori & Arakawa, 1989):

$$D = C_D(1/2)\rho U^2(\pi/4)d^2 \tag{10}$$

where C_D is the drag coefficient, ρ is the fluid density, and U is the fluid velocity. Similar to Swaminathan (Swaminathan et al., 2006), we assumed that ρ = 1,040 kg/m^3, U = 0.123 m/s, d = 5 mm, and Reynolds number, Re = 1,000. Moreover, using Re = 1,000, we obtained C_D = 0.4 (Tagori & Arakawa, 1989). Substituting these values into Eq. (10), we obtained D = 0.06 mN. Since the mass of the filter is 0.3 g, the gravity applied to the filter is 3 mN. Therefore, the force generated by the blood flow is much smaller than that generated by gravity, although the force depends on the size of the blood clot. On the other hand, since the friction model used in the present study is independent of the direction of the hook, we

evaluated the migration of the filter considering the safety factor when the gravity doubled (i.e., assuming a gravitational acceleration of -19.61 m/s^2 along the z-axis). Experiments in sheep (Greenfield et al., 1990) have demonstrated migration of the filter in both directions, and whether this migration is caused by gravity or blood flow remains unclear.
Based on the above assumptions, we calculated the Newton-Euler equations of motion (Eq. (1)) using the contact force at every finite time step, using numerical differentiation formulas (NDF). The time steps were not fixed in order to make the relative errors smaller than permissible values (10^{-3}) at each time step. When contact occurred within a time step, we divided the time step at the contact point. This numerical analysis was performed in a MATLAB/Simlink (Cybernet Systems Co., Ltd.) environment.

2.5 Calculation conditions

Complications after filter deployment include the migration of the filter, fracture of the wire legs, penetration of the filter, deployment of the filter in an improper position, and retroperitoneal hematoma (Ando & Kuribayashi, 2000). Moreover, it has been reported that there is no recurrence of pulmonary embolism when the GF is secured without tilting in 13 patients (Nara et al., 1995). Since the hook of the GF has been improved and is fixed as soon as the filter comes into contact with the blood vessel wall, some asymmetry of the limbs may result (Greenfield et al., 1991). Moreover, it is difficult to retrieve the GF once it has been deployed. Therefore, it is necessary to continue anticoagulation therapy and to deploy another filter when the deployed filter is inclined (Nara et al., 1995).
In the present study, we evaluated the effects of the parameters of the filter model and the deployment condition on the simulation system as follows. Cases *-1 and *-2 stand for cases without and with fixation of the hook to the blood vessel model, respectively. When there is no friction, the analysis shown in procedure 3 of Section 2.4 was not performed.

- Cases 1-1 and 1-2: Normal condition
  As a fundamental condition, we evaluated the motion of the filter when the axis of the introducer catheter is along the centerline of the blood vessel.
- Cases 2-1 and 2-2: The filter does not expand uniformly. Specifically, one wire cannot expand.
  The filter does not expand uniformly when a leg of the filter is captured by a blood clot that occurred in the catheter (Ando & Kuribayashi, 2000).
- Cases 3-1 and 3-2: The filter is deployed through a tilted catheter
  The filter may tilt according to the approach angle of the catheter, which depends on the shape and curvature of the blood vessel (Ando & Kuribayashi, 2000; Kinney et al., 1997). For example, in the case of right femoral approaches, a sheath caval angle of 10.3±4.7° results in a titanium GF caval angle of 4.1±5.8° (Kinney et al., 1997). Therefore, in the present study, the filter is deployed after being tilted and fixed at 10° with respect to the blood vessel, and the posture was then evaluated. As shown in Fig. 4, since the total length of the GF is 47 mm, angles of 10° and 4° correspond to the difference between the center of the blood vessel and the center of the head of 8 (= 47tan10°) mm and 3 mm, respectively.
- Cases 4-1 and 4-2: The filter is deployed through a catheter in which the axis is not same as that of the blood vessel.
  When the deployment sheath is close to the caval wall at the moment of filter release, the sheath slides along the lateral caval wall during filter deployment with the struts

instantly becoming attached to the adjacent wall. As a result, the filter cannot expand uniformly (Kinney et al., 1997). Therefore, we evaluated the condition in which the filter is deployed through a catheter for which the axis is not same as that of the blood vessel for a distance of 5 mm.

The results were evaluated based on the difference between the center of the blood vessel and the center of the head, and the migration of the head.

3. Results and discussions

3.1 Motion of the deployed filter

The difference between the center of the blood vessel and the center of the head after deployment of the filter is shown in Fig. 6. This difference indicates the tilt of the filter in the blood vessel. The distribution of the absolute value of the contact force after placement of the filter is shown in Fig. 7. When the difference in Fig. 6 is large (Case 3-2), the contact force in Fig. 7 is large and non-uniform. The ability to calculate the contact force distribution

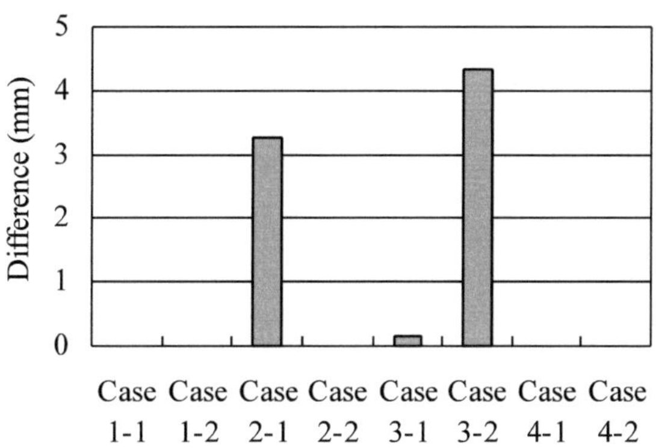

Fig. 6. Difference between the center of the blood vessel and the center of the head after deployment of the filter.

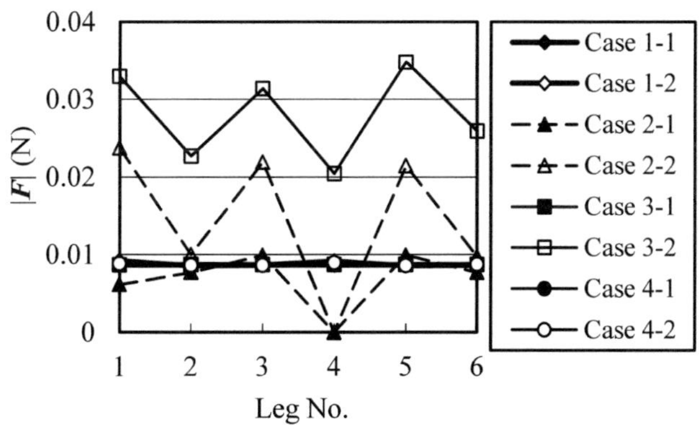

Fig. 7. Distribution of absolute value of contact force (F) after placement of filter.

is one of the advantages of numerical analysis, since it is difficult to determine clinically. In the following section, we described the results for each case in detail.

First, we evaluated the motion of the filter without friction when the axis of the introducer catheter is along the centerline of the blood vessel (Case 1-1). The trajectories of the head and the wire tips are shown in Fig. 8. In this figure, the initial and final positions are indicated by circle and square symbols, respectively. The wire tips expand uniformly from the center to the blood vessel wall in the directions shown by the arrows. As shown in Figs. 6 and 8, the head did not move from the center of the blood vessel and the filter could be deployed normally. Moreover, the final position for the case with friction (Case 1-2) did not change (Fig. 6).

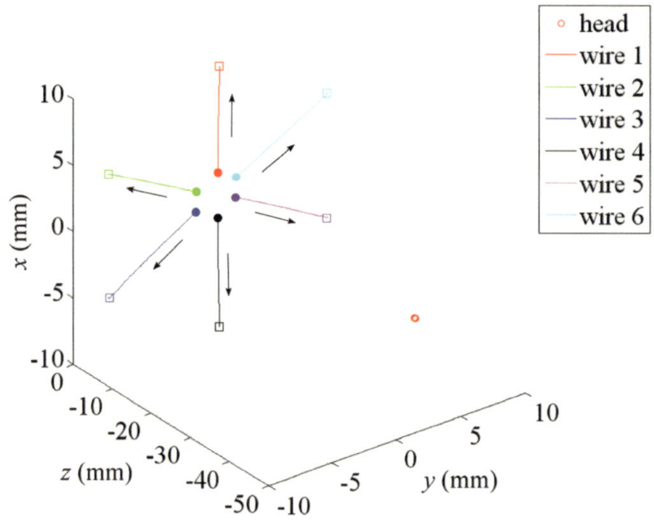

Fig. 8. Trajectories of the head and the tips of the wires (Case 1-1).

The motion of the filter was evaluated for the case in which the filter does not expand uniformly (Cases 2-1 and 2-2). The trajectories of head and the wire tips and appearance of the deployed filter are shown in Figs. 9 and 10, respectively. The transition of the contact force at the wire tips is shown in Fig. 11. The wire indicated by the arrows in Figs. 9 and 10 cannot expand. In Fig. 9, the initial and final positions are shown by the circle and square symbols, respectively. For the case without friction (Case 2-1), the head deviated from the center of the blood vessel (Fig. 9) and tilted and was fixed (Fig. 10). As the filter tilted, the values of all contact force except wire 4 approached closely (Fig. 11 (a)). On the other hand, for the case with friction (Case 2-2), the deviation of the head center of the blood vessel from was small even when one wire could not expand (Fig. 6). Namely, the filter did not move because the friction fixed the filter at the initial contact position. After the fixation, each contact force increased gradually (Fig. 11 (b)).

We evaluated the motion of the filter when the introducer catheter is not aligned with the axis of the vena cava (10°) (Case 3). The transition of the difference between the center of the head and the center of the blood vessel, and appearance of the deployed filter are shown in Figs. 12 and 13, respectively. For the case without friction (Case 3-1), the head approached the center of the blood vessel. On the other hand, for the case with friction (Case 3-2), the inserted filter tilted (Fig. 12) and stopped in the tilted position (Fig. 13). The angle of the tilt (difference: 4.3 mm) was similar to that for reported clinical results (Kinney et al., 1997). Moreover, when the filter was tilted, the contact force was large and non-uniform (Fig. 7). The transition of the contact force at the wire tips are shown in Fig. 14. The contact force increased gradually for the case with friction (Fig. 14 (b)) similarly to Fig. 11 (b), although the tilt with friction was larger than that without the friction contrary to Case 2. The transition of the distance between the wire tips and the center of the blood vessel is shown in Fig. 15. In this figure, the distance of the tip of wire 4 from the center of the blood vessel, as indicated by the arrow, first increased and then decreased abruptly. This phenomenon

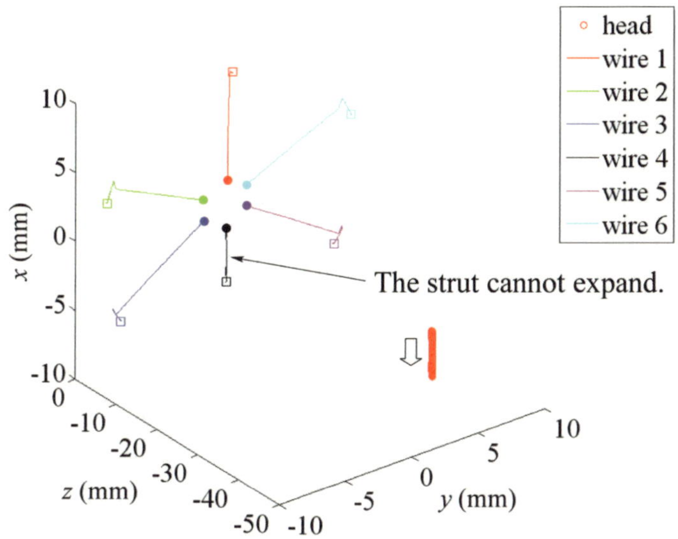

Fig. 9. Trajectories of the head and the tips of the wires (Case 2-1). The filter does not expand uniformly.

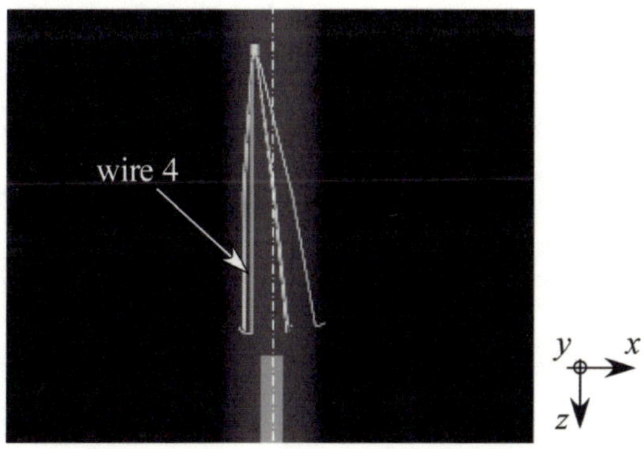

Fig. 10. Filter after deployment (Case 2-1). The filter does not expand uniformly. The arrow indicates a wire that cannot expand.

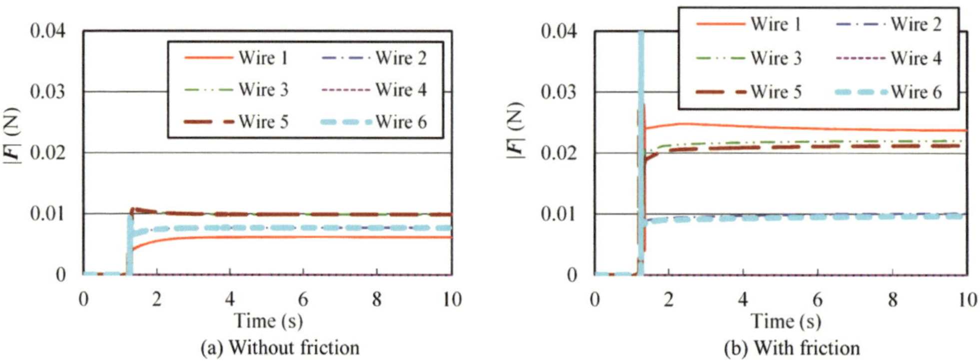

Fig. 11. Transition of the contact force (***F***) at the wire tip (Cases 2-1 and 2-2). The filter does not expand uniformly.

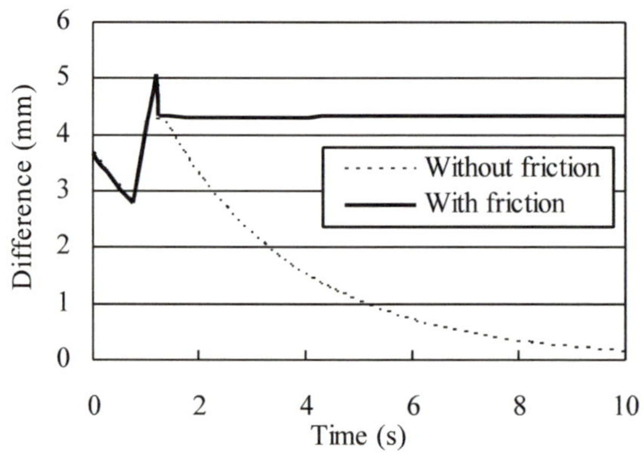

Fig. 12. Transition of the difference between the center of the head inserted through a tilted catheter and the center of the blood vessel (Cases 3-1 and 3-2).

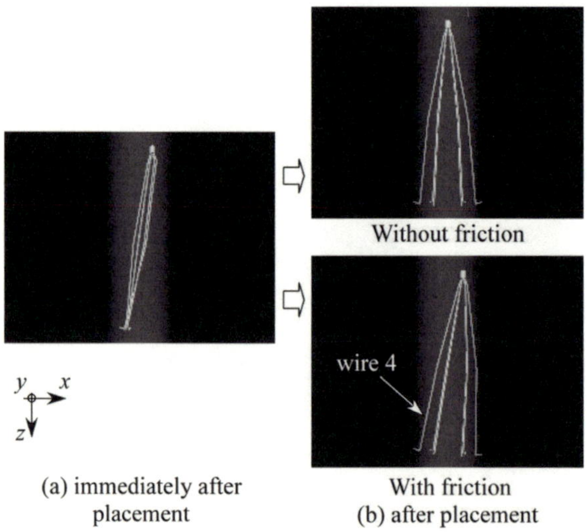

Fig. 13. Placement of the filter inserted through a tilted catheter (Cases 3-1 and 3-2).

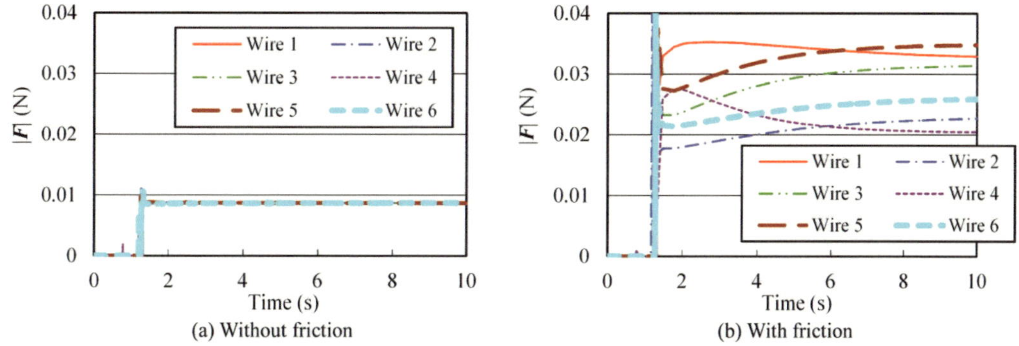

Fig. 14. Transition of the contact force (*F*) inserted through a tilted catheter (Cases 3-1 and 3-2).

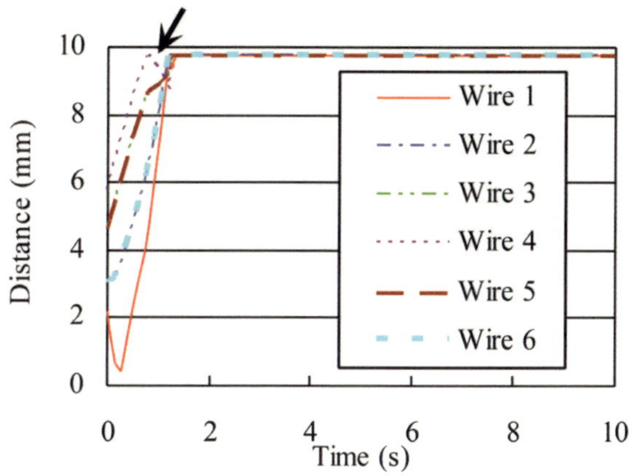

Fig. 15. Transition of the distance between the wire tips and the center of the blood vessel (Case 3-2). The filter was inserted through a tilted catheter.

indicates rebounding of the wire on the blood vessel. Moreover, after rebounding of the wire, all six wires came into contact with the blood vessel wall at the same time. Therefore, the tilt of the filter became smaller than that of the catheter.

When the axis of the catheter is not same as that of the blood vessel (5 mm) (Cases 4-1 and 4-2), the tilts of the filters with or without friction are small, as shown in Figs. 6 and 16. The transition of the distance between the wire tips and the center of the blood vessel are shown in Fig. 17. In this figure, after wire 1 (indicated by the arrow) first contacted the vessel wall and then rebounded, all six wires came into contact with the vessel wall at the same time. Therefore, similar to Fig. 13, the tilt of the filter was small (Case 4). Actually, the wire tip may bite and be fixed at the first contact point without rebounding. In this study, the force to keep contact was not defined. Therefore, it is necessary to investigate the contact force between the hook and the blood vessel experimentally.

As shown above, the difference between the center of the blood vessel and the center of the head after deployment of the filter is large when the filter does not expand uniformly or when the filter is inserted through a tilted catheter. Although it is unclear what constitutes a clinically significant filter tilt, in vitro studies suggested that the clot-trapping ability of the GF is reduced at angle of 14° or greater (Katsamouris et al., 1988, as cited in Rogers et al., 1998). This angle corresponds to a difference between the center of the blood vessel and the center of the head of 12 mm. As shown in Fig. 6, the maximum difference in the present study is 4.3 mm, which is smaller than this value. However, large tilt may occur for a variety of reasons. For example, the filter which cannot expand uniformly (Case 2) may be deployed through an inclined catheter (Case 3). Furthermore, although the difference between the center of the blood vessel and the center of the head was small for a catheter for which the axis was not the same as that of the blood vessel (Cases 4), the difference may become larger than that in Case 3 when the catheter tilts (Case 3) and close to the caval wall (Case 4) at the same time.

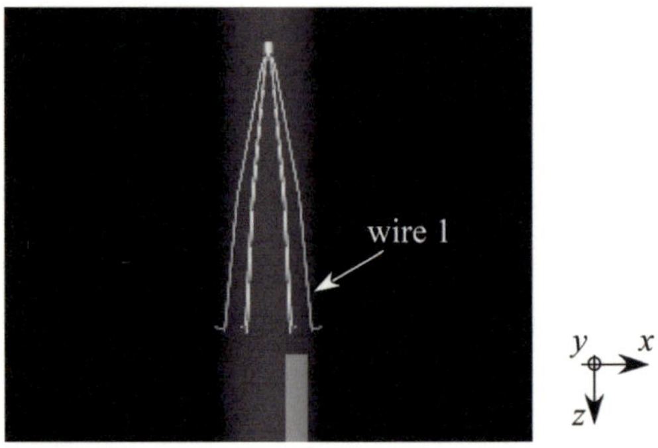

Fig. 16. Filter after deployment through a catheter for which the axis is not same as that of the blood vessel (Case 4-1).

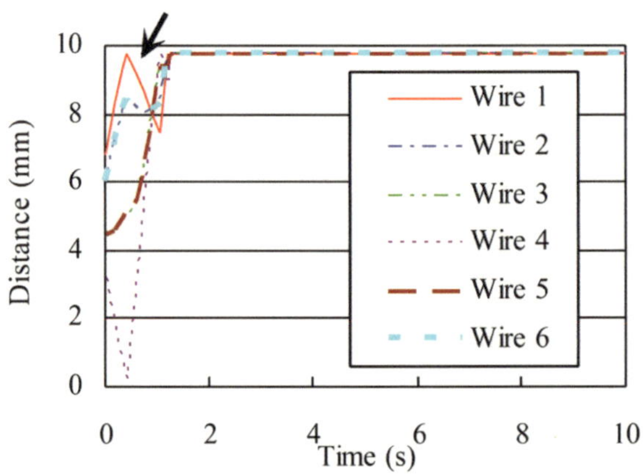

Fig. 17. Transition of the distance between the wire tips and the center of the blood vessel (Case 4-2). The axis of the catheter is not same as that of blood vessel.

3.2 Migration of the filter due to blood flow

Apart from the ability to precisely position and orient the filter, it is also important that it undergoes a minimal amount of migration. In this section, we evaluate the migration of the head for a fixed time under a constant force after deploying the filter, as described in the previous sections. The migration of the head for a fixed time (60 s) under a constant force along the *z*-axis is shown in Fig. 18. The migration was large in Cases 2-2 and 3-2. Significant migration is usually defined as caudal or cranial movement in excess of 1 cm (Streiff, 2000). Similarly, for example, Greenfield et al. defined as significant a change in vertical position of 9 mm or more at 30 days (Greenfield et al., 1991). However, the results of the present study are much smaller than these values.

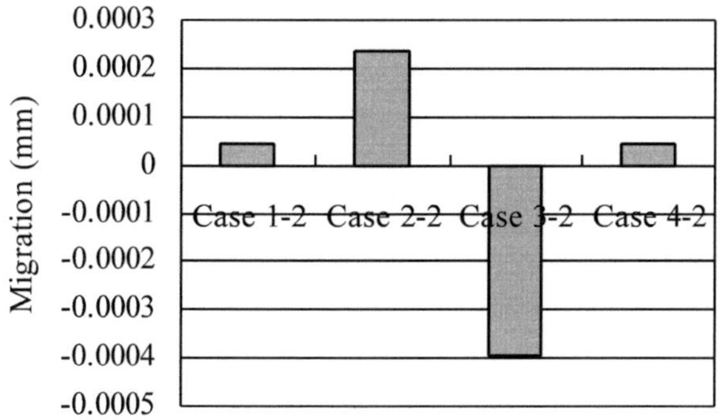

Fig. 18. Migration of the head for a fixed time (60 s) under a constant force.

In the present study, using Eqs. (8) and (9), the friction force is defined by springs at the contact points. Therefore, the friction force can change according to the spring constant. In this model, since there are six springs for which K_f = 32 N/mm, we obtain a migration of 3×10^{-5} mm when 2G is applied to the 0.3-g filter (6 mN). This value is similar to the values shown in the figure (Cases 1-2 and 4-2). In the future, it will be necessary to determine this parameter (K_f) exactly. Moreover, the filter will move when the friction force exceeds a certain value, and these effects must be considered. The contact force distribution is shown in Fig. 19. Comparing this figure with Fig. 7, the distribution was changed. The concentration of the contact force may cause the loosening of the hook actually.

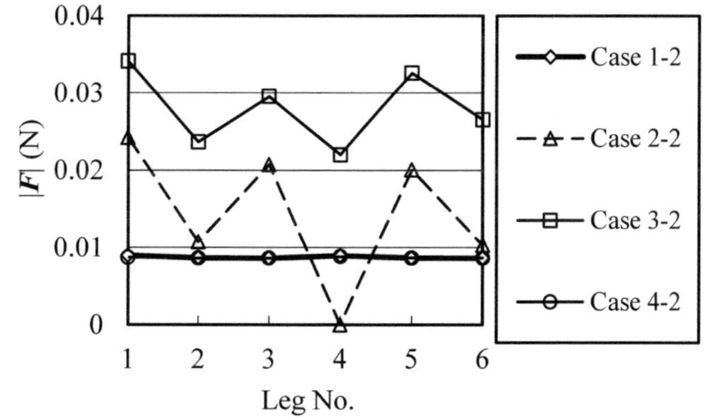

Fig. 19. Distribution of absolute value of contact force (*F*) for a fixed time (60 s) under a constant force.

3.3 Evaluation of parameters

As mentioned above, in addition to the GF, several other types of inferior vena cava filters have been developed. For example, although the Simon-Nitinol filter become popular because of its lower profile, a caval thrombosis rate of up to 50% has been reported for this filter (Decousus et al., 1998; Hawkins & Al-Kutoubi, 1992; Kim et al., 1992; Grassi et al., 1992; Simon et al., 1989, as cited in Swaminathan et al., 2006). In order to quantitatively compare different types of filters, numerical analysis is a very effective method because various filters can be compared under the same simulation condition, for example, the same vessel shape. Asymmetry of the limbs increases the possibility of impairment of filtration in the area of wider limb spread (Greenfield et al., 1991). However, theoretically, eccentric placement might be anticipated to impair performance, although no pulmonary embolisms have been linked to this finding (Streiff, 2000). Therefore, it is necessary to couple the present results with computational fluid dynamics results.

It is necessary to improve the simulation model in order to reproduce the motion in surgery. Although, in the present catheter simulator, the blood vessel is an artery, the filter is applied to a vein. In the present study, we used the same parameters in both conditions. However, since the mechanical properties of the artery and the vein are different, it would be necessary to measure the mechanical properties of the vein experimentally and to verify Eqs. (7), (8), and (9). Moreover, the diameter of the blood vessel model used in the present study is constant. However, there is some possibility of one of the limbs of the filter entering a tributary vein (Boston Scientific, 2007). Moreover, when the inner diameter is different, the applied force changes. Therefore, it is necessary to model the shape of the blood vessel exactly. Moreover, when the filter is released from the catheter, the friction between the catheter and the filter may cause the filter to tilt.

4. Conclusions

In this chapter, we describe the evaluation of the effects of the parameters of the simulation model on the deployment of the Greenfield filter. The results are as follows.

1. When the introducer catheter is not aligned with the axis of the vena cava, the inserted filter becomes tilted.
2. When the filter does not expand uniformly, the inserted filter also becomes tilted.
3. The friction between the filter and the blood vessel wall affects the tilt of the filter.

This simulation method can be used for surgical planning, intra-operative assistance, and the design of new filters.

5. Acknowledgment

The present study was supported by KAKENHI through a Grant-in-Aid for Young Scientists (B) (22700485).

6. References

Ando, M. & Kuribayashi, S. (2000). Placement of Inferior Vena Cava Filter: Indication, Technique and Results. *Japanese Journal of Phlebology*, Vol.11, No.1, pp.93–98, ISSN 0915-7395 (in Japanese)

Boston Scientific (2007). *Instructions for Use, Greenfield Vena Cava Filter System (5th edition)* (in Japanese)

Greenfield, L.J.; Cho, K.J. & Tauscher, J.R. (1990). Evolution of Hook Design for Fixation of the Titanium Greenfield Filter. *Journal of Vascular Surgery*, Vol.12, No.3, pp.345–353, ISSN 0741-5214

Greenfield, L.J.; Cho, K.J.; Proctor, M.; Bonn, J.; Bookstein, J.J.; Castaneda-Zuniga, W.R.; Cutler, B.; Ferris, E.J.; Keller, F.; McCowan, T.; Pais, S.O.; Sobel, M.; Tisnado, J. & Waltman, A.C. (1991). Results of a Multicenter Study of the Modified Hook-titanium Greenfield Filter. *Journal of Vascular Surgery*, Vol.14, No.3, pp.253–257, ISSN 0741-5214

Hahn, J.K.; Kaufman, R.; Winick, A.B.; Carleton, T.; Park, Y.; Lindeman, R.; Oh, K.M.; Al-Ghreimil, N.; Walsh, R.J.; Loew, M. & Sankar, S. (1998). Training Environment for Inferior Vena Caval Filter Placement, In: *Studies in Health Technology and Informatics*, Westwood, J.D.; Hoffman, H.M.; Stredney, D. & Weghorst, S.J. (Eds.), Vol.50, pp.291–297, IOS Press, ISBN 978-90-5199-386-8, Amsterdam, Netherlands

Kinney, T.B.; Rose, S.C.; Weingarten, K.E.; Valji, K.; Oglevie, S.B. & Roberts, A.C. (1997). IVC Filter Tilt and Asymmetry: Comparison of the Over-the-wire Stainless-steel and Titanium Greenfield IVC Filters. *Journal of Vascular and Interventional Radiology*, Vol.8, No.6, pp.1029–137, ISSN 1051-0443

Nara, S.; Moteki, K.; Kameda, T.; Ishitobi, K.; Kodera, K. & Kimura, M. (1995). Therapeutic Efficacy of Percutaneous Placement of the Inferior Vena Caval Filter, *Japanese Journal of Phlebology*, Vol.6, No.1, pp.39–45, ISSN 0915-7395 (in Japanese)

Petrini, L.; Migliavacca, F.; Massarotti, P.; Schievano, S.; Dubini, G. & Auricchio, F. (2005). Computational Studies of Shape Memory Alloy Behavior in Biomedical Applications, *Transaction of the ASME, Journal of Biomechanical Engineering*, Vol.127, No.4, pp.716–725, ISSN 0148-0731

Rogers, F.B.; Strindberg, G.; Shackford, S.R.; Osler, T.M.; Morris, C.S.; Ricci, M.A.; Najarian, K.E.; D'Agostino, R. & Pilcher, D.B. (1998). Five-year Follow-up of Prophylactic Vena Cava Filters in High-risk Trauma Patients, *Archives of Surgery*, Vol.133, No.4, pp.406–411, ISSN 0096-6908

Streiff, M.B. (2000). Vena Caval Filters: a Comprehensive Review. *Blood*, Vol.95, No.12, pp.3669–3677, ISSN 1528-0020

Swaminathan, T.N.; Hu, H.H. & Patel, A.A. (2006). Numerical Analysis of the Hemodynamics and Embolus Capture of a Greenfield Vena Cava Filter, *Transaction of the ASME, Journal of Biomechanical Engineering*, Vol.128, No.3, , pp.360–370, ISSN 0148-0731

Tagori. T. & Arakawa, C. (1989). *Fluids Engineering*, University of Tokyo Press, ISBN 4-13-062124-6, Tokyo, Japan (in Japanese)

Takashima, K.; Ota, S.; Ohta, M.; Yoshinaka, K. & Ikeuchi, K. (2006). Development of Computer-based Simulator for Catheter Navigation in Blood Vessels (1st Report, Evaluation of Fundamental Parameters of Guidewire and Blood Vessel). *Transactions of the Japan Society of Mechanical Engineers, Series C*, Vol.72, No.719, pp.2137–2145, ISSN 0387-5024 (in Japanese)

Takashima, K.; Shimomura, R.; Kitou, T.; Terada, H.; Yoshinaka, K. & Ikeuchi, K. (2007a). Contact and Friction between Catheter and Blood Vessel. *Tribology International*, Vol.40, Issue 2, pp.319–328, ISSN 0301-679X

Takashima, K.; Ota, S.; Ohta, M.; Yoshinaka, K. & Mukai, T. (2007b). Development of Computer-based Simulator for Catheter Navigation in Blood Vessels (2nd Report, Evaluation of Fundamental Parameters of Guidewire and Blood Vessel). *Transactions of the Japan Society of Mechanical Engineers, Series C*, Vol.73, No.735, pp.2988–2995, ISSN 0387-5024 (in Japanese)

Takashima, K.; Ohta, M.; Yoshinaka, K.; Mukai, T. & Ota, S. (2009). Catheter and Guidewire Simulator for Intravascular Surgery (Comparison between Simulation Results and Medical Images), *The World Congress on Medical Physics and Biomedical Engineering (WC2009)*, pp.128-131, ISBN 978-3-642-03897-6, Munich, Germany, September 7-12, 2009

Yamamura, N.; Himeno, R. & Makinouchi, A. (2003). Development of Catheter Simulator. *Proceedings of Riken Symposium on Computational Biomechanics*, pp.136–144, Tokyo, Japan, May 27-28, 2003 (in Japanese)